Chinese Herb Cultivation

Daodi Practices for Growing and Processing Chinese Herbs

Huang Lu-qi, Guo Lan-ping, Xie Xiao-liang

Chinese Herb Cultivation

Daodi Practices for Growing and Processing Chinese Herbs

Translated and Annotated by Thomas Avery Garran

Edited by Shelley Ochs

Passiflora Press

Authors of the Original Chinese Edition
Huang Lu-qi, Guo Lan-ping, Xie Xiao-liang

Translation and Annotation: Thomas Avery Garran
Editing and Proofreading: Shelley Ochs
Text Design and Layout: Thomas Avery Garran
Cover Photos and Design: Thomas Avery Garran

Copyright © Passiflora Press

Translation from the Simplified Chinese language edition:
道地药材特色栽培及产地加工技术规范
by Lanping GUO, Luqi HUANG, Xiaoliang XIE
Copyright © Shanghai Scientific & Technical Publishers 2016
All Rights Reserved.

Library of Congress Cataloging-in-Publication Data
Garran, Thomas Avery
Chinese herb cultivation : daodi practices for growing and processing chinese herbs /
Thomas Avery Garran

Includes index, NO
ISBN 978-0-9915813-1-3
1. herb-cultivation 2. Chinese herbs 3. Chinese medicine

This book is typeset in Gentium Book Basic.

Other than the original Chinese text and the work needed to communicated with authors
and contributors during the translation, all layout, formatting, art work, and other aspects
of the project were done on free, open source, software, including Scribus and GIMP.

Passiflora Press
www.passiflora-press.com

Table of Contents

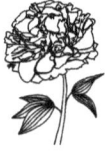

Photographs

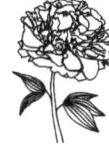

All photographs were taken by Thomas Avery Garran except those attributed to the people below.

Botanical Latin Binomial	Chinese Name	Page Number	Name & Institution
Achyranthes bidentata	*niúxī*	7, 9	Zhou Liang-yun, Lecturer at Guangdong Pharmaceutical University
Angelica sinensis	*dāngguī*	21, 26	Wang Xin, PhD Student at China Academy of Chinese Medical Sciences, Beijing, China
Aster tataricus	*zǐwǎn*	27, 30	Zhang Jing-li
Astragalus membracaceus var. mongholicus	*huángqí*	31	Zhang Jun, Systematic Botanist Yunnan, China
Atractylodes lancea	*cāngzhú*	35, 38	Zhang Jun, Systematic Botanist Yunnan, China
Aucklandia lappa	*mùxiāng*		From the original Chinese text with no further attribution
Belamcanda chinensis	*shègān*	49, 52	Zhang Jun, Systematic Botanist Yunnan, China
Bupleurum chinensis & B. scorzonerifolium	*cháihú*	53	Zhang Jun, Systematic Botanist Yunnan, China
Carthamus tinctorius	*hónghuā*	60	Zhang Jun, Systematic Botanist Yunnan, China
Chrysanthemum morifolium	*júhuā*	61, 64	From the original Chinese text with no further attribution
Cistanche deserticola	*ròucōngróng*	65, 68	Xu Xin-wen, Research Fellow at China Academy of Sciences in the Research Institute of Ecology and Geography, Xinjiang, China
Codonopsis pilosula	*dǎngshēn*	69	Zhang Jun, Systematic Botanist Yunnan, China
Coptis chinensis	*huánglián*	75, 79	Zhang Teng, Graduate student China Academy of Chinese Medical Sciences, Beijing, China
Curcuma phaeocaulis	*yùjīn*	84	From the original Chinese text with no further attribution
Dioscorea opposita	*shānyao*	89	Zhang Jun, Systematic Botanist Yunnan, China
Epimedium wushanense	*yínyánghuò*	95, 98	Li Xiao-dong, Botanist at China Academy of Sciences, Wuhan Botanical Gardens Herbarium
Forsythia suspensa	*liánqiáo*	99	Zhang Jun, Systematic Botanist Yunnan, China
Gastrodia elata	*tiānmá*	103	Wei Ze, Botanist at Chinese Academy of Sciences Institute of Botany
Gentiana rigescens	*lóngdǎn*	111	Zhu Xin-xin, Professor at Xinyang Normal University
Glehnia littoralis	*shāshēn*	115	Zhang Jing-li
Lilium lancifolium	*bǎihé*	125, 128	From the original Chinese text with no further attribution
Lonicera japonica	*yínhuā*	129, 132	Zhang Jun, Systematic Botanist Yunnan, China
Paeonia suffruticosa	*dānpí*	133, 138	Zhang Jun, Systematic Botanist Yunnan, China
Panax notoginseng	*sānqī*	139, 146	From the original Chinese text with no further attribution
Rehmannia glutinosa	*dìhuáng*	161	Zhang Jun, Systematic Botanist Yunnan, China
Trichosanthes kirilowii	*guālóu*	175	Zhang Hua-an, Botanist Henan, China
Trichosanthes kirilowii	*guālóu*	178	Wu Di-fei, Botanist Zhejiang, China
Trollius chinensis	*jīnliánhuā*	179	Zhou Liang-yun Lecturer at Guangdong Pharmaceutical University

🌸 FORWARD 🌸

The text *Chinese Herb Cultivation: Daodi Practices for Growing and Processing Chinese Herbs* translated and annotated by Thomas Avery Garran represents a milestone in the development of Chinese medicine. As the first full-length English text devoted to the concept of daodi medicinal material, it provides an authentic intro-duction to the rich history of quality discernment in Chinese herbal medicine. At the same time, it is among the first English texts devoted specifically to the cultivation of Chinese herbs, with detailed descriptions that will advance herbal production around the world.

By combining textual study with field research, Thomas brings his experience as both a scholar and a farmer to life, resulting in a unique text that is both inspirational and practical. As the first Western practitioner of Chinese medicine to undertake a PhD in the discipline of Chinese herbal pharmacy in mainland China, Thomas has a rare background that integrates agriculture, clinical practice, and academia. His work represents a bridge between East and West that will influence the field for decades to come.

Astute readers will appreciate the thorough discussion of factors that influence daodi medicinal material, which encompasses internal factors such as the influence of specific species and selected cultivar varieties, as well as external factors such as the climate, soil conditions, and processing practices that are fundamental for achieving superior quality. Throughout the text, Thomas models a respect for both inheritance and innovation, simultaneously aiming to preserve traditional knowledge while also advancing the discussion to fit the needs of the modern world. He explores techniques and considerations that illustrate how the concept of daodi material is continually expanding, resulting in a text that will be useful for herbalists and growers around the globe.

On the whole, the book aims to preserve valuable knowledge that has gradually accumulated for centuries in the Chinese world, much of which has never been previously translated into English. At the same time, Thomas integrates his own hallmark style of critical assessment and commentary, making the book much more than a summary of the work of others. Farmers will appreciate his detailed descriptions of soil requirements and cultivation practices, while clinicians will appreciate his comprehensive understanding of herbal quality and the factors that influence it.

Thomas stands out as one of the first Westerners to personally undertake the daunting task of commercial scale cultivation of Chinese herbs. During his long-term study in Beijing, Thomas had the opportunity to train with some of China's top experts in herbal quality assessment and cultivation, and over the years he has traveled throughout China to gain insight into the real situation on the ground. His proficiency in the Chinese language allows him to access literature and expertise that remains inaccessible to most Western enthusiasts, and his own direct experience with farming and research makes his work unrivaled on many levels. Throughout the text we find gems based on his own personal experience and his sophisticated understanding of organic and sustainable agricultural practices.

While no single book or individual can tackle the vast scope of issues that relate to herbal cultivation and daodi medicinal quality, the volume in your hands is without question the first step that we have all been waiting for. By standing on the shoulders of giants, Thomas has extended our vision and brought us a work that will advance the field for generations to come.

Eric Brand, PhD
May 2019

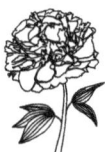

PREFACE TO THE TRANSLATION

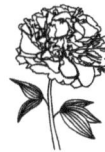

My grandfather was a great gardener. He always grew more food than the family could eat and he would share it with neighbors and friends. He died just before I started getting serious about studying European and North American herbal traditions and Chinese medicine, but I was struck when my grandmother told me he had said that if he could live his life again, he would be a farmer. Over the next couple years as I oriented myself toward plant medicine, I gave deep consideration to pursuing farming herbs as a path within this profession, but in the end, I went the clinical route. Life has a way of coming full-circle and after my wife and I lost our baby girl to SIDS we started a "learning garden" in her honor, which transformed into a full-scale farm over the next two years. This endeavor compelled me to search out information on growing Chinese herbs using traditional methods and to understand how this could be combined with modern information to expand the basis of knowledge passed down over the centuries.

Somewhat by chance, while at a conference here in Beijing, I met a professor, Guo Lan-ping (郭兰平), who literally wrote the book on the ecology of Chinese herbs and who is deeply connected to the research community focused on growing Chinese herbs informed by ecological science, something I had already begun to explore. This chance meeting eventually culminated in my decision to pursue PhD studies at the China Academy of Chinese Medical Sciences: National Center for Materia Medica Resources and Daodi Herbs. This translation is a fruit of the last four years at that institution under the tutelage of professor Guo, my advisor Huang Lu-qi (黄璐琦) (Director of the Center and President of the Academy), and many other experts in the field of Chinese herb agriculture.

I am deeply indebted to these two professors as well as professor Yuan Qing-jun (袁庆军), head of the Chinese herb ecology department, for supporting me and guiding me on my journey as I explored this subject in both the academic setting of the Academy, and the practical setting of my own farm and the many other farms I visited around the country. Of course, none of this would have been possible without the steadfast support of my lovely wife Wu Jiang-hong (吴江洪) who put up with me over these last four years while I became a student again. I am forever grateful to each and every one of you and the many others not mentioned here by name. Aside from those I have already mentioned, I want to thank three others who have helped to make this project possible. First, for her initial editing and comments, I would like to thank my apprentice Nately Ba, her comments and questions helped to shape the text. Next, my dear classmate, Ji Rui-feng (纪瑞锋), without whom I would not have made it through the PhD program and who helped in more ways than he knows. And finally, but certainly not lastly, my editor and friend Shelley Ochs, whose hand polished my translation so that it would be presentable to you the reader. With all that said, any and all mistakes, errors, and\or omissions lay entirely on my own shoulders.

The explosion in the use, and now cultivation, of Chinese medicinal plants since the mid-1990s has created a bustling industry around all that is Chinese medicine. A complete system of health dating back more than 2000 years, medicine in China, like nearly all pre-industrial cultures around the world, focuses its healing tradition around medicinal plants. These plants were, naturally, harvested from the wild and processed according to traditional requirements. However, over time, some of these plants were domesticated and plants like *dāngguī* (当归), have been under cultivation for approximately 1000 years. Moreover, the tradition of knowledge of this plant has been based on the cultivated product. In fact, until 2016, many decades had passed without any recorded sightings of wild *dāngguī* and it was considered extinct in the wild. Fortunately, through China's 4th National Survey of Chinese Medicinal Materials several wild stands were located and the process of integrating these wild genetics into the cultivated plant has begun.

Unfortunately, *dāngguī* is one of only a small number of plants that were brought under cultivation early. The vast majority of medicinal plants still come from wild sources. This has led to widespread wildcrafting of medicinal plants and a constant decline of wild populations. Aware of this fact, China began a serious agriculture project in the mid-20th century. This has led to the current situation in which more and more of the plants used in medicine are from cultivated sources. In fact, the National Survey mentioned above, as part of its charter, has also put an enormous amount of energy into medicinal plant agriculture with a goal of bringing all the major plants under productive cultivation by 2022. This text is part of that project and a second volume has recently been published in Chinese and will be the subject of our next project.

This text is the first book about daodi herb cultivation (see the Introduction for more information on daodi herbs) in any Western language. The term daodi is sometimes translated as "geo-authentic" suggesting a sense that location is what makes a specific herb "daodi." While this is true to a certain extent, there is more to the term "daodi" than simply location. For this reason, I have decided to leave this word untranslated, using the pinyin transliteration of the characters 道地 or daodi.

This text covers the growing and processing requirements for 39 herbs, including environment, weather conditions, soils, fertilization, field management, harvesting and more. This text was originally written in Chinese and was meant as a standard of cultivation and processing for the ever-growing medicinal herb industry, but was primarily intended for small landholders. While the number of herbs covered in this text is relatively small, the details needed to successfully grow and process these herbs are all included and are the fruit of the top experts from around China. The translation of this text was guided by many of those involved in the original project, ensuring accuracy as much as possible.

It is a great honor to bring this work to the English reading audience. I am humbled by the enormous amount of effort that went into the original work that allowed me to create the translation you now hold in your hand. I sincerely hope it will help to lead a new chapter in Chinese medicine history.

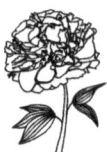

PREFACE TO THE ORIGINAL

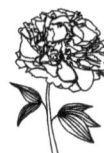

Xie Zong-wan, a senior pharmacist in China, stated, "Daodi herbs refer to herbs from the region in specific natural conditions and ecological environments. The herbs produced in daodi regions are relatively concentrated in production and the cultivation techniques, harvesting, and processing also have special requirements. All this produces better quality and greater clinical effectiveness compared to those same herbs grown in other regions. This is the origin of how daodi herbs got their name, based on long-time recognition by people. The medicinal materials produced in daodi regions are of good quality, good curative effect, and are recognized by the world for their long-standing reputation." Among the 500 commonly used Chinese herbs, the quantity of daodi herbs is the highest. Of these 500 herbs, about 200 have defined daodi characteristics, which accounts for approximately 80% of total herb use.

Daodi herbs is a unique standard developed by the ancients to evaluate the quality of Chinese herbs. The formation of daodi herbs is influenced by the combination of genetic variation, environmental influences, and human factors. The selection of seeds, seedlings, cultivation, harvesting, and processing of finished products is the perfect combination of hard work of the local people and the natural environment for hundreds of years. Therefore, the excellent quality of daodi herbs can be said to be the "combination of heaven, medicinal plants, and humans." Humans have had significant influence on the formation of daodi herbs.

Cultivation and local processing techniques are an important part of the formation of daodi herbs. In the process of standardization of Chinese herbal medicine, it has been found that the unique cultivation methods and techniques from the daodi area have played a critical role in the formation of daodi herbs. For example, research shows the formation of daodi dānshēn has a close relationship to the history of local processing, cultivation methods, breeding, and seed selection during the cultivation process. During the course of cultivation, long-term breeding of varieties shaped the consistency of the genetic background, which eventually brought about uniformity of quality, making the Zhongjiang region of Shandong province the daodi area for dānshēn.

Another example is the whole cultivation process of daodi Chuanxiong, which is divided into two stages: alfalfa cultivation and medicinal cultivation. Alfalfa is cultivated in the mountain at 1000 m elevation, the medicinal materials are cultivated in the dammed area (plain), which shows the special requirements for daodi herbs to grow. Another example is the Sanqidao District in Wenshan county in Yunnan province, which has formed comprehensive traditional and intensive cultivation techniques, such as choosing land, seed low-temperature germination, shading treatment, pest control, etc. To summarize, the quality of most of the cultivated herbs has a close relationship to the unique cultivation methods.

In the traditional Chinese medicine processing and production, the local herb farmers have formed locally unique processing methods according to their own processing habits and sales needs. For example, in the process of producing sānqī, the use of buckwheat polishing gives it a unique character. Over hundreds of years of cultivation, Mianxian County of Gansu Province has established a unique smoke processing method for dāngguī including digging, piling, covering, softening, tying the roots willow bark, piling up, and smoking.

However, over history, small-scale farming production methods of Chinese medicinal plants have led to most of the special cultivation and processing methods being taught and learned orally, organized recording have been missing. This resulted in the cultivation and processing techniques from daodi areas not being promoted and applied. At the same time, large-scale application of modern agricultural technology in the cultivation of daodi herbs has greatly accelerated the modernization and scale of production of daodi herbs. However, some traditional cultivation and processing methods have been impacted significantly. Moreover, some traditional cultivation and processing methods have gradually faded from use, which had serious negative impacts on the quality of daodi herbs.

This book is a key project of the National Natural Science Foundation of China, "Study on the Environmental Mechanism of Chinese Medicine and Its Formation" (81130070), "Twelfth Five-Year Plan" Supporting Project "Technology and Environment-Based Quality Control Technology for Natural Medicines Fan Research" (2012BAI29B02), the State Administration of Traditional Chinese Medicine Industry Research Project "Twenty Kinds of Daodi Materials Training and Standardization and Application of Training and Processing Technology (201107009) and Chinese Medicine Supporting Project of Ministry of Industry and Information Technology

Supported by the project "Safety Production of Chinese Herbal Medicine and Construction of Demonstration Cultivation Technology and Demonstration Base," based on the needs of the industry, it systematically sorts out the special cultivation and local processing techniques of 39 kinds of daodi herbs, and the corresponding technical regulations. There are three purposes: one is to pass-on and promote the characteristic cultivation, production, and processing techniques of authentic medicinal materials to ensure the quality of herbs from the source as well as the safe use of the herbs. Second, in the process of promoting the modernization of Chinese medicine agriculture, this book serves as a good reference for realizing the unique advantages of traditional Chinese medicine, inheriting, developing, and leveraging the treasure from our ancestors. Third, given the fact that daodi herbs are usually found in under developed areas of central and western China, this book can play an important role of technical support in developing cultivation and local processing of daodi herbs, which will support local farmers through herb growing. This is in line with the State Council's "Precise Aid-the-Poor Program" and would help solve the "Three-Rural-Issues."

The Center for Chinese Materia Medica Resources and Daodi Herbs of the China Academy of Chinese Medical Sciences and the Chinese Medicine Research Institute of China Academy of Chinese Medical Sciences participated in the preparation of this book. The Research Institute, Beijing University of Chinese Medicine, Chinese Medicine Company, Nanjing University of Traditional Chinese Medicine, China National Medicine Group Chengde Medicine Co., Ltd. Responsible company, Tianjin University, Inner Mongolia University of Science and Technology Baotou Medical College, Inner Mongolia Daxie Biological Co., Ltd., Inner Mongolia Alxa League Mongolian Medical Hospital, Hebei College of Traditional Chinese Medicine, Hebei Institute of Agriculture and Forestry, Institute of Economic Crops, Hebei Plant Protection, the Agricultural and Animal Husbandry Bureau of Shexian County, Hebei Province, Shanxi Medical University, Shanxi University, and the Agricultural Comprehensive Development Bureau of Lingchuan County, Shanxi Province, Shandong Provincial Academy of Sciences Analytical Testing Center, Anhui University of Traditional Chinese Medicine, Wuhan Light Industry University, Guiyang College of Traditional Chinese Medicine, Guizhou Tong Jitang Pharmaceutical Co., Ltd., Southwest Jiaotong University, Chongqing University, Institute of Medicinal Plants, Yunnan Academy of Agricultural Sciences, Kunming Ming University of Technology, and other units also contributed to the production of this text.

Abbreviations

Throughout the book several abbreviations are used, mostly specific to weights and measures. The following is a key to those abbreviations.

m	meter
cm	centimeter
mm	millimeters
kg	kilogram
l	liter
ml	milliliter
C (°C)	centigrade
NPK	nitrogen, potassium, phosphorus
lx	lux

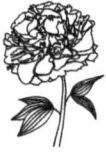

Introduction and Explanation of Text

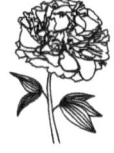

This text is about growing Chinese herbs in their *daodi* locations, using *daodi* processing methods, with the resultant material being deemed the *"daodi herb."* However, as a translation, it assumes that readers are not within the "daodi location" but instead will be trying to mimic, as best as possible, the daodi locations' ecological influences. This text is not aimed at gardeners, although the information found within will certainly be helpful if you are growing Chinese herbs in your garden. Instead, this text is aimed at the growing number of farmers outside of China who are showing interest in growing Chinese herbs. The text has all the technical specifications for growing commercially viable volumes of any of these plants with the hope that some farmers will have an opportunity to make a reasonable living or supplement their current income by growing Chinese herbs. Farming is hard work, requiring more than 24 hours in a day, and although this book cannot do the work for the farmer, it does provide the most authentic information available in the English language.

So, what is daodi? In a very general sense, daodi is a descriptor term that designates an herb as coming from a specific region known traditionally as the location where the highest quality of that particular herb comes from. However, in the strictest sense of the word, daodi also includes the techniques used to grow, harvest, and process harvested material so that it becomes what is "officially" a daodi medicine in China. The Chinese pharmacopoeia does not require herbs to be daodi in order to be official but they are generally considered to be the highest quality.

The term daodi herb came to be during the mid-Ming Dynasty (1368–1644) and has been sporadically used since that time to describe a region or herb that was considered of the highest clinical efficacy. However, location specific descriptive names have been added to herb names since at least the time of the *Shennong Bencao Jing*, written sometime around 200 CE. This was done by using a character (or more than one) at the beginning of the herb name to describe the origin of that herb. Although many of those characters are not used in everyday Chinese medicine, some still remain and are critical ways of distinguishing herbs.

Two herbs that any Chinese medicine practitioner in the West would be familiar with that still use these descriptor characters are; *chuān bèimǔ* (川贝母) where *"chuān"* suggests the herb comes from the province of Sichuan in southwest China. On the other hand, *zhè bèimǔ* (浙贝母) suggests this type of *bèimǔ* comes from Zhejiang province in southeast China.

The region an herb originated in is very important for a number of reasons, which are described below in more detail. However, the daodi region has not always been the same in every text. There has been an evolution over time that has led to wide agreement with regards to the general region for most herbs and specific regions for many herbs. The current theory concerning daodi herbs is that they are a combination of genetics and environmental conditions, which produce regional genotypes. Thus, it is not only the region that makes an herb daodi, but also the genetics that have evolved within that herb while growing in a specific region under the environmental stressors of that region. Current Chinese law states (of daodi herbs): "Daodi Chinese herbal medicines refer to the long-term application of traditional Chinese medicine, which is produced in a specific area. Compared with other Chinese herbal medicines produced in other regions, the quality and efficacy are better, and the quality is stable. These Chinese herbal medicines are famous."

When purchasing herbs, sellers will frequently state or sometimes write out that one or more of the company's herbs are "daodi." Furthermore, in the minds of some, herbs must be grown in their daodi region. While this may be excessive in the minds of some people, there is little doubt regarding the growing importance of this concept as China works diligently to standardize certain aspects of Chinese medicine. The fact remains, if the genetics of the seeds planted are not from the daodi region, then the herbs grown, even if in the daodi region, could not be called daodi.

China has invested significant amounts of research funds and time into the concept and promulgation of daodi. The largest hurtle is probably understanding why past generations considered a particular herb from a particular region to be daodi. This is mostly based on the writing of past doctors and their understanding of the clinical efficiency of each of these herbs. However, the issue is extremely complicated. For example, when using chemical markers (a standard for nearly every pharmacopeia around the world), these markers are not necessarily higher in the daodi region, they are sometimes lower; there does not seem to be any particular pattern. So, for now we must accept what tradition says and continue to look deeply at daodi herbs and try to uncover the mysteries of this ancient concept.

The text in your hands takes the most current research and combines it with the knowledge base that has developed over hundreds of years to offer the best methods to grow, harvest, and process herbs using daodi procedures. For growers outside of China, some of the most important information is the ecological conditions necessary to grow good quality material and should be given significant weight when making decisions regarding appropriate herbs to grown on your farm. Basic information such as local average weather conditions combined with soil requirements form the basis for choosing an appropriate location. Noting the time of year that rain comes or number of frost-free days can be essential to success. And, while many of these plants will grow outside of the climatic conditions stated herein, a growing body of research is showing that the ability to grow a plant in a particular area does not necessarily correlate with good quality medicinal herb material. In fact, plants can appear to be quite vibrant while growing and yet have vastly different chemical make-up when tested in the lab. And, while laboratory tests should not be the only means of testing the quality of medicinal plants, when there are consistently different results, it is worth pausing and evaluating the situation.

Finally, as explained below, because of significant soil issues in China and relatively fertile soils in North American and other regions, many of the deficiencies and diseases Chinese farmers struggle with may be of less consequence when growing the herbs in these more fertile soils. Furthermore, the organic and other progressive agriculture techniques used in the West have a much longer history and are far more developed than they are in China. Taken together, this is a great opportunity to use these potential advantages to test and learn new and innovative ways to produce these medicinal plants. However, when introducing a plant to a new environment there is no way to be sure it will thrive, in fact, it might very well succumb to a local disease or insect pest. Keeping that in mind, it is generally wise to start with a relatively small plot, perhaps no more than a ¼ acre and observe how the plant you choose grows. Observe how it responds to its new environment and take notes, both on how it is similar to what is described in this text and what might be different. This may yield valuable information if you choose to embark on a more committed venture of growing Chinese herbs and can be added to the growing body of information via *Passiflora Press*'s discussion group on the topic. (www.passiflora-press.com/daodi-discussion-group/)

IMPORTANT NOTES ABOUT THIS TEXT

Use of Chemicals in Cultivation of Herbs in China

There are many aspects of this text that made translation challenging, or at the very least require further explanation. One of the primary problems rendering this text in to English is the use of chemical fertilizers, pesticides, antifungals, etc. are common in the cultivation of Chinese herbs. While this is changing ever so slowly, the text represents the standard for using these chemicals. Keeping in mind that the vast majority of growers interested in growing Chinese herbs in the West are unlikely to employ these methods of cultivation, and the simple fact that many of the pesticides discussed in the original text are not available to Western growers, most of this information has not been translated here. However, mentions of using chemicals, e.g. the use of iso-fenphos-methyl and carbendazim for the pre-treatment of *danggui* seedlings prior to transplanting, are included as a reference and perhaps as a cautionary note that commercial production of these plants may be challenging without using these chemicals. There are other occasions when "natural" pesticides, chemicals extracted from plants, are used and considered "biological controls." I have retained most of these although I personally do not recommend them and urge growers to find solutions that do not include single compound pesticides that can have significant disadvantages to a farm ecosystem and beyond.

Fertilizers proved to be more difficult because most the text includes information about the use of NPK fertilizers without any other measure for adding compost or other "non-chemical" fertilizers. Furthermore, there is almost never a reference to ratios of these three compounds and unless it is stated otherwise, it should be assumed that a 15–15–15 (NPK) fertilizer should be used. Although I strongly support the used of non-chemical fertilizers, I have retained this information as a standard reference for those using other methods of cultivation to help in understanding what might be required to amend the soil in order to grow these crops. This information almost always includes a range of application rates, e.g. 180–300 kg per acre. This range should be used as a guide when considering the needs of your site. If your soil is relatively healthy and organic matter is high, many of these applications will be either unnecessary or can be applied at the lowest end of the scale, or less. It is important to remember that these herbs grow naturally without the use of any fertilizer applications but those natural conditions also provide it with a range of soil qualities, including but not limited to the native soil biota, which may be difficult to mimic in cultivated ecosystems, especially in areas far from the plants' native habitat. Therefore, it is reasonable to think, at least to some extent that some of these or similar applications will be needed to grow commercially viable crops. It is probably also important to note that many of China's agricultural lands have soil that is "tired," which means it is seriously depleted of soil organic matter and thus lacks much of what is needed for plants to grow as they once did, i.e. abundance and diversity of soil microbiota, ability to hold water, etc. However, it would be improper to think that just because your soil has a higher level of organic matter or more of any particular mineral nutrient(s) that you can grow a higher quality Chinese medicinal. The reason(s) for this are difficult to be certain of but could be due to specific environmental requirements, skill level of farmers, soil biota only present in its daodi location, or execution of processing techniques; among other potential issues. While it may be possible to overcome some of these issues, some may be difficult, if not impossible, to overcome. Therefore, it is prudent to carefully study this text and do ones best to approximate ALL the requirements in an attempt to bring the best and most representative crop to market. Remember, these techniques are often hundreds of years old or have been built on the experience of generations of farming these specific plants.

There is a significant movement in China to find solutions to many problems facing herb farmers. Many farmers are already growing Chinese herbs without chemicals, some even complying with international organic growing standards. However, this is an area where Western farmers may be able to add a significant contribution to this field of study. I urge anyone using this book who is interested in closely monitoring and measuring results to contact me and join the discussion group at the *Passiflora Press* website.

Regarding pesticides discussed in the original text

As noted above, most of these have not been translated but it seems appropriate to briefly discuss some of them here. Matrine is the most frequently cited chemical pesticide in this text, however it is not approved for use in either the US or Europe. This compound is an alkaloid from the plant *Sophora flavescence*, a Chinese medicinal plant, and is approved in China for organic agriculture. There is little data on the environmental impact of this compound but it is still used as a natural, non-synthesized, product. Pyrethrins are also frequently mentioned in this text. This should be distinguished from pyrethroids, which are synthesized compounds and have a more deleterious environmental impact. While these compounds – there are several related compounds under this general name – are considered relatively safe, they are known to be extremely toxic to aquatic life and bees are very sensitive to them. Therefore, if you choose to use these products it is strongly advised to apply them at night after bees and other pollinators have left the area and make sure that they are used responsibly and run-off is controlled if there is a possibility of it ending up in any body of water.

Language and Translation

Chinese language uses "characters," which are not pictographs, to represent "words" as we understand them in English. Like any language, time has created a number of different ways in which these characters are used, including adding layers to meaning or, in some cases, adding entirely different meanings to the same characters. One of the characteristics of modern Chinese is that words are almost always a contraction of two characters; this was not always true. In the case of herb names, while most are represented by two characters, some may have three characters, or rarely even four characters. However, these combinations of characters constitute a single "word" as we would understand it in English. Keeping this in mind, it is common for the transliteration of characters to be combined as follows: Latin binomial - *Angelica sinensis*, Simplified Chinese - 当归 where 当 = *dāng* and 归 = *guī*, thus giving us "*dāngguī*." Some readers might look at this and say, "Well, we separate "*Angelica*" and "*sinensis*" why should be keep "*dāng*" and "*guī*" together?" The answer is that botanical Latin is based on the hieratical system designed by the Swedish botanist Carl Linnaeus, the Chinese have no such native system of division. Therefore, a name is just a name, it does not have any connection to other related plants from the same genus. For example, other species of *Anglica* are not called "*dāng* sp." in the same way that we would say *Angelica* sp., which we can use if we are unsure of what particular species of *Angelica* is being referred to in a text. However, in the case of *dāngguī* there is, probably because of the fame of the medicinal plant, some similar ways of naming other species such that many, but not all, species of *Angelica* are called "something" *dāngguī*, e.g. *dàyè dāngguī* (big leaf *dāngguī*).

Common names in Chinese are not capitalized just as common names are not capitalized in English, e.g. purple cone flower is *Echinacea purpurea*. Finally, in sticking with convention of italicizing "foreign" words within a text, all pinyin is italicized and diacritic tone marks are used on all plant names, however they have been omitted from any other pinyin terms in the text such as daodi and this word is only italicized at the beginning of the text, from there on, it remains unitalicized. It is the translator's hope that this might be beneficial to those interested in studying Chinese language and will at least help with the communication with those who do speak Chinese.

In this text I have tried to avoid using pinyin as much as possible, a primary exception being plant names. Plant names are given in Hanzi characters, pinyin transliteration (including the entire name for the daodi herb), common English name, and botanical Latin in the introduction of each plant. From that point forward the plant is identified using the pinyin name only, including diacritic tone marks. While this may cause some confusion, there is no standard for an English "common" name of these plants and in an effort to reduce the chances of further confusion I have decided to stick with the common names used in China, which are, more or less, standard. In addition to these issues, all plants in this text have one, or sometimes two, characters added to the beginning of the name. These characters denote the daodi location for the herb and are much less frequently used in everyday discussion of herbs unless one is attempting to differentiate it from the same plant grown in a different location. For this reason and for the sake of flow and readability, I have only included this part of the name in the title for each monograph and in the first paragraph when introducing the herb, otherwise this part of the name is not used in the main body of the text. There are many websites and texts that discuss pronunciation of Mandarin and I encourage you to learn how to properly pronounce the herbs you grow.

A final language note about the Chinese characters found in the text. While I have chosen to include some, these are only for names of plants and a few oddities in the text. Names are given as characters in two places, in the title of each monograph and then again in the introduction at the very beginning of the monograph, which introduces the plant and its use in medicine. While I have chosen to use the simplified characters for the title heading, I have included the traditional characters along-side the simplified characters in this introductory material for each monograph. If there is only one set of characters, this is because the simplified and traditional characters are the same.

Measurement of Time and Space

In the Chinese system of time, months are divided into three parts; first-third, middle-third, and last-third. In this text the use of this division is common for planting, cultivating, weeding, fertilization, harvesting, etc. Because this artificial division is unfamiliar to Western readers I have decided to simply translate these divisions as (using "June" only as an example), "early June," "mid-June," and "late June." It is my belief that this subtle difference is not of major importance when it comes to performing most farm work since there is always a range of time to perform such tasks and most of them are weather dependent. However, these times should serve as a guide and should be followed as closely as possible. For those interested in the strictest sense of these terms they are as follows: first 10 days of a month (*shàngxún* 上旬), the middle 10 days of the month (*zhōngxún* 中旬), the last ten days of the month (*xiàxún* 下旬).

A note on weights and measures. Like the rest of the world, excluding the United States, China uses the metric system. Because this text is meant for use anywhere outside of China including North America, South America, Europe, Africa, and beyond, I have left all weights and measures using the metric system. I apologize to my fellow Americans who might find this challenging, but it's time to join the rest of the world and use a system that makes sense and is easy; for those not familiar with the metric system, I have included the following table for conversion of length, weight, volume, and temperature (see below).

Like many places, China still uses a traditional system of measure for agricultural area called "*mǔ*" (亩). A mu is equivalent to 667 square meters or approximately 1/6 of an acre or 1/15 of a hectare. I have calculated all applications of mu into acre since this is likely the easiest for most readers of this text.

I have added, for the sake of clarity or from personal experience, notes or short phrases in brackets [] as "Translator's Notes." Ultimately, most of these original notes were, after consulting with the authors of the monographs, integrated into the text. However, some of these remain, primarily because they are specific to the English reading audience this book has been designed for and they are based on my 7 years of growing Chinese herbs commercially in China and visiting other farms around the country.

Notes on Organization of the Text

Each plant has a section titled "*Principles of Prevention and Treatment*." In almost all cases, the original text is exactly the same. For this reason, I have placed it here in one single location for ease of reading without the need to repeat it over and over again in the text. However, there are some plants that have some specific information, in those instances, the text was translated and can be found within the monograph of that plant. This section is relatively simple and was written as follows: "When growing from either seed or transplanting, plants that appear weak or sick should be removed, prescribed methods of application of fertilizer, field management, proper encouragement or application of biological controls should be adhered."

Another section of the book that constantly repeats itself is the "*Packaging*" heading at the bottom of each monograph. As above, I have included any herb-specific information in the main body of the text but the primary information is the same for all herbs and is as follows: "All medicinal plants can be packaged in standard thick-walled plastic bags, or, where available, the use of environmentally friendly packaging is suggested. Be sure to label properly with the name of the product, weight, specifications (e.g. plant part, etc.), location of production, lot number, and date of harvest."

Photographs are very helpful when using this type of text, unfortunately the resolution of most of the photos submitted for this publication was too low to use in book format to adequately represent the plant or process pictured. Therefore, *Passiflora Press* has dedicated a page on its site (www.passiflora-press.com) where photos for everything from plant pictures to photos of specific processing techniques can be found. While this may be somewhat inconvenient, it does help to keep the price of the book low and access to the photos on the website is and will always be free. Furthermore, using this system allows the publisher to continue to add new photos and keep farmers up-to-date on any new developments or important information.

METRIC TO U.S. CUSTOMARY UNITS

1 meter (m) = 1.094 yards
1 meter (m) = 3.281 feet
1 meter (m) = 39.370 inches
1 centimeter (cm) = 0.3937 inches

1 liter (L) = 0.26 gallons
1 liter (L) = 1.06 quarts
1 kilogram (kg) = 2.20 pounds
1 gram (g) = 0.035 ounces

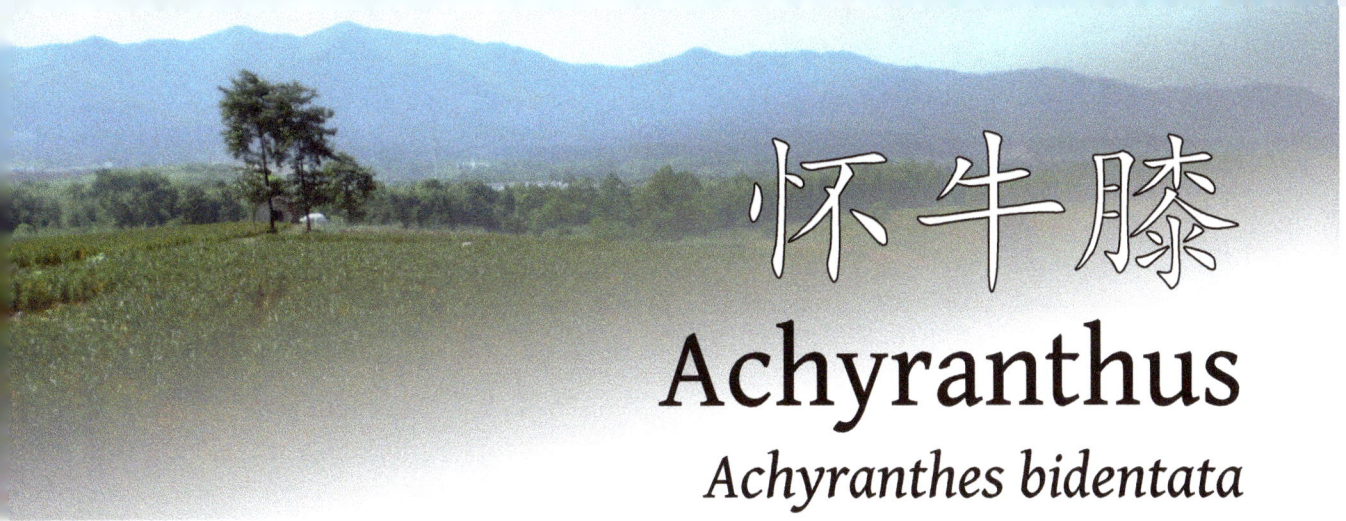

怀牛膝

Achyranthus
Achyranthes bidentata

DISTINGUISHING FEATURES

The dried root of the daodi medicinal *huái niúxī* (*Achyranthes bidentata* Bl.) is commonly known as *niúxī* or *huái niúxī* (懷牛膝 \ 怀牛膝) in China. The addition of "huái" is important to delineate it from a plant from a different genus, that is native to Sichuan province also known as *niúxī*. The latter is called *chuān niúxī* (*Cyathula officinalis* 川牛膝) to clarify its origins in Sichuan. *Huái niúxī* is a member of the Amaranthaceae family and is in a genus of approximately 15 species that are spread across the tropical and sub-tropical regions of the planet. This species grows on hillsides throughout much of China from 200–1800 m elevation. The plant is also native to most of Southeast Asia, Japan, Korea, and India. The daodi location for this plant is in the Jiaozuo district of Henan province.

Traditionally this plant has been used primarily to quicken the blood to relieve almost any kind of pain from menstrual pain to joint pain. The herb is commonly used to treat pain from trauma and is a main ingredient in "martial arts formulas" used to treat injuries. It is also known to supplement the liver and kidney so it is frequently used for arthritic pain, including knee pain, hip pain, lower back pain, and other similar pain syndromes in the elderly.

Modern science has determined that this herb has pharmacological activities including antitumor, anti-inflammatory, antiarthritis, antioxidative, anti-aging, and positive affects on the immune system, nervous system, bone metabolism, and blood circulation. Some research has suggested this herb may be helpful for treating post-menopausal bone loss and painful arthritic conditions in the elderly.

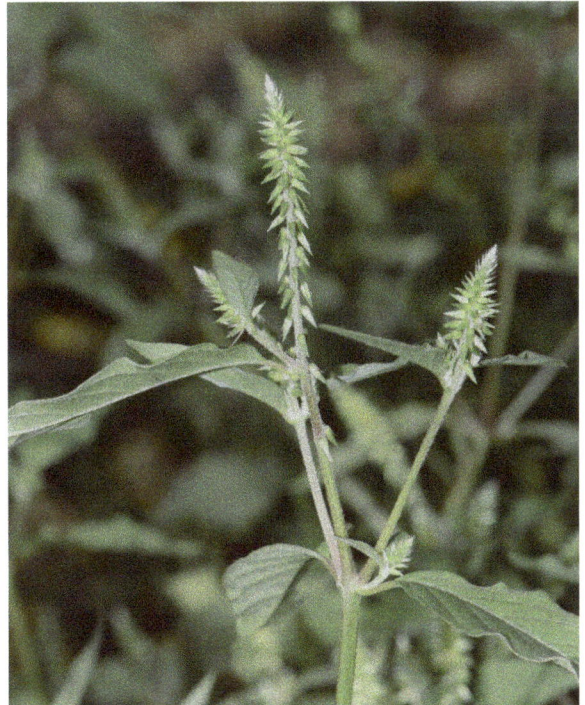

Contributing Authors

Liu Ming, Wen Chun-xiu, Xie Xiao-liang, Huang Lu-qi, Hao Qing-xiu, Guo Lan-ping, Liu Ling-di, Gu Dong-sheng, Tian Wei

7

PRODUCTION SITE ECOLOGY

Elevation

Huáiniúxī is cultivated between 50–500 m elevation.

Temperature

A frost free period of at least 197 days is suitable.

Photo Period

Annual sunshine hours should range between 2500–2757 hours. Average daily sunshine of 35-70% is suitable.

Moisture

The average annual rainfall range is 500–1000 mm with an average humidity of 34–55%.

Soil

A loose sandy soil with a pH of 5.5–6.5 is best. A thick soil layer greater than 30 cm is recommended.

Topography

Level fields and slopes up to 15° are suitable. If the land is sloped it should be from the south-east facing the north-west. Good wind circulation and water drainage are important.

FIELD MANAGEMENT

Site Selection & Soil Preparation

Amend a loose sandy soil with 3000 kg per acre of organic fertilizer and a NPK fertilizer. Plow at least 30 cm deep then harrow smooth.

Sowing Seeds

Seeds are planted 0.5–1.0 cm deep in rows spaced 15–20 cm apart. After sowing seeds, cover with soil and press down gently. Each acre requires 9–12 kg of seed.

Cultivation and Weeding

After seedlings have emerged, use cultivation to keep soil loose and maintain a weed-free environment.

Irrigation and Top-Dressing

Irrigate during dry periods and after top-dressing. Make sure that water drains well after heavy rains. In early August a 15–15–15 NPK fertilizer is used to top-dress at a rate of 210 kg per acre.

Trimming

During the time of the plants most vigorous growth (June and July), a sickle or other appropriate tool is used to cut the top 20 cm or so off the plant. When the plants grow quickly, they develop branching and fibrous material that causes the roots to be more woody; this reduces the quality of the herb material. By cutting of the tops of the plants they grow more slowly and the roots stay more supple and are of higher quality.

PREVENTION AND TREATMENT OF DISEASE AND INSECT PESTS

Principles of Prevention and Treatment

Huáiniúxī is relatively free of diseases and pests. The pests discussed here may not be problematic in your location, however the potential for similar pests should be monitored in your fields. Most of the disease problems are associated either directly or indirectly with water drainage problems. Therefore, good water drainage is critical for successful cultivation of this plant.

Silver Looper Moth (*Ctenoplusia agnata*)

Prevention and Treatment

During larvae and early worm stage the bugs are removed by hand.

Biological Controls

During the early worm stage, 100 million spores per gram of Bt can be sprayed on the plants.

Beet armyworm (*Spodoptera exigua*)

Treatment for this pest is the same as the Silver Looper Moth (above).

Bean Blister Beetle (*Epicauta gorham*)

Prevention and Treatment

Autumn deep plowing is employed to destroy over-wintering insects.

Leaf Spot (*pathogen not identified*)

Prevention and Treatment

Crop rotation with a grass family plant is done every 2–3 years to prevent this disease.

Wilt Disease (*Fusarium* sp.)

Prevention and Treatment

Crop rotation every 3–5 years is done to prevent this disease. Diseased plants should be immediately removed from the field.

Root Rot (*Fusarium* sp.)

Prevention and Treatment

Proper field management, including fertilizer application (amending the soil to strengthen the plant if necessary), and timely removal of diseased plants all will help to prevent or slow further spread of this disease.

HARVESTING

Harvest Season

Huáiniúxī is harvested in the autumn of the first year after spring sowing. Plants are dug when the leaves have withered, usually from late October through early November before the first freeze sets in.

Harvest Method

Hand digging: The above ground portions of the plants are cut away with a sickle, then plants are dug with a shovel or digging fork. Be sure to avoid damaging the root. Mechanized digging: This is used for large tracts of flat land in the same manner as *cháihú* (chapter 11).

ON-FARM PROCESSING

Drying Method

When digging, shake to remove as much soil from the root as possible. Roots are immediately put in the sun to dry and are flipped in the morning and evening to ensure even drying. Avoid dropping or throwing the roots as this may damage the skin and allow mold to grow on the roots.

Straightening the Roots During Drying

When the roots reach 70% dry, carefully straighten them by hand, then allow them to complete the drying process in the sun. Finished roots should not exceed 15% moisture.

Flower bud of *huái niúxī* just emerging in Henan province, China.

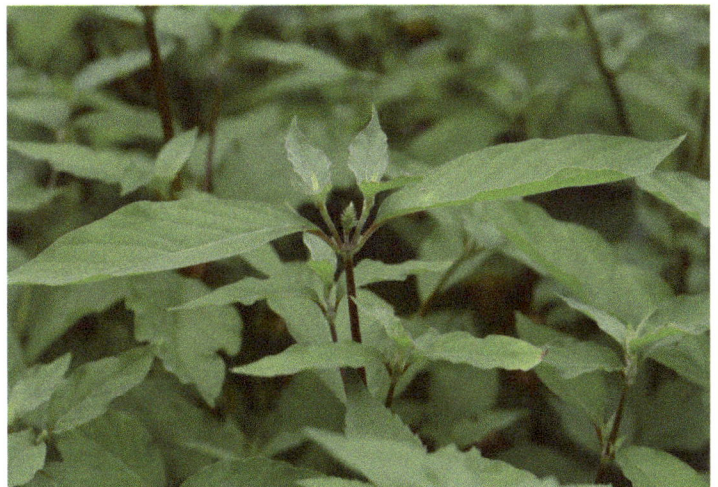

西陵知母

Anemarrhena

Anemarrhena asphodeloides

DISTINGUISHING FEATURES

The dried rhizome of the daodi herb *xīlíng zhīmŭ* (*Anemarrhena asphodeloides* Bge.) is commonly known in China as *zhīmŭ* (知母) and is a single species genus within the lily family (Liliaceae). The plant can grow to about 60 cm tall with a scape (flowering stalk) that extends to 100 cm. Flowers are relatively inconspicuous but quite attractive up-close. In its native habitat (most of northern China, Mongolia, and Korea) it grows in scrub, grassy slopes, steppes, and hillsides from near sea level up to about 1500 m. The daodi location for this medicinal is in Yi County and its surrounding area of Hebei province.

Traditionally this herb is classified as a clear heat and drain fire medicinal. It is a major herb in one of the most famous formulas for treating qi aspect heat (White Tiger Decoction *Baihu Tang*) and can be found in many other similar formulas. However, *zhīmŭ* is special in that is also can nourish and enrich yin. Since repletion heat can deplete yin fluids, this herb's ability to both drain fire and supplement yin gives it a special place in the material medica. It can be used for lung, stomach, and kidney heat in both replete and vacuity heat patterns.

Modern science has looked extensively at this plant's anti-inflammatory action finding that is can act to protect neurons by decreasing cell death (aptosis). This research has also shown potentially positive outcomes for the treatment of Alzheimer's disease. Several compounds found in the herb have been shown to enhance learning and memory abilities in aged rats. Other compounds have been the object of Parkinson's disease research and some models show positive results. The herb also exhibits antioxidant, antidepressant, antidiabetic, antihypertensive, antimicrobial, and anti-osteoporosis activities.

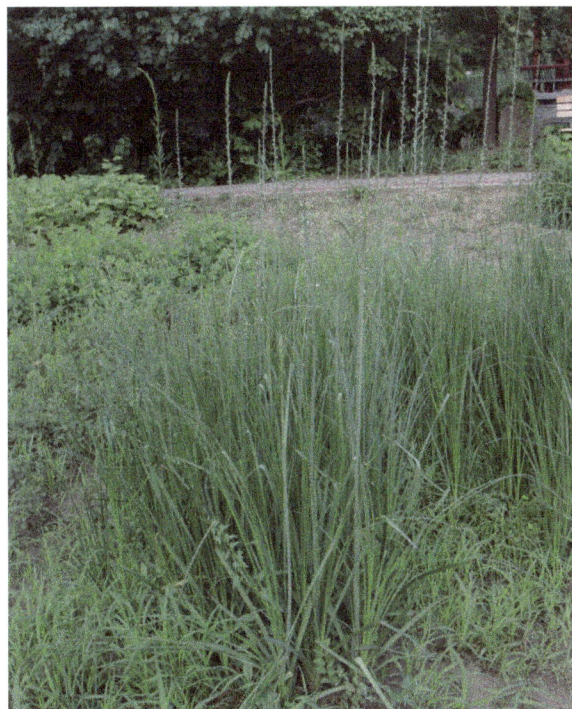

Contributing Authors

Wang Wen-quan, Chen Qian-liang, Hou Jun-ling, Zhong Ke, Xie Jing

PRODUCTION SITE ECOLOGY

Elevation

Zhīmǔ is cultivated between 100–1000 m elevation.

Temperature

An annual mean temperature of 8–12°C is suitable.

Moisture

Annual average rainfall 150–300 mm, concentrated in the months of July-September.

Soil

Zhīmǔ can be cultivated in a range of soils including; chestnut soil, brown calcic soil, gray calcic soil, light carbonate brown soil, black humus-rich soil, and by using recovered land from pastures. The soil should have a high enough sand content to allow for good drainage. The soil should be slightly alkaline (pH 8–9).

Topography

A south facing or southeast to southwest facing gentle mountain or hilly slope (<15 degrees) is appropriate. The area should be grassland or prairie, reclaimed woodland is not appropriate. Shaded areas or low-laying areas are not appropriate for growing *zhīmǔ*.

Site Selection

The site should be sunny with good drainage, loose humus and sandy soil, and have a gentle hill or mountain slope.

Soil Preparation

Manure and\or compost should be added prior to cultivation. This should then be plowed in using a 20–30 cm deep disking tool. Finally, the field is harrowed smooth.

SOWING SEEDS & RAISING SEEDLINGS

Seed Quality Requirements

The seed is black and has three ridges that run from tip to tip. It should be full and plump without disease or insects. There are four grades of *zhīmǔ* seed. Grade I: 1000 seeds should weigh at least 7.52 g and have a germination rate greater than 67%; grade II: 1000 seeds should weigh at least 6.52 g and have a germination rate greater than 58%; these two grades are suitable for growing medicinal material. Grade III: 1000 seeds weigh between 5.01-6.52 g and have a germination rate between 41-58%. This grade must be cleaned further and shriveled seed and other materials must be removed before it can be reevaluated and used. Grade IV: 1000 seeds weigh less than 5.01 g and has a germination rate less than 41%. This grade of seed should be discarded and not used for planting.

Saving and Storing Seed

Seeds are generally ripe from the middle of August through the middle of September and should be collected from vigorous plants that are at least 3 years old, without disease or insects. Seeds are born in capsules and often are partially or wholly contained within these capsules when harvested. The entirety of the harvested material is spread out to dry in the sun (or another suitable drying environment). Once dried, capsules are easily broken\ threshed either by hand (tools, or feet) or by machine. After winnowing select the plumpest seeds for saving (see above). Seeds should be saved in a well ventilated, cool, dark, dry area indoors. Containers should be air-tight.

Selection of Seedling Area

An area that is level, with adequate sunlight, with a good source of irrigation, but also good drainage. Soil should be loose with a loose humus\sand (20:80) mixture. Avoid using vegetable garden soil or other soils that may contain grubs or other insects, including apple, pineapple, apricot, etc., as orchards are places where insects tend to assemble.

Seed Pre-Sowing Preparation

Pre-soak seeds by pouring 60°C water over them and allowing them to sit for 8–12 hours; remove and allow to air-dry until they are visibly dry on the exterior. Meanwhile dig a hole 4-5 cm deep and large enough to place all the seeds inside at approximately 1 cm thickness. After the seeds appear to be dry, mix with 2 times their volume of moist, fine sand, place in the hole, cover with 3–4 cm soil, and cover with agricultural plastic. When most of the seeds have sprouted, they may be planted. Seeds will begin to sprout after three days and the peak sprouting time is six to eight days. After 10 days, more than 90% of the seeds that will sprout, should have already done so.

Sowing Seeds

Zhīmǔ seeds may be sown in the autumn or spring. Autumn sowing is done before the first frost. Spring sowing is done during early April. Rows should be 25 cm apart and a furrow 1.5 cm deep should be dug. After the seeds are sown, they are covered by 1.5–2.0 cm soil and gently patted. Beds should be mulched with straw to protect the seeds and soil for becoming dry and the new seedlings from receiving direct sunlight. Soil must be kept moist after sowing seeds.

TRANSPLANTING

Transplanting Seedlings

Transplanting may be done during spring, autumn, or a rainy season. *Zhīmǔ* is most commonly transplanted in the spring. Spring transplanting is done with one-year old seedlings with rhizomes that have grown to 6–10 mm in diameter. Rows should be spaced at 15–20 cm and plants should be placed 25 cm apart. Dig a small trench 5–6 cm deep for transplanting. Cover plants with soil and press firmly, making sure to mound the soil so the height of soil exceeds the existing soil by approximately 2 cm. Allow soil to dry (on the surface only) after transplanting, then irrigate once. When transplanting during autumn or during the rainy season, leaves should be trimmed to approximately 10 cm, otherwise use the same techniques as spring transplanting.

Propagating by Division

Propagating by division is best done in the spring prior to the emergence of leaves, or in the late autumn when the plant has begun its dormancy phase. Choose plants that are at least 2 years old to dig. Rhizomes should include roots. Slice into 5 cm sections; it is best for each section to include 1–2 buds. Transplant into 6 cm trenches in rows 25 cm apart with cuttings spaced every 15–20 cm. When propagating by cuttings in the autumn it is best to cover cuttings with a 6 cm mound of soil to ensure their survival through the winter; in the spring, level off the mound to facilitate sprouting. In order to economize planting and propagation, this method can be used during harvest by cutting off the sections

of the rhizome without buds for processing and using the sections with buds for propagation. This will result in shortening the growing period before harvest. To simulation wild-cultivation, space rows 25–30 cm apart and plant divisions 15–20 cm apart.

FIELD MANAGEMENT

Thinning and Final Singling of Seedlings

When planting seeds, once seedlings have reached 4–5 cm they should be thinned to 5–7 cm apart; remove weak plants and keep the strong plants. Once plants reach 6–10 cm they are ready for transplanting. Generally, thinning is done 2–3 times when direct seeding in the field, and it is best to do this early rather than late. Loosening the soil and weeding can also be done during this period.

Cultivation and Weeding

Cultivating the soil and weeding are generally done on sunny days when the soil moisture is low. Weeding should be done before weeds get established. It is best to weed the first time when *zhīmǔ* has reached a height of 7–8 cm and therefore the soil can be shallowly loosened (4–6 cm) without damaging the young plants. Weeding young plants should be done by hand; careful use of hand tools is permitted. Application of fertilizer is best done following weeding.

Irrigation

During the peak growing season when watering is done in mid-June and mid-August, weeding and application of fertilizer are also performed. This is advantageous for the even distribution of nutrients from the fertilizer. If during this period it is raining and the soil moisture is at approximately 60%, then irrigation is not necessary. *Zhīmǔ* does not like extended periods of water saturated soil. During periods of high temperatures, especially if there is also extensive rain, care should be taken to drain water by trenching. Do not allow water to accumulate in the planted area, because, if this occurs the chance of root rot increases significantly.

Application of Fertilizer

Thoroughly composted manure or other compost should be applied to the soil prior to sowing seeds at a rate of 7500–12000 kg per acre. During the growing season composted manure or plant ash can be applied by top-dressing 1–2 times at a rate of 6000 kg per acre, after which time the soil is loosened with hand cultivators to hasten the integration of the material. During July and August *zhīmǔ* is at its peak vegetative period. During this period a potassium dihydrogen phosphate fertilizer may be applied as a foliar feeding at a rate of 600 kg per acre; this will strengthen the plant, help it to resist disease, and promote the growth of the root system. The best timing for this spray application is in the afternoon starting at approximately 4pm.

Scape Removal

When planting from seed, the following year, at approximately the spring equinox, *zhīmǔ* begins to bolt. Unless saving seed is a priority, the scape is always cut off to improve growth of the plant.

PREVENTION AND TREATMENT OF DISEASE AND INSECT PESTS

Principles of Prevention and Treatment

Generally, *zhīmǔ* is not prone to diseases or pests. Damping-off is most often seen in seedlings when they are over watered or the soil does not offer proper drainage. Below-ground pests can be problematic, but don't often cause significant crop loss. Because this is a perennial needing 2-4 years to maturity, intercropping to attract predatory insects to control aphids is recommended.

Blight Diseases (*Fusarium* sp.)

Prevention and Treatment

Remove diseased plants and dispose of them properly. Proper top-dressing, watering, and good drainage are all important to avoid damping off. Cover cropping is an important method for avoiding disease associated with damping off.

Damping-off (*Rhizoctonia solani*)

Prevention and Treatment

Remove any infected plants and properly dispose of them. Water at a time when leaves will dry quickly

(generally morning). Be sure that the soil is draining properly, especially after heavy rains. Using cover-cropping with cereals and legumes for one year after harvest helps to reduce disease. Heavy mulching (minimum 2.5 cm) has also been shown to reduce the occurrence and spread of this disease.

Aphids (Aphidoidea)

Prevention and Treatment

Aphids are naturally attracted to the color yellow. Deploying "sticky yellow board" or construction of areas with yellow painted boards will attract aphids to places where they can be killed. Close monitoring of plants is important when using biological controls. At the first sigh of aphid infestation lady bugs should be used to control the infestation.

Grubs (*Holotrichia* sp.)

Prevention and Treatment

Fields with grub problems should be plowed deeply before winter to reduce the numbers of grub larva. Use *Bacillus popilliae*, *Beauveria bassiana*, or other similar biological controls according to the manufacturers' instructions.

HARVESTING

Harvest Season

When growing from seed, the plant may be harvested starting in the 3rd or 4th year. When propagating from rhizome stock, harvesting can begin after 2–3 years. Spring harvest should commence prior to the emergence of new growth, which is usually March or April depending on weather and other environmental conditions. Autumn harvest is carried out after the above-ground portion of the plant has withered; generally in September or October depending on weather and other environmental conditions. Every 3–4 kg of fresh rhizome yields 1 kg of dried medicine.

Harvest Method

The entire root and rhizome structure is dug up from the beds with a pick-axe or digging fork. These tools are best because they generally cause less damage to the rhizomes. Avoid using shovels as they are likely to cut rhizomes. In larger operations, a modified plow may be used to unearth the rhizomes. When using either method it is important to clean the plow and/or other tools to avoid cross-contamination of diseases from other fields.

ON-FARM PROCESSING

Initial Processing and Sorting

Remove any plants that may have been growing with the *zhīmǔ* such as grasses or other weeds, including their roots. Discard any sections that are rotten or show any signs of disease. Any remaining withered leaves or flowering stocks may also be removed at this time. Take care to remove as much dirt as possible before transporting to an appropriate area for further processing.

Processing Prior to Drying

Remove any remaining above-ground portions and roots with hand shears. During this process discard any other foreign matter and diseased or rotting rhizomes. The upper portion of *zhīmǔ* is covered with remnant fibers from old leaves which must be removed. This can be done by hand or mechanically. The machine used is a cylinder that should be filled half full with the rhizomes and spun at 400 revolutions per minute for 30 minutes. At the end of this period the roots are removed with the fibers. This process is generally repeated once to remove all but a small percentage of the fibers; the remaining fibers are removed by hand when the root bark is scrapped off. While still fresh, the thin root bark is scrapped off with a knife, being careful not to cut too deeply. During this process there will be sections of the rhizome for which it is difficult to remove the outer skin. These sections can be left and sold as "*hairy zhīmǔ*." However, this is generally considered an inferior product and commands a lower price; this is not recommended. Do not use water to wash the rhizomes. Rhizomes should not be stacked in piles above 50 cm high. Rhizomes not immediately processed should be allowed to dry in the sun, however they must be processed relatively quickly because, if left whole, they will rot.

Drying Method

Traditionally *zhīmǔ* was dried in the sun or with the use of heat from a fire. Modern drying technology is, however, far superior to these methods and yields a better product. Rhizome should be dried at 50°C until they reach a uniform moisture content not to exceed 12%.

Final Preparation, Grading, & Packaging

Once dried, rhizomes are graded according to size and quality. Grades should be of a uniform size and quality. Each grade should be packaged separately and sold accordingly.

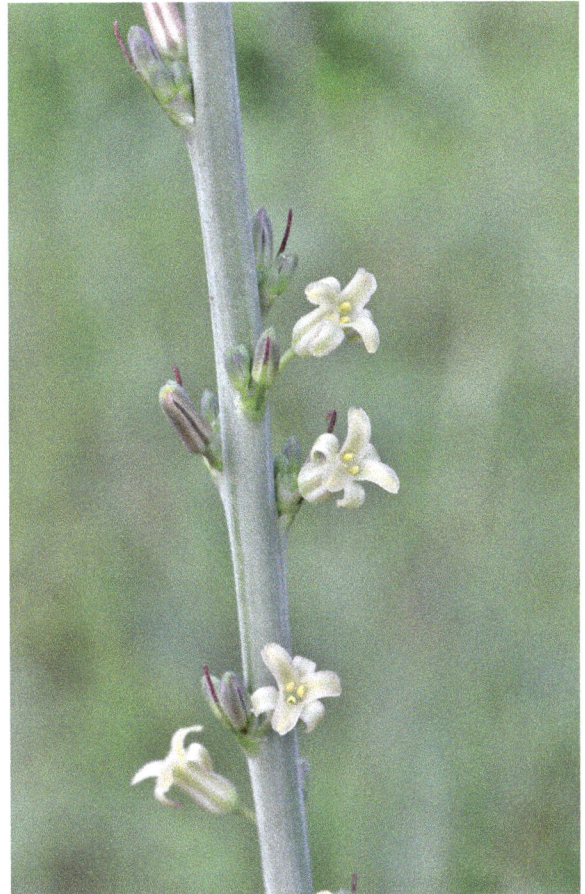

Flowers of *zhīmǔ* at our farm in Beijing, China.

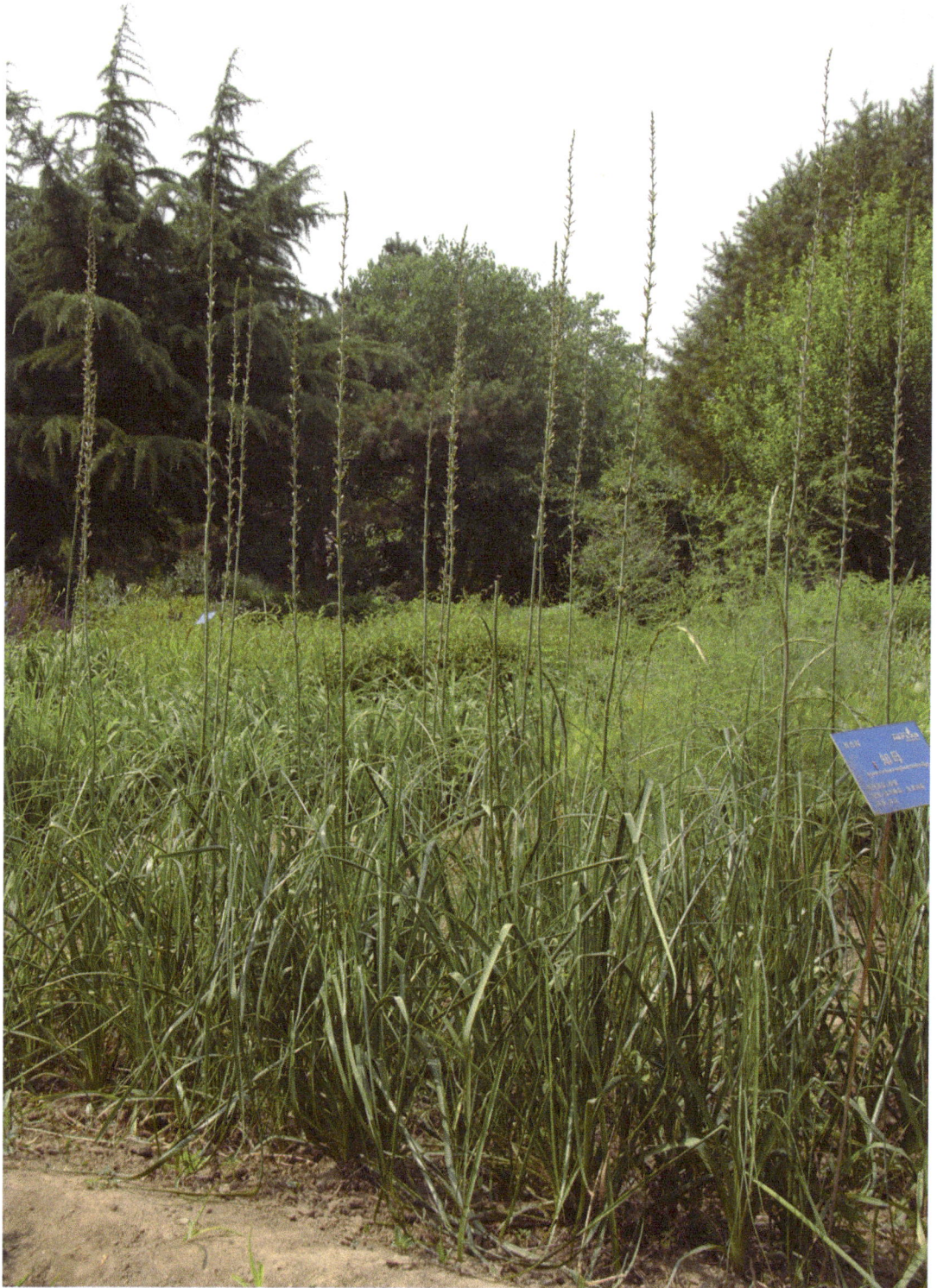

Zhīmǔ at the Institute of Medicinal Plant Development in Beijing, China

祁白芷

Dahurica Angelica

Angelica dahurica

The dried root of the daodi herb *qíbáizhǐ* (*Angelica dahurica* Fisch. Ex Hoffm.) commonly known as *báizhǐ* (白芷) in China is a member of the carrot family (Apiaceae). This species of Angelica grows to 1–2.5 m tall. The plant is perennial and generally flowers from the second year on, however 12–25% will flower in the first year. It grows along forest margins, in valley grasslands, and stream-banks between 500–1000 m elevation. The herb is native to Hebei, Heilongjiang, Jilin, Liaoning, and Shaanxi provinces as well as northern Taiwan, Japan, Korea, and far eastern Russia. Daodi *báizhǐ* refers to the herb that is produced in the area of Anguo in Hebei Province.

Báizhǐ is used traditionally as an herb to eliminate wind and stop pain. It is exceptional for treating headache and sinus congestion caused by external wind-cold invasion. This herb enters the yang-ming channel and therefore treats toothache. *Báizhǐ* is an important herb to treat abscesses, both externally and internally. It can be applied externally for abscesses and boils, eliminating pus and stopping pain. Finally, this herb is commonly used for cold-dampness pathogens caus-ing copious white vaginal discharge.

Modern science has confirmed many of the traditional uses for *báizhǐ*, showing that it has significant antibacterial activity and new research suggests it could be a candidate for some types of cancer therapy. The roots have shown antioxidant, anti-inflammatory, and antiproliferative activity, which is mostly due to the phenolic and terpenoid compounds. The chemical constituents responsible for its antioxidant and anti-inflammatory actions are mostly alcohol soluble and therefore hydro-ethanolic extracts are the best way to administer this herb for these functions.

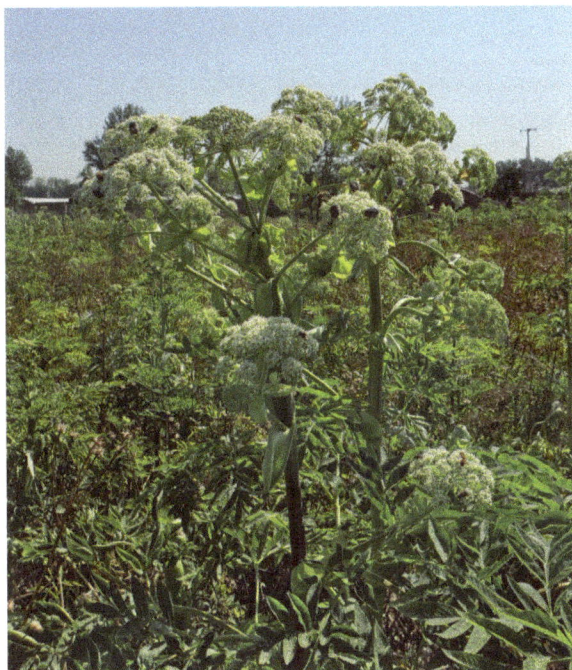

Contributing Authors

Zheng Yu-guang, Xie Xiao-liang, Guo Lan-ping, Huang Lu-qi, Hao Qing-xiu, Liu Ming, Song Jun-nuo, Wen Chun-xiu, Liu Ling-di, Gu Dong-sheng, Tian Wei

PRODUCTION SITE ECOLOGY

Elevation

Báizhǐ is cultivated between 50–500 m elevation.

Temperature

At least 190 frost free days. Average annual temperature is 12.4°C. January is the coldest month with average temperatures below 3°C and July is the hottest month with average temperatures between 18–27°C.

Photo Period

Annual sunshine hours range from 2500–2757 hours. Daily sunshine percentage range is 35–70%.

Moisture

Average annual rainfall should be 500–1000 mm with relative humidity of 34–55%.

Soil

A loose sandy soil with a depth of at least 30 cm is ideal with pH in the 5.5–6.5 range.

Topography

Field can be either level or have a slope up to 15 degrees. If the field is sloped it should be facing either southeast or northwest to allow for proper drainage and wind-flow.

PRODUCTION AREA ENVIRONMENTAL REQUIREMENTS

Site Selection

A sunny location with good drainage, loose humus and sandy soil, and level or sloped land is acceptable.

Soil Preparation

Manure is spread at a rate of 12000–18000 kg per acre, or fertilizer at a rate of 2400–3000 kg per acre. The field is then plowed to at least 30 cm, leveled, and 2 m wide beds are built.

SOWING SEEDS & RAISING SEEDLINGS

Seed Quality Requirements

According to the *Pharmacopoeia of the People's Republic of China* (2015) seeds for *Angelica dahurica* (fisch. Ex Hoffm.) Benth. et Hook. f. is the original source for the herb *báizhǐ*. Seeds should be full and plump, free of insects or damage by insects, they should be stored at normal atmospheric temperature for up to one year.

Sowing Seeds

Spring planting should be around the first week of April. Autumn planting should be during the last two weeks of August or the first week or September. Autumn planting is best for plant development, harvest volume, and herb quality.

Space rows at 30 cm and hoe a channel 1–1.5 cm deep. Distribute seeds evenly in the furrow, cover with soil and press gently. Seed at a rate of 12 kg per acre.

FIELD MANAGEMENT

Thinning and Final Singling of Seedlings

When the seedlings have reached 5 cm thin to 5–8 cm apart. When the seedlings have reached 15 cm space to 12–15 cm apart. When performing final singling of seedlings, eliminate plants that are either too large or those that are weak and small. Final distance apart should be 30×15 cm.

Cultivation and Weeding

Pull any weeds during the thinning process. The first time you thin, loosen the soil shallowly, after this the soil can be loosened more deeply. The best time to cultivate is after irrigation or a period of rain, this ensures that the soil stays loose and free of weeds. Be careful not to disturb the roots during this process.

Irrigation and Top-Dressing

The first time fertilizer is added to the edges of the beds at a rate of 210 kg per acre. Then, in August when the root is growing rapidly, a urea fertilizer is added at a rate of 120 kg per acre.

Irrigation and Water Drainage

When using the autumn seed sowing method, the field should be watered once prior to the emergence of the seedling. Plants should be watered after top dressing. There are no rules regarding watering prior to harvest, water as necessary. Good drainage is important, if the field gets water logged it should be drained if possible.

Removal of Flowering Plants

Plants that bolt in the first year produce woody roots that are considered inferior medicine. These plants should be removed from the field. Farmers can expect 12–25% bolting and thus loss.

PREVENTION AND TREATMENT OF DISEASE AND INSECT PESTS

Principles of Prevention and Treatment

Generally, *báizhǐ* does not have significant disease problems. Following the recommedations below should minimize potential continuous cropping issues. Excessively dense planting should be avoided to minimize spread of potential aphid or red spider mite infestation. Proper management of soil, encouraging diverse soil biology, should minimize root rot disease problems.

Leaf Spot (*Septoria dearnessii*)

Agricultural Controls

Crop rotation after 2 years is an effective method for prevention and treatment of this problem.

Gray Leaf Spot (*pathogen not identified*)

Agricultural Controls

Crop rotation, using a grass as a cover crop for 2 years after harvest of *báizhǐ* and being careful not to plant too close together can also help with prevention, as well as appropriate watering and drainage of the field, but excessive humidity can contribute to the problem. Diseased leaves should be removed immediately to reduce the possibility of the disease spreading to other plants. Increasing management of weeds and soil, including increasing the soil organic matter to improve the soil will help the plant resist the disease.

Root Rot Disease (*Macrophomina phaseoliua*)

Agricultural Controls

Crop rotation, using grass as a cover crop, every 3-5 years. Reasonable application of fertilizer with appropriate nitrogen, and increases in phosphorus and potash, to improve plants' resistance to disease. Timely removal and burning of diseased plants, and use lime in the hole where the plant was removed.

Purple Root Rot (*Helicobasidium mompa*)

Agricultural Controls

Improve field management with better drainage of any stagnant water. Pull and dispose of any diseased plants. Apply lime (5%) in holes where plants were removed to kill disease in the soil.

Aphids (Aphidoidea)

Prevention and Treatment

Aphids are naturally attracted to the color yellow. Deploying "sticky yellow boards" or construction of areas with yellow painted boards (60×40 cm) will attract aphids to places where they can be killed. The surface of these boards can be covered with oil so the aphids get stuck there. Check to see when the board is coated with aphids, then scrape the board and add more oil. These boards are deployed at a rate of 180 per acre.

Biological Controls

Introduction of lady bugs early can be a very effective control of aphids (lady bugs should be put out in the evening). A 0.3% solution of matrine diluted to a concentration of 0.07–0.1% in water; or natural pyrethrins diluted to a concentration of 0.01% in water and sprayed according to manufacturer's instructions.

Striped Shield Bug (*Graphosoma rubrolineata*)

Prevention and Treatment

Till the soil to reduce winter survival rates. During the early stages of development of eggs and larvae, physical elimination by hand can be used to reduce populations. Eliminate withered plant debris, fallen leaves, and eradicated weeds.

Biological Controls

A 0.3% solution of matrine diluted to a 0.1–0.5% concentration in water or natural pyrethrins diluted to a concentration of 0.01% in water; sprayed according to manufacturer's instructions.

Spider Mite (*Tetranychidae*)

Biological Controls

A 0.36% solution of matrine diluted to a 0.07% concentration in water, or natural pyrethrins diluted to a concentration of 0.01% in water and sprayed according to manufacturer's instructions.

Common Yellow Swallowtail (*Papilio machaon*)

Prevention and Treatment

Elimination of the larvae in the early stage, this is generally done by hand.

HARVESTING

Harvest Season

Báizhǐ is harvested in the autumn of the second year in late September when the leaves have withered. Plants from spring sown seeds can be harvested in October of the first year after the first frost.

Harvest Method

Choose a fine sunny day after the leaves have withered and remove the dead leaves and stems, most of these should be easily removed without the need for cutting. Then carefully dig the entire root and shake off as much soil as possible but be careful not to damage the exterior of the root. In large commercial operations, tractor-powered root diggers are employed for this operation.

ON-FARM PROCESSING

Drying Method

After digging and removal of dirt, roots are sliced fresh and dried either in open air or with low-temperature processes; drying temperature should not exceed 45°C. When done in the open air, or in the sun, turning or mixing of the material is important to prevent mildew. Dried *báizhǐ* should not exceed 14% moisture.

Final Inspection

When the slicing and drying are completed the outside of the root should be grayish, the inside whitish, and it should have a strong aromatic quality; the root should not have any black coloration in the center and it should be free of bugs.

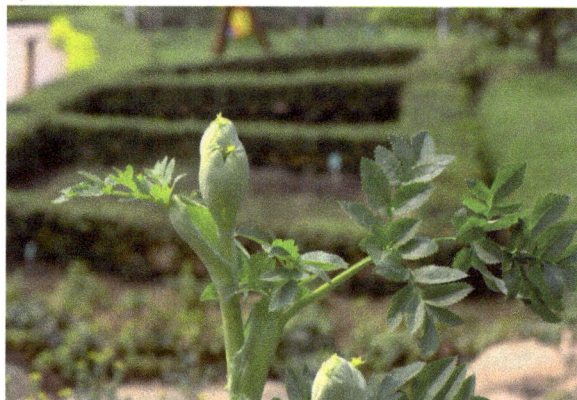

Báizhǐ budding out on our farm in Beijing, China.

20

岷县当归

Dang Gui

Angelica sinensis

DISTINGUISHING FEATURES

The root of this daodi herb, *mínxiàn dāngguī* (*Angelica sinensis* Oliv. Diels.), commonly known in China as simply *dāngguī* (當歸 \ 当归), is a member of the carrot family (Apiaceae) in the genus *Angelica*. The Angelica genus has 90 species, 45 of which are present in China and 32 are endemic. Many medicinal plants from this genus are used around the world, including three official species in China. The daodi location for this herb is Min county in Gansu Province. Once thought to be extinct in the wild, discoveries of several wild stands in 2014 have led to extensive research and cultivation experiments to help integrate the wild genetics into the cultivated plant, thus protecting this extremely valuable medicinal resource.

Dāngguī is one of the most famous of all Chinese herbs and has an extensive history, including a cultivation history of over 1000 years, which is quite rare. This medicinal herb is used to supplement the blood for any condition of blood vacuity. It is also known for its ability to quicken the blood and is revered as a first-choice herb for the treatment of nearly all menstrual disorders. Because of this, it is sometimes called "woman's ginseng," however it is not botanically related to ginseng.

Modern science has identified many pharmacological activities for *dāngguī* including; anticancer, neuroprotective, anti-Alzheimer, nephroprotective, hepatoprotective, antioxidant, immunoregulative, and anti-inflammatory. Most of these findings support traditional knowledge about the plant.

While there have been numerous studies on the chemistry of this medicinal plant, some recent work has been devoted to investigation of polysaccharides found in the root, which have been shown to have hepato- and neuro-protective activities.

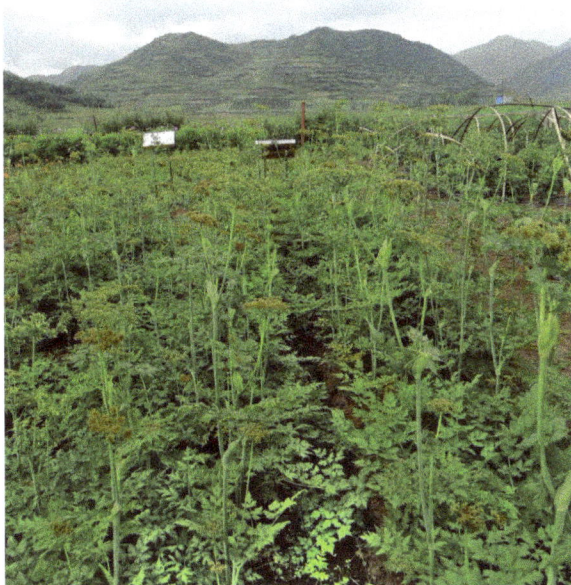

Contributing Authors

Duan Jin-ao, Yan Hui, Qian Da-wei

PRODUCTION SITE ECOLOGY

Elevation

Dāngguī is cultivated between 2000–2500 m elevation. Seedlings should be raised between 2500–2700 m elevation.

Temperature

Average annual temperature between 4.5–5.7°C in a mountainous region.

Rainfall

Average annual rainfall is 570–650 mm.

Soil

Loose soil, rich in organic matter (black to grayish-brown). Weak alkaline soils are most appropriate.

Topography

Seedlings: *see below.* Mature plants can be planted on level fields and up to 15° slope.

PRODUCTION AREA ENVIRONMENTAL REQUIREMENTS

Seedling Site Selection

Dāngguī seedlings are raised at an elevation of 2500–2700 m in virgin soils, or soils that have rested for 5 to 10 years. The soil should be very deep, fertile virgin soil is best. North slopes of 5–25° are shady and moist, sunshine is very limited, this is ideal for raising seedlings.

Preparing Soil for Seedlings

Soil must be very deep, sandy, fertile, rich, and loose, with significant organic matter, and a neutral pH. The soil should be plowed at least 25 cm deep. Soil is prepared with 2500–3000 kg of composted manure thoroughly tilled into the soil, then high beds are built to ensure adequate water drainage. Generally, ditches are dug every 1.3 m creating pathways between beds 30–40 cm wide and 25 cm deep. These pathways help to ensure that all sides of the beds have adequate water drainage.

SOWING SEEDS & RAISING SEEDLINGS

Saving Seed

Dāngguī originates in the high mountains where it is a cool to cold moist environment. The history of cultivation is very long, ~1000 years! To improve seedling quality and reduce early bolting, raising seedlings has traditionally been done at high elevation. When choosing plants, selection of larger roots has taken priority, along with the growth and development of healthy/strong above-ground portions of the plant, ripening of seed in a relatively even manner, and uniform fruit production for sowing. It is most appropriate to gather seeds during the month of July when they are ripe. At this time the fruit coating is slightly pink and the peduncle droops. When harvesting, the entire peduncle is cut off. Because *dāngguī* seeds do not ripen simultaneously, the harvesting of seeds must be done in stages, as the seeds mature, and this generally starts on the tallest peduncle. Begin by choosing the fullest, plumpest seeds for harvest, but avoid cutting the entire stem when harvesting. After harvest, place seeds in a shaded, dry, well-ventilated area. Once seeds are properly dried, thresh and store.

Sowing Seeds

In Min county (southern Gansu province), and the surrounding area, seeds are sown from early to mid-June.

Seeds are generally soaked before sowing in order to ensure fast and complete germination. Seeds are soaked for 24 hours in water at approximately 30°C. After 24 hours, the seeds are removed from the water and placed in the sun to dry. Once dried, they are mixed at a 1:10 ratio with plant ash.

Generally, seeds are broadcast evenly across planting beds. A thin layer of rich soil (0.5 cm) is used to cover seeds, beds are then compressed with a weighted bed roller to ensure seeds and soil are in complete contact with each other. Seeds are sown at a rate of 24–30 kg per acre, with an expected germination rate of over 70%.

After seeds are sown, beds must be kept moist. Beds are mulched with grass or hay to help preserve soil moisture.

Mulching to Preserve Moisture

When plants reach 1–2 cm tall, select a shady day, or work just before nightfall, and gently fluff the mulch over the plants to 3 cm thickness. Be sure to be careful when the mulch is fluffed because the sprouts will have come up through the cracks in the mulch and hasty fluffing could damage the young plants.

Shade

Once the plants have reached a height of 4–5 cm the straw mulch is removed and a structure must be constructed to ensure 50–65% shade. This structure should be approximately 60 cm tall. Alternately, a simple inverted "V" structure (approximately 1 m tall) can be built to shade the beds. Tree branches or other plant material can be used to create the shade. Be conscious not to create an overly shady area to avoid the situation where cloudy or rainy days render the beds too dark, as this will inhibit the health and overall growth of the plants.

Cultivation and Top-Dressing

Keep the area free from weeds during the period while they are still in the seedling bed. During this time, work such as thinning, eliminating weak plants, and keeping the strongest plants, aiming for a spacing of about 1 cm, can be performed. A quick acting nitrogen-rich fertilizer is best during this period.

OVER-WINTER STORAGE

Digging Seedlings for Winter Storage

Dāngguī seedlings frequently will not survive through the winter, so for this reason they are dug prior to winter and stored in an appropriate environment. Seedlings are dug from late September to early October, when the leaves begin to whither and yellow. Generally, this represents about 110 days of growth and each root should weigh approximately 40 g. Plants are dug with a small shovel or other appropriate tool; it is very important to remove the entire root system as an intact whole. Excess soil is gently shaken off and leaves are removed, leaving approximately 1 cm of the petiole. Plants are divided into small and large, then bundled into groups of 100 plants. At this time the plants are placed in a cool, shady, dry location and allowed to dry for 5–7 days, until the root

epidermis is slightly dried. At this time the root morphology begins to change and the root moisture content is 60–65%. Once the petiole is withered, the roots can be stored. After digging avoid leaving them in the sun for extended periods of time, as this can quickly reduce the water content in the roots and kill the plant.

Winter Storage

There are two methods of storing plants over the winter, one is to store them in a cellar or pit, the other is known as piling. Regardless of the method chosen, it is important to ensure that plants are neither allowed to be in the sun for extended periods, nor allowed to get too hot or damp; the latter conditions could cause the plant to begin to bud out prematurely.

Cellar or Pit Storage

The area chosen to dig the pit should be dry, shaded, and cool. Avoid using any areas that are prone to flooding. An area free of pests, such as rodents and other animals, should be chosen. The pit should be dug according to the number of roots needed to be stored, both rectangular and circular pits are used. After the pit is dug, 3 cm of clean sand/clay (not soil) is laid on the bottom of the pit and a layer of roots is laid on top. The roots are covered with dirt and another layer of the roots is added, alternating the direction of the head of the root so that the arrangement is neat. This is repeated 6–7 times to a thickness of 65–75 cm. When completing the burying process, use dirt to raise the area of the pit above the level of the soil around it.

Pile Storage

There are several methods of storage by piling. This method is always done in an out-building where there is no heating of any kind. There are two basic methods: 1) In this method a rectangular brick form is built with dimensions of 100×100 cm. The bottom is covered with 3 cm of sand/clay (as above) and the roots are laid inside in a circular pattern with the crown of the root facing toward the walls of the structure and the tails of the roots facing toward the middle (there should never be less the than 6 cm between the crown of the root and the outside wall). As above, after each layer of root is laid, a layer of sand/clay is added (1 cm) until the structure is full, at which point a thick layer (4–6 cm) of sand/clay is added to the top creating the look of the back of a fish. 2) Alternatively, one can forgo the bricks and simply pile the roots in the same manner as above, ensuring that the roots are covered by at least 10 cm on the outside and piling up the sand/clay on top to look like a steamed bun. Smaller amounts can simply be placed in a basket and buried in the same manner as the latter method.

TRANSPLANTING

Selecting Suitable Land

Dānggui cultivation is best done at 2000–2500 m elevation with deep, fertile (black-grayish), loam-sand, soil; convenient irrigation; and a slope of less than 15 degrees. Prior to planting *dānggui*, a grain crop is usually planted on the land, and this crop rotation is repeated after 3 or more years depending on the needs of the land.

Soil Preparation

After the grain crop is harvested, the field is plowed to a depth of approximately 30 cm and allowed to sit for the remainder of the summer, then in the autumn the field is shallowly plowed. Prior to planting, 24000–30000 kg per acre of well composed manure, 300–600 kg per acre of balanced NPK, or 1800–3000 kg of organic fertilizer should be shallowly plowed into the soil. Then the land is harrowed into slightly elevated beds 10–15 cm tall, 60 cm wide, with 30 cm between beds; the beds should be flat and smooth.

Selection of Seedlings

Before planting it is critical to choose healthy plants for planting. The standard for this is a taproot that is whole and measures 3–5 mm in diameter with 100 seedlings weighing approximately 110 g. Plants are transplanted into the field between late March and mid-April, early April is generally considered the most optimal time.

Transplanting

In Min county and the surrounding area (Gansu province) *dānggui* cultivation utilizes plastic bed covering to protect soil temperature and conserve water. The bed is formed to slant toward the pathway and the plastic bed covering covers the bed and extends into the pathway. The high-pressure polyethylene plastic is usually 40 cm wide and 0.015 mm thick, but 0.008–0.010 mm thickness can also be used. The beds are 60 cm wide and 10–15 cm tall, and the pathways are 30 cm wide. The plastic bed covering should be pulled tightly over the bed and the edges covered with soil every 2 m to prevent the plastic from being blown away by the wind. Before transplanting, combine 40% isofenphos-methyl and carbendazim, each 250 g, with 10 L water and soak plants for 10 minutes. After soaking allow them to air dry; once dry they should be immediately transplanted. Each bed is planted with two rows of *dānggui* 25 cm apart in the bed. Holes are dug through the plastic to 15 cm and 2 plants are placed in each hole, which is recessed 2–3 cm below the level of the soil. After planting, the plants are covered with soil to the level of the surrounding soil. Wait for early bolting of the plants, during the third weeding period, to thin plants to one per hole; one acre should have 36,000–48,000 plants.

Cultivation and Removal of Bolting Plants

Proper field management must include timely weeding. When growing *dānggui* weeding is generally done 2–3 times in May and June, and it must be done at least 3 times during the season. The first time is done in mid-May with shallow hoeing. The second time is done in mid-June with deeper hoeing. The third time is done in mid- to late July, again with shallow hoeing. During the period of mid- to late June, early bolting plants are pulled during the thinning process.

IRRIGATION AND FERTILIZATION

Top-Dressing

Dānggui requires significant amounts of fertilizer. Apart from general fertilization, top-dressing is generally used twice per season. The first application is when the above-ground plants are in full growth (early July), during this period urea is added at a rate of 30 kg per acre. The second time is early August when urea is applied at a rate of 30 kg per acre and potassium dihydrogen phosphate at a rate of 12 kg per acre is used. When applying fertilizer as top-dressing it should be spread about 8 cm from the plants, and after application the soil should be covered with a light layer of soil from the pathways.

Watering and Water Drainage

Watering is done in autumn before the first freeze, then again in the spring before planting, and then again in the event of insufficient rain. Flood irrigation is most commonly used, but it is important not to over-water. Toward the end of July when there are generally long stretches of continuous or repeated rains, care should be taken to drain off excess water to avoid root rot.

PREVENTION AND TREATMENT OF DISEASE AND INSECT PESTS

Cultivated *dāngguī* is generally relatively free of pest and diseases. Potato rot nematode can be very destructive. However, it is not common. Root rot is a far more common problem, especially when cultivation is on farmland without slope. There are no known pest, but farmers growing this herb outside of China should be aware that they may have native pests in their area that could be problematic.

Potato Rot Nematode (*Ditylenchus destructor*)

Prevention and Treatment

Ditylenchus destructor is a pathogenic nematode commonly called "potato rot nematode" and can be found in many regions of the northern hemisphere. It can infect a wide range of crops, including weeds, and is difficult to manage if it becomes a serious problem. Maintaining strict control over equipment, plants, and soil movement from one field to another is important if there is any threat of an out-break. Cover-cropping is highly recommended as a control.

Agricultural Control

Crop rotation with a grass family plant is used every 3 years or so. When using organic fertilizer, it is important to be sure it is properly composted and matured. During transplanting, select only plants without disease or mechanical damage to the roots. They should have only a few lateral roots, root bark that is smooth and glossy, and a diameter of 3–5 mm, and 100 seedlings should weigh approximately 110 g. Be sure to keep fields clear of diseased plants and ensure they are well-drained during heavy or prolonged periods of rain.

Root Rot Disease (*Fusarium* sp.)

Prevention and Treatment

Use crop rotation with a grass family plant after 3 years. Be sure to eliminate any diseased plants immediately and dispose of them properly. After removal of diseased plants, 100 g of wood ash or 200–300 g of quick lime is added to the holes. Be sure that water is properly drained during periods of heavy or continuous rain.

HARVESTING

Growing Period Before Harvest

Dāngguī requires three years of growth before it produces mature seeds, meaning that it must go dormant through two winters and three summers of growth. We can conceptualize the development of the plant over three years in the following way: raising seedlings (1st year), attainment of value as a medicine (2nd year), and ability to produce viable seed (3rd year). In Min county most plants are harvested for medicine in the autumn of the year they are transplanted (end of the 2nd year).

Harvest Season

The optimal time for harvesting is from mid- to late October when the leaves have begun to yellow and whither.

Harvest Method

Select a sunny day and a time when the weather will remain pleasant and sunny for at least several days. Before digging the roots, the leaves are cut off from the petiole (leaf stem) and the roots are left in the ground to allow petioles to be exposed to the sun for 3–5 days; it is important to take care not to damage the petiole in this process (cuts should be clean). When digging be careful to keep the entire root system intact, and avoid cutting or breaking the roots. Roots are laid out on a clean dry surface (tarps are mostly commonly used) to partially dry in the sun; turned over once a day to ensure even drying. As the roots dry, any soil that remains attached can be relatively easily shaken off. Once the roots become soft, they can be transported back to an appropriate area for further processing.

ON-FARM PROCESSING

Initial Drying

Once *dāngguī* has been transported back to the processing area it should never be piled and should not be allowed to freeze or mold as this will adversely affect the quality. Select a dry, shady, cool area with good air circulation and promptly spread the harvest out for several days until the remaining petiole is dry and withered and the lateral roots are mostly dried but still soft. Avoid any exposure to the sun during this period because this could cause the root resins to become red. During the drying period the root should be turned 1–2 times per day, carefully checking for any mold, mildew, or other rot. Any root found with mold, mildew, or rot should be promptly discarded.

Binding

Once the roots are half dried, any soil should be shaken free and the remaining petiole cut off. The root is then placed on one's legs, or on a board or table, and vigorously rolled to bind together the lateral roots with the main root. Strips of cloth are used to bind the entire mass together in groups of 2–3 roots (large roots) or 4–6 roots (small roots) forming a bound mass of roots that should weigh approximately 0.5 kg.

Shed Drying

Wood shelving is built to the following specifications. Wooden shelves are constructed to fit with a 1.2–1.5 cm lip around the edge rising from the platform. A bamboo mat is placed inside and the *dāngguī* is stacked on top in 2–3 layers; a thickness of 30–50 cm is suitable. The shed must be left open to ensure proper air flow. (See photographs at www.passiflora-press.com) [Translator's Note: Length and width of your shelves are dependent on your shed size.]

Heating Process for Drying

Stalks from lima beans, stems from willow or poplar trees, etc. can be used as fuel for heating. Use water to spray-moisten. Make a fire that creates smoke, giving the surface of the *dāngguī* a smoke cure. Smoke should be distributed across the roots and the fire should be kept moderate; avoid a brightly burning fire. After 10–15 days when the root skin has a golden yellow to light brown appearance. Take care to control the temperature inside the shed, keeping it between 30–70°C. After 10 days the roots should be flipped over. After flipping the roots, the roasting should continue for 8–20 days, bringing the root moisture content to 20–30%. Once the roots have achieved this moisture content the fire is extinguished and the roots remain in the cool shade for another 3–5 days; this allows the moisture toward the center of the roots to move to the outside. When the outside of the roots becomes moist again after this waiting period, the fire is stoked again for another 5–7 days. During this heating period all the root hairs must fall off, the body of the root becomes hard, and, using a bit of force the tails can be broken into small pieces. This process takes 30–60 days to complete, rendering the raw root into the medicine known as *dāngguī*. At the end of this period the skin of *dāngguī* should be yellowish-brown to sepia in color, the material should be pliable and tough, and cutting to reveal the inside should confirm that it is light-yellow to light sepia in color, with a strong aromatic odor. Any material that is light and flimsy or is excreting oils should be rejected.

Special Storage Details

Roots should not be stored above 20°C or 65% humidity.

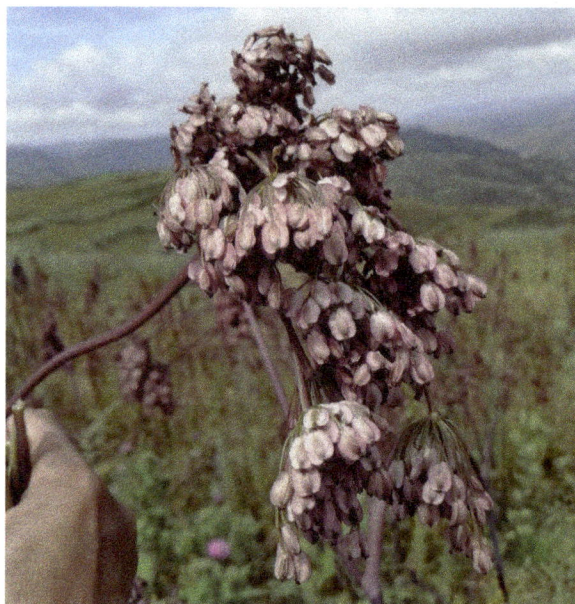

Fresh *dāngguī* seeds in Gansu province, China.

祁紫菀

Chinese Purple Aster

Aster tataricus

DISTINGUISHING FEATURES

The dried root of the daodi herb *qí zǐwǎn* (*Aster tataricus* L.f.), commonly known as *zǐwǎn* (紫菀) in China, is a member of the aster family (Asteraceae). This is a perennial herb grown from rhizomes. It forms a rosette with flowering stems that are 10–150 cm tall with blue or pale lavender to purple ray flowers and yellow disc flowers. It grows from 400–3300 m elevation and is native throughout much of China as well as Japan, Korea, Mongolia, and Russia. It is an introduced weed in many eastern states in the United States. Daodi *zǐwǎn* refers to the production of this herb is the area of Anguo in Hebei Province.

Chinese medicine uses *zǐwǎn* primarily to stop coughing and calm panting, but it can also eliminate phlegm. One of the primary clinical applications for this herb is to treat cough and/or panting that is accompanied by phlegm. Although this herb is considered warming, it is commonly used for conditions with either heat or cold symptoms, and is well-known for being effective for both patterns. Likewise, it is also somewhat moistening to the lungs and therefore can be used when there is lung dryness. The combination of being acrid, warm, and moistening makes this a primary herb for dry cough marked by cold.

Modern scientific research has confirmed traditional uses of this plant with proven antitussive, anti-inflammatory, and expectorant activities. Although the triterpene shionone has long been considered the active compound in the plant and is, in fact, the chemical marker used in the *Pharmacopoeia of the People's Republic of China* (2015) to measure quality, more recent research has suggested that caffeoylquinic acids, saponins, and aster peptides are likely working synergistically to create these pharmacological activities. These and other compounds have also shown antitumor, antioxidant, antiviral, and other actions.

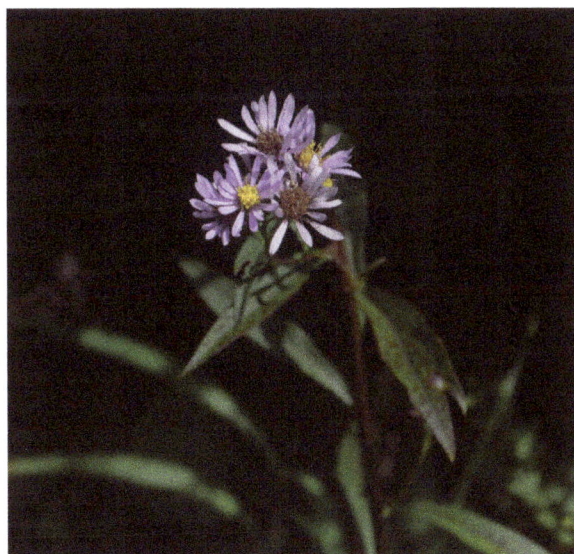

Contributing Authors

Zheng Yu-guang, Xie Xiao-liang, Huang Lu-qi, Hao Qing-xiu, Guo Lan-ping, Liu Ming, Wen Chun-xiu, Wang Qian, Liu Ling-di, Jia Dong-sheng, Tian Wei

PRODUCTION SITE ECOLOGY

Elevation

Zǐwǎn is cultivated between 50–500 m elevation.

Temperature

At least 197 frost free days. The coldest month is January with average lows below 3°C. July is the warmest month with average temperatures between 18–27°C.

Photo Period

Growing *zǐwǎn* requires annual sunshine around 2500–2757 hours. Sunshine percentage range 35–70%.

Moisture

Suitable average annual rainfall is 500–1000 mm with relative humidity of 34–55%.

Soil

A loose sandy soil with a depth of at least 30 cm is ideal with pH in the 5.5–6.5 range.

Topography

Field can be either level or have a slope up to 15 degrees. If the field is sloped it should be facing either southeast or northwest. The site must allow for proper drainage, wind-flow, and have irrigation available.

Soil Preparation

Other than overly acid or alkaline soil, all soils are acceptable for growing *zǐwǎn*. Soils should be loose\sandy and have a large humus content. Well-composted manure can be added at a rate of 12,000–18,000 kg per acre. This is plowed in, then leveled, and 2 m wide beds are built.

DIGGING RHIZOMES AND TRANSPLANTING

Digging and Preparing Rhizomes

Rhizomes can be dug during the last 7–10 days of October and immediately transplanted (see below for details). Rhizomes chosen for transplanting should be free of disease, rot, or insect damage. Fall harvested rhizomes may also be kept in moist sand and buried in a pit or kept in a cool cellar over the winter for spring planting. Rhizomes may also be dug in the early spring (March and April) before they begin to sprout. When planting the rhizomes, they should be cut with a clean sharp knife or scissors into 6–10 cm sections, each with 2–3 buds.

Transplanting Method

Transplanting is done during the months of March and April. In level beds prepare furrows 3–5 cm deep and 30 cm apart, 2–3 sections of roots are laid every 15–20 cm. Cover with soil and gently press, making the soil level. Rhizomes are transplanted at a rate of 300 kg per acre.

FIELD MANAGEMENT

Cultivation and Weeding

Cultivation and weeding are done after watering or after a rain. Do not hoe too deeply. It is important, especially in the initial period after transplanting, to keep the soil loose and free of weeds.

Irrigation and Water Drainage

Water appropriately during early stages not allowing the ground to dry out. During the month of June, the leaves become long and growth is vigorous, watering should be increased if there is a lack of rain, and soil should be kept loose. During the month of September, the roots are maturing and extra water can be given if necessary. Be sure that plants have good drainage during heavy or continuous rains.

Top-Dressing

During the months of June or July an NPK compound fertilizer is applied at a rate of 210 kg per acre. This is done by digging a shallow furrow between rows and sprinkling the fertilizer into it before covering with soil.

Removing Flowers and Buds

When the plant begins to bolt and flower buds appear, these should be carefully removed with sharp clean scissors, do not use hands to pull or tear the stem. This is done to focus the plant's energy on root production.

PREVENTION AND TREATMENT OF DISEASE AND INSECT PESTS

Principles of Prevention and Treatment

Cultivation of *zǐwǎn* mostly has two classes of pest and disease problems, fungal infections and insect pests. Generally, fungal infections first affect the root system, although they may manifest in the leaves, i.e. black spot and spot blight diseases. These diseases are most commonly prevented by regular crop rotation with a grass family plant, intercropping with a grass may be an alternative to rotation. Insect pests are most treated manually with traps but can also be treated with bacterial sprays. Attracting insect predatory birds may help to lessen these pests.

Black Spot Disease (*Alternaria* sp.)

Prevention and Treatment

Use a grass family plant in crop rotation after 2 years. Remove and clear the field of debris in the autumn. Destroy any diseased plants and be sure that water is properly drained during heavy or prolonged rain; never allow standing water or sodden soil.

Spot Blight Disease (*pathogen not identified*)

Prevention and Treatment

Use a grass family plant in crop rotation after 2 years. Remove and clear field of debris in the autumn. Deeply bury or burn any diseased plant material and till or plough the land immediately after roots are removed for transplanting to discourage the growth of the fungus.

Root Rot Disease (*Fusarium* sp)

Grass family plant crop rotation every 3–5 years. Use fertilizer appropriately. Apply nitrogen fertilizer and increase phosphorus and potash fertilizer to strengthen plant's ability to cope with disease. Finally, diseased plants should be removed in a timely manner and immediately and properly disposed of.

Silver Lined Noctuid (*Argyrogramma agnata*)

Prevention and Treatment

During seedling and young plant growth, watch closely for the larvae stage and manually eliminate them.

Biological Controls

During larvae and early life stages use 100 million spores per gram of *Bacillius* (Bt) at a 0.5% concentration in water and apply accordingly. Natural pyrethrum (5%) at a 0.1–0.05% concentration in water can also be used. These treatments should be applied once a week for 2-3 weeks to kill the insects.

Black Cutworm (*Agrotis ypsilon*)

Biological Controls

During the adult stage, black light traps are used to attract and kill them. While the adults are active a combination of sugar, alcohol, and vinegar at a ratio of 1:0.5:2 is placed in pans at a rate of 30–36 pans per acre, 1 m above the ground in the field to lure and kill them.

Grubs (*Holotrichia* sp.)

Prevention and Treatment

Before winter deep plowing and extensive harrowing are employed in an effort to reduce the winter survival rate of the insect. Utilize phototaxis for the adult insects by employing black or green lights, or a combination of the two to lure them to traps. If using both black and green lights, they can be either alternating or keep both on at the same time. Generally, using one of these traps per 8 acres is sufficient.

Biological Controls

Use *Bacillus popilliae* and spores of *Beauveria bassiana* as biological control. *B. popilliae* should be used at a rate of 9 kg of the powder per acre, while *B. bassiana* is used at an application rate of 2.0×109 spores per square meter.

HARVESTING

Harvest Season

When rhizomes are transplanted in the spring, roots are harvested in October of the same year, or March of the second year.

Harvest Method

Roots are harvested after the above-ground portions have withered. First, remove the withered above-ground portions, then carefully dig up the root and rhizome, including all new rhizome growth. Rhizomes with joints that have little to no roots are reserved for replanting, and heavily rooted sections are harvested for dry herb.

ON-FARM PROCESSING

Drying Method

After initial sun drying of 1–2 days, plants are dried in one of two ways. The most appropriate method is to put them in a cool, dry, shady area with good air circulation. After the roots have dried but are still soft, i.e. not hard and brittle, they are braided for further processing. The other method is to continue the sun-drying method, but when using this method, the roots should be turned every day and inspected for mold and mildew, any roots showing signs of mold or mildew should be removed immediately. Dried roots should not exceed 15% moisture content.

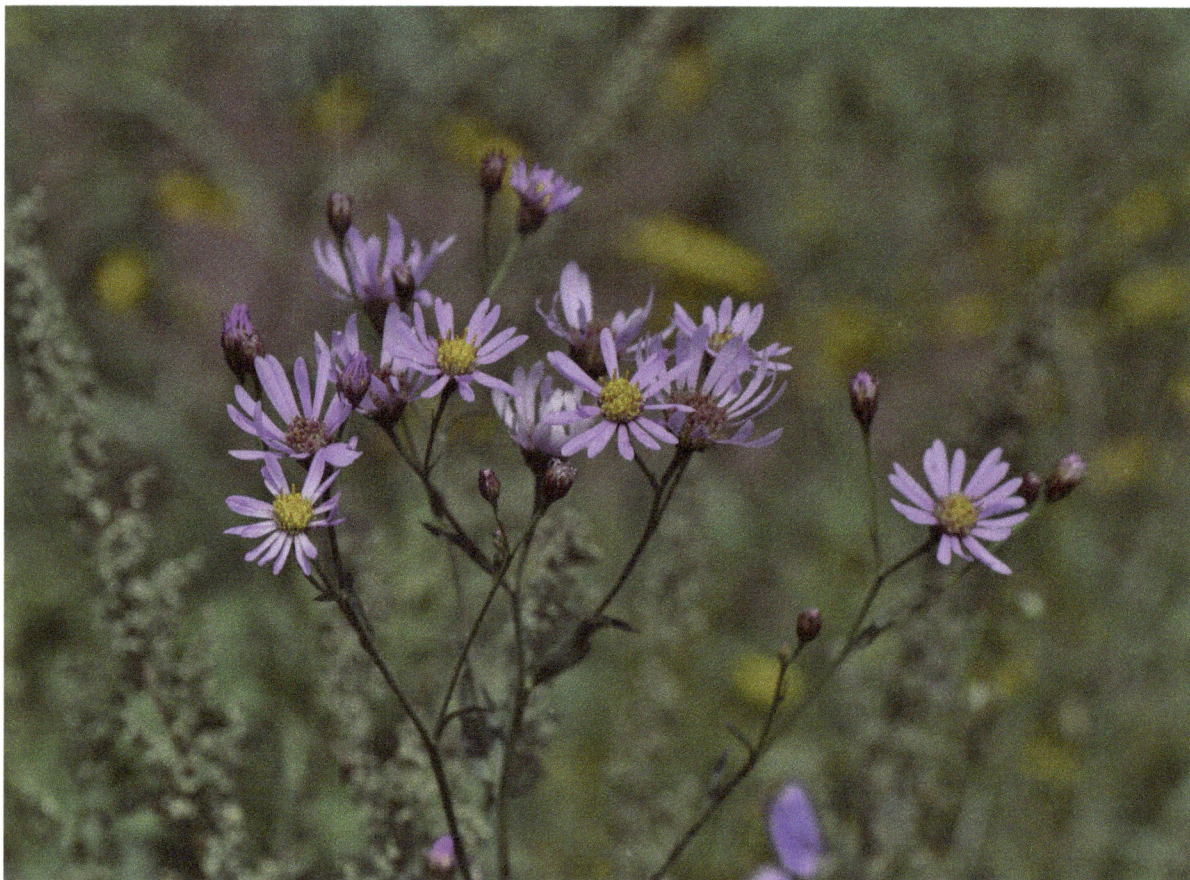

Wild *zǐwǎn* in the mountains of Hebei province, China.

蒙古黄芪

Astragalus

Astagalus mongholicus

The dried root of the daodi medicinal *měnggǔ huángqí* (*Astragalus membracaceus* var. *mongholicus* (Bunge) P. K. Hsiao), which is commonly known as huángqí (黄芪 \ 黄芪) in China, is a member of the pea family (leguminaceae). The very large *Astragalus* genus has around 3000 species, around 450 of which are endemic to China. The material produced in Guyang county, Wuchuan county, Tu Mo Te You Qi, and the surrounding areas in Baotou, Inner Mongolia is considered the daodi medicinal. [Translator's Note: This variety has been renamed to *A. mongholicus*, however the most current Chinese Pharmacopoeia (2015) doesn't yet reflect this change.]

Huángqí is, without a doubt, one of Chinese medicine's most famous herbs. In ancient times some authors considered it to be even better at supplementing qi than the highly-coveted Asian ginseng. This herb is most commonly used to supplement qi, specifically for spleen and lung qi vacuity. *Huángqí* has the ability to lift the clear yang qi from the spleen to the lung as well as to "lift the sunken." When used for these applications, it should be used in its processed "honey mix-fried" form. The raw herb is also used to improve urine flow when spleen qi is vacuous and fluids are not being transformed properly. Because qi governs blood, when there is excessive blood loss, *huángqí* is a very important herb to supplement qi and nourish blood, it is generally combined with *dāngguī* (see page 21). This is based on the principle that qi is necessary to help the body produce blood, especially because increasing blood is a slower process that increasing qi.

Modern science has studied this plant extensively, particularly for its pharmacological activities related to the human immune system. Various markers showing improved immunity have been shown to increase with moderate doses of the herb over at least a 2-week period. The herb is also commonly used in the treatment of cancer patients with positive results. It has shown cardiovascular activity, in particular cardiac performance shows marked improvement after ingestion or injection of the herb or its extract. Finally, this herb has shown positive hepatoprotective, antiviral, and antioxidant activities, as well as improvement of sperm mobility.

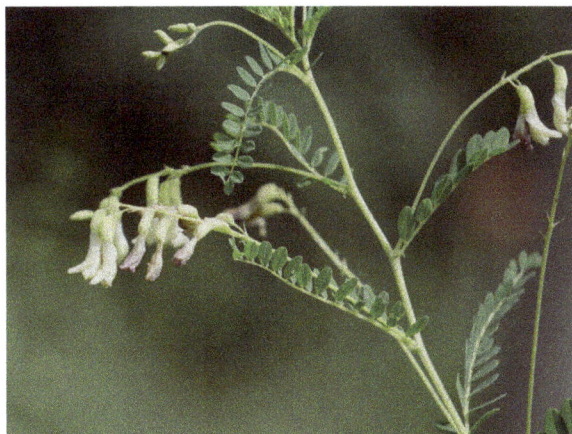

Contributing Authors

Li Min-hui, Zhang Chun-hong, Zhang Ai-hua, Xu Jian-ping, Wang Jie

PRODUCTION SITE ECOLOGY

Elevation

Huángqí is cultivated between 1000–1500 m elevation.

Temperature

Suitable average annual temperature is 2–5°C, with more than 95 frost free days. January is the coldest month with temperatures ranging between -35--11°C. July is the warmest month with high temperatures ranging between 22–30°C.

Photo Period

Average annual sunshine ranges from 2500–3100 hours; average daily sunshine is 70–75%.

Moisture

Suitable average annual rainfall is 250–350 mm with an average humidity of 50–60%.

Soil

A sandy, gravelly, alluvial soil is preferred.

PRODUCTION AREA ENVIRONMENTAL REQUIREMENTS

Site Selection

Level ground at the proper elevation with good water drainage and excellent penetration of water; the water must penetrate deeply through the sandy loam or alluvial soil. South facing mountains or level areas within the mountains are suitable. Soil should be deep, loose, and fertile. Remains of wheat or corn in the field are suitable; avoid continuous cropping. Fields that previously grew legumes, beets, millet, and rapeseed, as well as newly reclaimed wasteland are all unsuitable for growing *huángqí*.

Soil Preparation

Soil should be prepared in the autumn prior to transplanting. Irrigate the soil so that there is good penetration of water, then plow to about 30 cm deep. Spread well composted manure at a rate of 12000–18000 kg per acre or organic fertilizer at a rate of 1800–3000 kg per acre, and a balanced NPK fertilizer at a rate of 300–600 kg per acre, then harrow the soil to mix in the compost and fertilizer. In hilly areas build beds according to the contour of the land. Beds should be 40–80 cm wide and 25 cm tall with 25 cm pathways between the beds.

SOWING SEEDS & RAISING SEEDLINGS

Seed Quality Requirements

Use the previous year, autumn harvested, seed. Seeds should have no more than 10% foreign matter, greater than 60% germination rate, and seeds that germinate should have greater than 90% survival rate.

Seed Storage

Seed should be harvested from 3–4-year-old healthy plants. Plants kept for seed production should be maintained in fields at least 200 meters away from production fields to avoid crossbreeding. Starting in early to mid-September, when seed pods begin to turn yellow but are still somewhat translucent, seeds may be collected. Pods are dried in the sun, then seeds are threshed and foreign matter is removed. Seeds selected for storage should be full and plump, and brown with a lustrous shine.

Boiling Seed to Accelerate Germination

Seeds are placed in boiling water and vigorously stirred for one minute, then immediately plunged into cold water. Re-heat to bring the water, with the seeds, to 40°C and soak for 2–4 hours, then scoop out into a moist cloth, wrap or cover the cloth and keep moist in this fashion for 8–12 hours. Seeds should be inflated and ready for sowing at the end of this process. After this soaking process, seeds must be scarified. There are many methods to accomplish the desired result. Seeds should be processed until they turn from shiny-brown to a gray-brown color. Large quantities of seeds can be processed using a rice mill or other similar machinery. Small quantities can be rubbed between the hands with 2–3 times the volume of fine sand added; the seed/sand combination can then be sown together.

Nursery and Seedling Bed Preparation

The area should have excellent drainage and beds should be a sandy soil. In the autumn after tilling the soil, prepare beds approximately 5 m long, 2–4 m wide, and 10–15 cm tall. Then add composted manure at a rate of 18000 kg or organic fertilizer at a rate of 3000 kg per acre as a base fertilizer; this is then tilled into the soil and the beds are raked level.

Sowing Seeds

Seeds are sown during the months of April and May. Seeds are sown using a seed drill set at a depth of 3 cm and should be covered by 1.5–2.0 cm of soil in rows 30 cm apart. Originally seeds were sown in trenches, then covered with earth and the land was leveled with a *lào* (a type of rake dragged across the bed). It is inappropriate to use a drill to sow seeds on a mountain slope, so in those sites seeds can be broadcast then raked or plowed very shallowly to evenly distribute the seeds, then the land is leveled as above. Seeds are sown at a rate of 30–36 kg per acre.

Nursery Bed Management

After sowing seeds check seed beds once per day, observe soil moisture and progression of seed germination. If the beds are dry, water with a sprayer or sprinkler irrigation to protect the soil moisture. Remove weeds in a timely manner. Once seedlings have 6–7 compound leaves, thin to 4–5 cm apart, which should give you 120,000–210,000 seedlings per acre. After thinning is complete, plants may be top-dressed with 21–42 kg ammonium sulfate and 21 kg calcium phosphate per acre.

Transplanting

Transplanting is done from late April through mid-May. The best time is from early to mid-May. Roots to be transplanted should be greater than 30 cm long and 0.5 cm wide just below the crown. The root should be shiny with no sign of disease or physical damage. Ditches 30 cm apart and 10–15 cm deep are dug and seedlings are laid in the ditch in one direction 15–18 cm apart. Roots are covered with soil and pressure is applied to press the soil evenly. Seedlings are transplanted at a rate of 75,000–96,000 per acre. Water in after transplanting is complete.

FIELD MANAGEMENT

Cultivation and Weeding

Cultivation and weeding should be done as needed.

Irrigation and Fertilization

During the initial growth period, the soil must not be allowed to become dry. Timely watering during its vigorous growth period is essential. After the plants have become established, 300 kg per acre of compound fertilizer can be applied prior to a scheduled irrigation. After rain, be sure not to let water accumulate, if it does take measures to immediately drain off the excess water.

Pinching

During early June inflorescences should be removed from plants being grown for root production. In fields being used for seed production, only the larger inflorescences should be allowed to mature.

PREVENTION AND TREATMENT OF DISEASE AND INSECT PESTS

Principles of Prevention and Treatment

Huángqí has several common diseases that should be monitored during its life cycle: root rot, root-knot nematode, and powdery mildew. Pests are primarily above-ground including: blister beetle, larva of the snout moth, and stinkbug, as well as aphids and small cutworms, pest diseases affecting this plant .

Root Rot (*Fusarium* sp.)

Prevention and Treatment

Crop rotation with a grass family plant for two years between harvests. Avoid fields with known root rot problems and do not transplant any seedlings with any sign of root rot. Use appropriate application of fertilizer. Apply suitable amounts of organic fertilizer and a phosphorus\potash fertilizer. Remove any diseased plants in a timely manner during the early stages of plant growth; use lime in the holes after removing diseased plants.

Powdery Mildew (*Oidium* sp.)

Prevention and Treatment

Use appropriate spacing when transplanting into the field; do not plant too close. Improve air circulation in the field. Use organic fertilizer, paying particular attention to nitrogen, phosphorus, and potassium; use suitable methods to increase the amounts of these trace nutrients in the soil. Use a grass family cover crop.

Snout Moth Larva, Blister Beetle, and Stinkbug

Prevention and Treatment

Crop rotation and deep plowing are common methods. Avoid planting soy, milk vetch, and other leguminous plants in the same field as *huángqí*, they should not be used as either a cover crop or as interplanting.

Aphids (Aphidoidea)

Prevention and Treatment

Aphids are naturally attracted to the color yellow. Deploying "sticky yellow boards" or construction of areas with yellow painted boards will attract aphids to places where they can be killed.

Biological Controls

Close monitoring of plants is important when using biological controls. At the first sigh of aphid infestation lady bugs should be used to control the infestation. [Translator's Note: Lady bugs should be set out around dusk for best results.]

HARVESTING

Harvest Season

Huángqí can be harvested after 2–3 years, 3 years is best. *Huángqí* is harvested during the months of October and November.

Harvest Method

Hand digging (or small machinery) is necessary when fields are in mountainous areas. It is important to do one's best to dig deeply and remove the entire root system. When grown in level fields, *huángqí* can be dug using machinery to excavate the roots.

ON-FARM PROCESSING

Sorting

Fresh roots are sorted by removing any foreign matter including roots from weeds and cutting off the withered stems of the plants. Any roots showing signs of disease, rot, insect damage, or other physical damage are discarded.

Pruning the Roots

After any soil is cleaned from the root, all remaining areal portions are cut off at the crown, and lateral roots are trimmed away.

Freeze Drying

The time to dig roots is in late October and early November, when the weather is already cold. Roots are dried in the sun until they are 70–80% dry. Then, the roots are tied in small bundles of 3–5 kgs, stacked to a height of 70–80 cm in a place with good air circulation with cold air coming from outside to allow the natural cold dry air to freeze dry the roots. Each layer of roots should have a separator to allow for good air flow, flipping the bundles regularly to ensure even dryness and to guard against mold is strongly advised.

Sun Drying and Hand-Rolling

The choice of methods is based on local weather conditions and either is suitable to produce daodi material. Roots are dug from late October through early November and laid in the sun to dry. When the roots reach 20, 30, and 50% dryness they are rubbed in the hands until the skin is taut. Roots are allowed to finish drying in the sun until they are below 12% moisture content.

ADDENDUM

In the counties of Hunyuan, Yingxian, and Wuzhai in Shanxi province, the scale is small, but it's also known as a *daodi* area for *huángqí*. *Huángqí* produced in that region is named *húnyuán huángqí*, *héngshān huángqí*, or *zhèngběi qí*. *Héngshān huángqí* is cultivated in an simulatated wild environment, direct seeded at an altitude of 1200–1800 m, on 10–35-degree slopes, and plants are grown for 5 or more years.

茅苍术

Green Atractylodes

Atractylodes lancea

DISTINGUISHING FEATURES

The dried rhizome of *máo cāngzhú* (*Atractylodes lancea* (Thunb.) DC.), generally known as *cāngzhú* (蒼术 \ 苍术) in China, is a member of the aster family (Asteraceae) in a small genus of about eight species centered in Asia. This plant grows natively in the eastern central part of China from 200–2500 meters elevation, however wild populations are extremely rare. A very closely related species, *Atractylodes japonica* Koidz. ex Kitam. (or *běi cāngzhú* 北苍术 , which is listed as *Atractylodes chinensis* (DC.) Koidz. in the *Pharmacopoeia of the People's Republic of China* 2015), is frequently used as a substitute for this herb and is an official species in China. The daodi location of this medicinal is Mao Mountain in Jiangsu province and its surrounding area.

A medicinal plant with a long history of use, *cāngzhú* and its cousin *báizhú* (*Atractylodes macrocephala*) originally were not differentiated, simply going under the heading "zhu." This herb is, however, exceptional at drying dampness while fortifying the spleen. *Cāngzhú* lacks the strong supplementing action of *báizhú* but of all the medicinals in the Chinese materia medica, it may have the greatest ability to dry dampness when the spleen is overwhelmed or underfunctioning. Although it is a warm herb it is often combined with cool or cold herbs to treat replete heat conditions in the middle and lower burner. *Cāngzhú* can also be used to treat impediment syndrome but is best when it is due to cold dampness patterns.

Modern science has looked extensively at this plant and its essential oils for potential therapeutic actions. Alcoholic extracts of *cāngzhú* have shown promising anti-cancer activity both *in vitro* and *in vivo*, significantly reducing lung metastasis in rat models. The herb shows cardiac activity with a hypotensive effect and neurological activity as a muscle relaxant. It has a significant positive effect on gastric ulcers and is both anti-inflammatory and antibacterial, making it an excellent herb for the treatment of gastric ulcers.

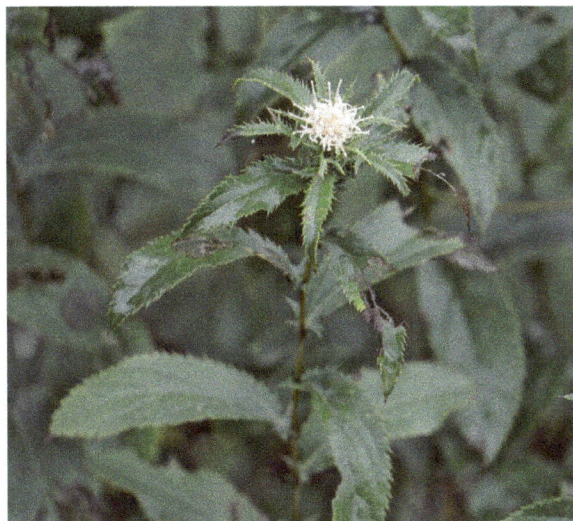

Contributing Authors

Guo Lan-ping, Huang Lu-qi, Zhang Yan, Zhao Dong-yue, Hao Qing-xiu, Sun Hai-feng, Zhang Xiao-bo, Kang Li-ping, Zhu Shou-dong, He Ya-li, Wang Ling

PRODUCTION SITE ECOLOGY

Elevation

Cāngzhú is cultivated between 100–1000 m elevation.

Temperature

Frost free period should be approximately 220 days. Annual average temperature of approximately 15°C. The coldest month is January with an average temperature around 0°C, and the warmest month is July with an average temperature round 30°C.

Photo Period

Annual sunlight averages 2000 hours.

Rainfall

Average annual rainfall around 1000 mm is suitable.

Soil

A loose sandy soil with an acid pH between 3–7 is suitable.

Topography

A hill with good drainage or gentle slope is best for growing *cāngzhú*.

PRODUCTION AREA ENVIRONMENTAL REQUIREMENTS

Site Selection

The most suitable area from growing *cāngzhú* is in a hilly mountainous zone with a deep, well-drained soil (soil layer should be at least 40 cm deep). It is critical during the rainy season that water does not accumulate but is easily drained through the sandy soil and via slope. Clay or alkaline soil is inappropriate for growing this plant. Areas facing either east or west are most suitable as *cāngzhú* prefers a habitat offering 30% shade. Avoid continuous cropping; rotations of wheat, corn, onion, garlic, coix, castor, etc. are all appropriate. Medicinal plants, when the root is not the medicinal part, can also be used. Likewise, *cāngzhú* can be grown in orchards, but should not be grown with leguminous plants or other medicinal root crops.

Soil Preparation

In October the soil is plowed to at least 30 cm deep with 12,000–18,000 kg of well-composted manure per acre or 1800–3000 kg of organic fertilizer per acre. This can be raked clean of large clods of soil to prepare for building beds. Beds are built according to the topography, but the standard beds are 40–80 cm wide, 25 cm tall, with 25 cm pathways; all pathways must have clear drainage so that water will never be left standing.

SOWING SEEDS & RAISING SEEDLINGS

Seed Quality Requirements

Seeds should be from the current year's harvest. The weight of 1000 seeds must be greater than 10 g and have no more than 5% foreign matter. Germination rate should be at least 85%.

Seed Saving Requirements

Seeds should only be gathered from healthy, robust plants which are free from disease or insect damage.

Nursery Soil and Bed Preparation

The area should have a sprinkler system installed. Sandy, well-drained soil, plowed at least 30 cm deep with 18,000 kg of well-composted manure (or 3000 kg of organic fertilizer) added per acre. Rake smooth.

Sowing Seeds

Seeds can be sown in winter or spring. Winter sowing is generally done in late November, before the ground has frozen. Spring sowing is done during early March. Seeds are planted at a rate of 21–30 kg per acre. Seeds are scattered evenly on the soil and raked in before covering with 1–2 cm of fine grain soil. Water in and keep the surface of the soil moist. The soil surface should remain moist at all times and weeds should be removed in a timely basis.

Seedling Development

Generally, plant dormancy is during the period of November through December. Planting at any other time is fine. Once plants have emerged, they should have a shady area to develop, and any sub-standard seedlings should be discarded.

Transplanting to Field

Before transplanting carefully examine all roots for any sign of disease or pests, immediately quarantine rhizomes showing any signs of disease to avoid cross-contamination with other plants. At this time also separate the large and small rhizomes and plant some of each in each section to guarantee the final product will be similar in any particular area; each rhizome should have 2–3 shoots. Then use a 50% solution of broad-spectrum carbendazim at a 0.2% concentration and soak for 25 minutes before removing and drying in the shade. Following this soak the rhizomes in a 0.067% solution of phoxim for 30 minutes, followed by drying in a cool shaded location. After the plants are dry, moisten the shoots with water, scatter plant ash on them, and prepare to transplant. Transplant with the rhizomes all facing in the same direction, shoots toward the sky, and cover with about 1 cm of soil.

FIELD MANAGEMENT

Cultivation and Weeding

Cultivate and eliminate all weeds in a timely manner. Generally, weeding is done during the month of April when *cāngzhú* sprouts, then again in June (according to the rate of growth of the weeds), and then at the end of the rainy season (late August to early September).

Irrigation and Top-Dressing

Watering is done according to the needs of the plant and weather conditions; if it is dry, the plants should be watered. After rains care should be taken to ensure that fields are draining properly. When the rhizome is growing fastest (at the time flower buds are developing) top-dressing can be done before watering. Avoid using nitrogenous fertilizer or compost that is not fully decomposed.

Removing Flower Buds

During the months of June and July, when the flowering stem emerges and begins to show signs of producing buds, remove the entire pedicle except for two of the healthiest buds, leaving at least 40 cm of the plant intact.

PREVENTION AND TREATMENT OF DISEASE AND INSECT PESTS

Principles of Prevention and Treatment

When growing from either seed or transplanting, plants that appear weak or sick should be removed, and prescribed methods of application of fertilizer, field management, proper encouragement or application of biological controls should be followed.

Root Rot Disease (*Fusarium* sp.)

Prevention and Treatment

Use crop rotation with grass family plants for at least three years. Keep fields clean, reduce sources of disease by burning dead leaves and any diseased material. Ensure that soil used for seedlings is free of disease and that planting beds are tall to ensure good drainage, do not allow water to be left standing. Use plant ash when planting. Do not over-fertilize, and use organic fertilizer to increase phosphorus.

Southern Blight (*Athelia rolfsii*)

Biological Controls

During transplanting the use of *Trichoderma harzianum* has been found effective against this disease. For agricultural controls see root rot disease above.

Leaf Spot (pathogen not confirmed)

Prevention and Treatment

See root rot disease above for appropriate controls. Pathogen may be *Cercospora salviola* and/or *Alternaria zinnia*.

Root-knot Nematode (*Meloidogyne* sp.)

Biological Controls

Use *Pseudomonas syringae* [a saprotrophic strain] (200,000,000 million spores\g) to irrigate the roots.

Generally done two times, with an interval of seven days between treatments. For agricultural controls see root rot above.

Aphids (Aphidoidea)

Prevention and Treatment

Remove weeds, withered plants, rotten leaves, etc., in a timely manner. Use appropriate winter plowing, and only use fully composted manure. Utilize ash-tea to treat aphids. Use 10–15 kg of plant ash per 50 kg water, soak for 24 hours, then use the clear water at the top to spray on the plants.

HARVESTING

Harvest Season

Plants are harvested 2 years after being planted in the field. Plants are generally harvested during the months November and December.

Harvesting Method

Rhizomes are harvested with either hand tools or small machinery. [Translator's Note: Rhizomes tend to have significant small fibrous roots that hold soil, so it is best to harvest when the ground is relatively dry so that the soil easily falls away. As the rhizomes dry, the small fibrous roots will dry and break off, allowing any remaining soil to be easily cleaned from rhizomes. Although rhizomes are not washed in China because exposure to water may lead to mold growth, the small fibrous roots that hold soil are difficult to clean and the use of a pressure washer may be useful to thoroughly clean the rhizomes prior to drying.]

ON-FARM PROCESSING

Grading

Rhizomes are separated by size while still fresh for sun-drying. Any non-medicinal materials, including, plant tops, weeds, and soil should be removed at this time.

Drying Methods

Rhizomes should be spread out loosely in thin layers and frequently turned to avoid mold. During the drying process, plants should be protected from rain or damp weather. A mechanical drier can also be employed. The temperature should be set at 45–50°C. Using either method, once the rhizomes have reach approximately 80% dryness, they are placed in a plastic bag for 48 hours to sweat (moving the moisture from the middle to the outside), then returned to the drying area until they reach less than 11% moisture. At this time, any remaining small fibrous roots are removed either by hand or mechanically.

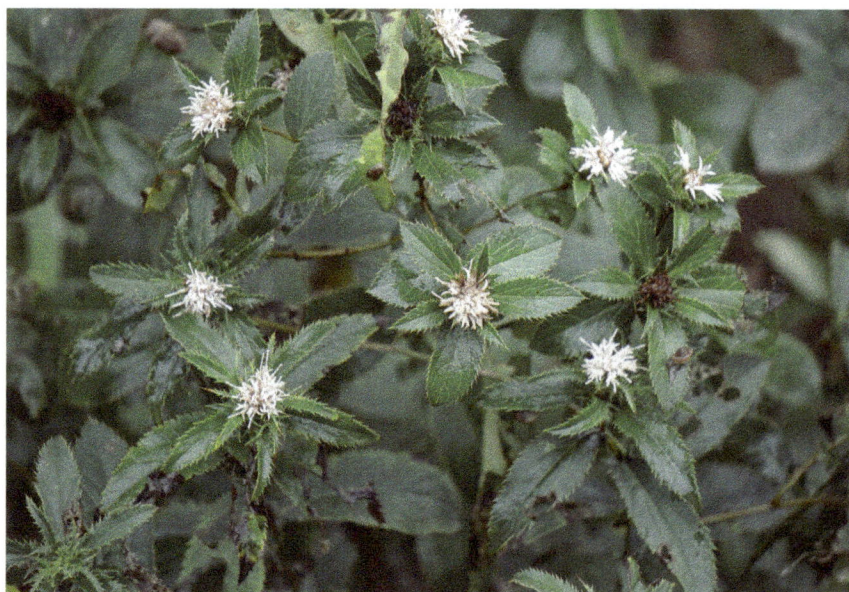

A rare stand of flowering wild *cāngzhú* on Mao mountian in Jiangsu province, China.

杭白术

White Atractylodes
Atractylodes macrocephala

DISTINGUISHING FEATURES

The herb, *hángbáizhú* (*Atractylodes macrocephala* Koidz.), which is generally known as *báizhú* (白术 \ 白术) in China, is a member of the Asteraceae family in a small genus of about eight species that are centered in Asia. This species is native to the eastern and central parts of China, growing in grasslands and forests from 600–2800 meters elevation. The root is the medicinal part and daodi herb cultivation occurs in Panan in Zhejiang province and its surrounding area.

A medicinal plant with a very long history of use, *báizhú* and its cousin *cāngzhú* (*Atractylodes lancea*) originally were not generally differentiated, simply going under the heading "zhu," and used interchangeably. However, we can be reasonably sure that it has been used for at least 2000 years. This medicinal plant is one of the primary herbs used to supplement spleen qi in Chinese medicine and is often considered the most important herb for this purpose because it also dries dampness. Therefore, *báizhú* supplements qi, fortifies the spleen, dries dampness, and disinhibits urine. However, although this herbs supplements qi, it is also commonly used for water swelling even when there is no spleen qi vacuity. *Báizhú* is also used in combination with other herbs to help stop sweating and to "settle a restless fetus" during pregnancy.

Modern science has identified the following pharmacological activities in *báizhú*: improving gastrointestinal function, anti-tumor activity, anti-inflammatory activity, anti-aging activity, anti-oxidative activity, anti-osteoporotic activity, anti-bacterial activity, gonadal hormone regulation and tocolytic effects, neuroprotective activity, immuno-modulatory activity, and energy-enhancing metabolism. While some of these activities are consistent with traditional use, the research suggests a much wider understanding of the plant and also may help to elucidate the basic theory that is used in Chinese medicine to explain its therapeutic actions.

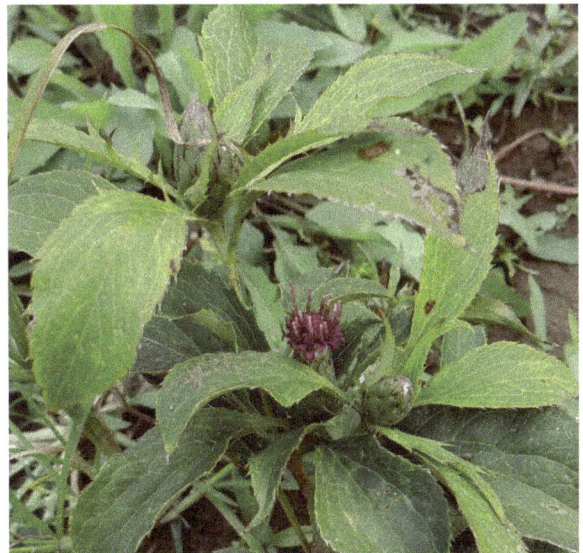

Contributing Authors

Zheng Yuguang, Wang Qian, Hou Fangjie, Li Jing, Liu Zhenyi

PRODUCTION SITE ECOLOGY

Elevation

Báizhú is cultivated between 500–800 m, but seedlings are raised between 100–300 m elevation.

Temperature

The counties of Panan, Xinchang, and Tiantai form a belt of production area where the average temperature ranges from 13.9–17.4°C and has a frost-free period of 200–260 days. The plant prefers cool clear days and does not favor very hot weather, although it can withstand low temperatures up to -10°C. Ideal average summer temperature ranges from 26–28°C in this region. However, when temperatures rise above 35°C the growth and development of the plant is slowed.

Photo Period

Annual sunlight averages 2000 hours.

Moisture

Average rainfall is between 1200–1500 mm. Soil must maintain a moisture content of 30–50%. The average annual humidity is 75–80%. These factors play a major role in the growth and development of the plant.

Soil

Preferred soils are sandy, yellow, or an iron rich-red soil, but with poor organic matter content. The plant prefers loose soil with a pH of 4.5–6.

Topography

Level land with good drainage and a deep fertile soil layer is most appropriate for growing *báizhú*. If growing in mountainous or hilly areas, the slope should be between 3–5 degrees.

PRODUCTION AREA ENVIRONMENTAL REQUIREMENTS

Site Selection

The best choice for land is an area that either has never been under cultivation, or at least has not had *báizhú* grown on it within the previous 5 years. Previous crops that included the grass family are appropriate, but the site should not have had peanut, cabbage, *shānyao* (*Dioscorea* sp.), tobacco, or melons cultivated on it.

Soil Preparation

In the autumn of the year before planting, plough the soil to a depth of 30 cm, remove any plant matter on the surface, and harrow. After this initial ploughing, only shallow tilling is necessary. Seedling nursery areas require more fertile soil than the main planting areas. 1200 kg per acre of "burnt earth ash,"* composted manure 9000 kg per acre should be added to the seedling nursery beds. Drainage ditches should be dug around all four sides of the beds.

* "Burnt earth ash" (火土灰) is a traditional process of burning barnyard manure for application as fertilizer. This simple process reduces manure to an ash, making application simple and removing any possibility of introducing disease or weeds through its application. This process also concentrates minerals so that higher concentrations can be applied with little effort. However, this process is used less and less because it causes smoke pollution. Therefore, the use of thermal compost is strongly recommended to replace this process and its application in the field.

SOWING SEEDS & RAISING SEEDLINGS

Nursery Soil and Bed Preparation

Nursery soils should be deeply ploughed during the autumn prior to the year they will be planted. Prior to planting they are shallowly tilled with 15000 kg / acre of thoroughly composted manure, then harrowed. Beds are built 1.2–1.5m wide with paths 25–30 cm wide and 15–20 cm deep around all sides of each bed to ensure good drainage.

Sowing Seeds

Seeds are planted during late March and early April. Only sow seeds with a full and plump appearance. Prior to sowing, soak seeds in water (25–30°C) for 24 hours. Once the seeds swell, they can be sown. Furrows are dug every 20 cm, 5 cm deep and 10cm wide, for scattering the pre-soaked seeds. Seeds are covered by 3 cm of soil then covered with mulch to protect the soil moisture content. Seeds are sown at a rate of 30 kg per acre, and 1/4 acre of nursery beds can plant out 10–15 acres.

Nursery Bed Management

Seeds should sprout in 10–15 days. After the seeds have sprouted, the mulch should be gently removed from the planting area and only allowed to cover the spaces between the planted rows. Weeding must be done in a timely manner. As the seedlings get larger, they should be thinned to 5 cm apart. Generally, by June plants should be growing strong and healthy, at this time a moderate top-dressing of 3000 kg per acre of composted manure can be added. During the rainy season pay close attention to not allow water to remain standing anywhere, including the pathways. Remove any diseased plants in a timely manner; lime can be added to the hole where the diseased plant was removed to kill the pathogen in the soil.

Storing Seedlings

Seedlings should be dug and stored before freezing temperatures arrive prior to the first winter. First the plants are dug and placed in a cool, shaded, area with good air circulation for 3–5 days until the exterior of the root is dry. Sand is generally used to store the roots; it is recommended to inspect the roots every 15–30 days for disease and rotting, any such roots should be removed immediately. If there are signs the roots are sprouting, the sand/root pile should be turned over, moving the top roots to the bottom and vice versa. Be careful not to break or damage any sprouts as this will affect the quality of the plant.

Transplanting to Field

Before planting out seedlings be sure that all plants are healthy and without signs of disease. Plants sizes, large and small roots, should be evenly distributed through the field. Before planting, roots are placed in cool, clean water and gently agitated before being removed to be air-dried. Then, the roots are soaked for 1 hour using 0.17–0.33% concentration in a 40% solution of broad spectrum of carbendazim or 80% solution at a concentration of 0.17–0.2% thiophanate ethyl. The roots are removed from the fungicide and allowed to dry in a shaded area until dry on the outside before planting. Holes for planting are dug 7 cm deep in a pattern of 20×30 cm. Plants are placed in the hole so that roots are not tangled and buds are facing upward, then covered with 6–8 cm of soil.

FIELD MANAGEMENT

Cultivation and Weeding

Cultivation prior to *báizhú* sprouts emerging is helpful, especially if the ground surface is hard, but care must be taken not to cultivate too deeply to avoid damaging emerging sprouts. Cultivation is done after the plants have sprouted to remove weeds. In late May, when the stems of the plants are strong, cultivation is repeated to remove weeds, this can be done mechanically, but care must be taken not to damage the plants, therefore this is generally performed using hand tools.

Irrigation and Top-Dressing

Generally, organic fertilizer is added three times during the season. The first time is about 20 days after the plants are transplanted (March/April) adding 9000 kg per acre of composted manure. The second time is late May at a rate of 12000 kg per acre. Finally, in late August, when the flower buds have all emerged, they are removed, and another 15000 kg per acre is added. Approximately 50 days prior to harvest, the plants should be irrigated. Also, if there is a dry period during July and August, which is the time when the rhizomes are expanding, plants should be watered. It bears repeating that care must be taken to always be sure that water is draining properly and that water is never allowed to stagnate.

Removing Flower Buds

Most buds are removed from early July through early August. This process can be done 2–3 times, and with the final time make sure to remove all the buds except the bud on the central leader. If you are planning to save seeds, leaving 3–5 buds per plant is generally recommended.

PREVENTION AND TREATMENT OF DISEASE AND INSECT PESTS

Principles of Prevention and Treatment

When growing from either seed or transplanting, plants that appear weak or sick should be removed, prescribed methods of application of fertilizer, field management, proper encouragement or application of biological controls (including but not limited to diversity of species) should be followed. There is a variety of *báizhú* that is short with thick, wide leaves that is good quality and is disease resistant.

Root Rot Disease (*Fusarium* sp.)

Prevention and Treatment

A rotation of a grass family plant should be used every 5 years or so. Be sure that proper amounts of compost and fertilizer are applied. Increase organic fertilizer, phosphorus, and potash. Do not use weak seedlings or remove those that do not thrive. Remove any diseased plants in a timely manner.

Sheath blight (*Rhizoctonia solani*)

Prevention and Treatment

Make sure you have selected land that is high enough and relatively dry with good sandy soil; all these factors contribute to good water drainage, which is a major issue with this and most *báizhú* diseases. Plow deeply (minimum 30 cm) in the early winter, allowing the soil to be weathered over the winter. This also can bury and kill disease while reducing the source of the fungi. After the harvest, collect all the withered plants and burn them to reduce the origin of the fungus. Any plants that show signs of disease during the growing season must be removed immediately, being careful to manage all the diseased plant matter. Use appropriate fertilizer, and focus on the use of organic fertilizer while increasing phosphorus and potash in the fertilization formula to strengthen the plants. Use at least a 5-year crop rotation.

Aphids (Aphidoidea)

Prevention and Treatment

Yellow sticky boards can be used to attract and kill aphids when they are in their winged stage.

Biological Treatment

During the early stages when aphid populations are still low, the introduction of lady bugs can be very helpful. Other natural treatments such as 0.3% matrine or pyrethrins can also be used during the winged stage to kill aphids.

HARVESTING

Growing Period Before Harvest

Plants are harvested 2 years after being planted in the field.

Harvest Season

Roots are harvested in late October and early November after the aerial portion of the plants has turned from green to withered yellow-brown.

Harvesting Method

Plants are harvested on sunny days. The entire plant is dug up, all dirt is removed, and the withered stem/leaves are cut off. Any rotten or damaged roots are discarded.

Digging by hand is usually done in hilly or mountainous areas when larger machines can't be used. When digging try to dig deeply to keep the entire root system intact without damage.

Larger root digging machinery is generally used on flat fields where larger volumes of *báizhú* are being cultivated.

ON-FARM PROCESSING

The traditional processing method used is to first dry, then cure, using smoke, then sweat, then dry completely, inspect, and finally package.

Cleaning

Clean until completely free of any dirt, foreign matter, and any roots that are unfit to be used for medicine.

Curing with Smoke

Roots are toasted on a fire that is dying down; a blazing fire or one with an open flame can't be used. If using an oven, the roots must be separated by 2–3 levels; do not pack them too densely in the oven. The roots are covered by straw or a gunny sack to assist the curing process. A fire is built in the oven with firewood until it reaches a temperature of 780°C. Roots should never be allowed to come in contact with the flames. Roots are roasted under these conditions until the small rootlets of the herb burn and fall off. When these fibrous roots fall off, this assists the smoking process. Roots should be turned every 6 hours until all the small fibrous roots have fallen off; this should take 18–24 hours and the root should be evenly dry.

Sweating

After the above process is completed, the roots are dried at 60–70°C until they are approximately 80% dry. The roots are then removed and piled in bamboo baskets for 6–7 days and allowed to sweat. This allows the water to move from the inside to the outside and the skin will become soft.

Re-Drying

After the skin of the rhizome has become soft, the rhizomes are covered with hemp and then re-dried for 12 hours at 50–60°C. The roots are deemed dry when a sharp sound is heard when dropping them on a hard surface; moisture content must not exceed 15%.

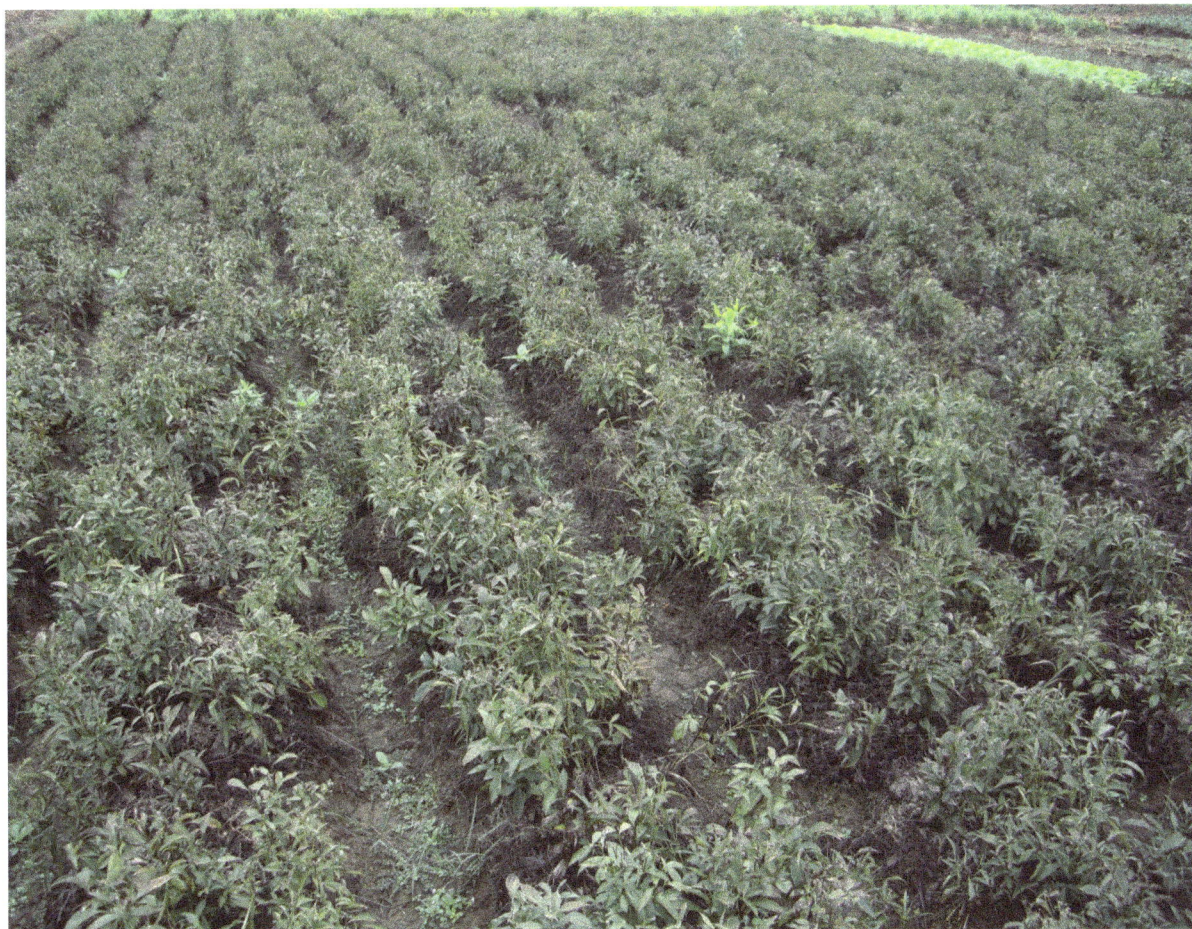

Báizhú growing in Zhejiang province, China.

云木香

Aucklandia Root

Aucklandia lappa

DISTINGUISHING FEATURES

The dried root of this daodi herb, *yún mùxiāng* (*Aucklandia lappa* Decne.), is commonly known as *mùxiāng* (木香) in China, it is a member of the aster family (Asteraceae) in a monotypic genus (only one species). However, the naming of this plant is somewhat confusing because different sources may list it as *Auklandia lappa*, *Auklandia costus*, *Saussurea lappa*, or *Saussurea costus*. *Saussurea* is a very large genus with over 300 species and *Auklandia* is a single species in a monotypic genus, the genus is very closely related to *Saussurea*. This plant is not native to China. It is native to northwest India, northeast Pakistan, and Kashmir and is threatened in the wild. Due to its rarity in the wild, it is listed by the *Convention on the International Trade of Endangered Species* as a protected plant, which means the wild plant cannot be legally traded internationally. The daodi location for this herb is northwestern Yunnan around the city of Lijiang, Diqing Prefecture, Dali Prefecture, and Nujiang Prefecture in Yulong, Weixi, Xianggelila, Deqin, Jiangchuan, Heqing, Lanping, Fugong counties, and the surrounding area.

[Translator's Note: *Aucklandia lappa* is the old scientific name for this species, which is also found in the *Pharmacopoeia of the People's Republic of China* (2015). The current scientific name is *Aucklandia costus* Falconer.]

Mùxiāng has been used in Chinese medicine for about 2000 years, mostly coming from cultivated sources in Guangdong province until the 20th century when cultivation was moved to northwest Yunnan. *Mùxiāng* is used to move qi and stop pain, almost exclusively for pain in the abdominal region, although the cause of the pain may have developed from a number of different patterns.

Modern science has identified anti-inflammatory, antitumor, hepatoprotective, choleretic, anti-gastric ulcer, antispasmodic, and analgesic functions in *mùxiāng*. It also promotes or inhibits gastric emptying in an dose dependent manner.

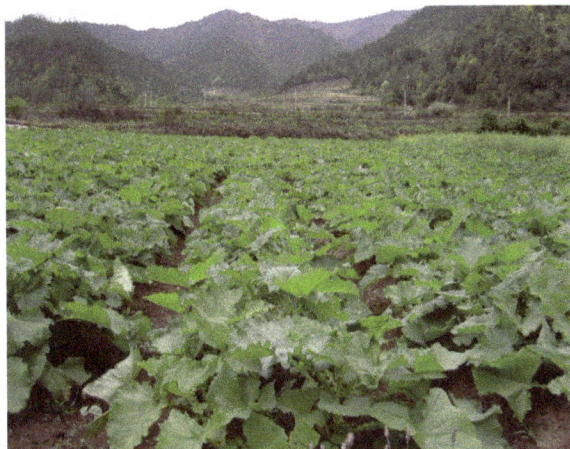

Contributing Authors

Li Lin-yu, Li Shao-ping, Yang Li-ying, Guo Lan-ping, Yang Bin, Wang Xin, Dong Zhi-yuan, Ma Wei-si, Yan Shi-wu, Li Jia, Zuo Zhi-tian

PRODUCTION SITE ECOLOGY

Elevation

Mùxiāng is cultivated between 2700–3300 m elevation.

Temperature

An average annual temperature between 7–10°C is suitable, with summer-time highs not exceeding 25°C and winter lows not exceeding -14°C. The site should have between 150–180 days of frost free weather.

Moisture

Annual rainfall should be between 800–1000 mm and average humidity between 60–80%.

Soil

The soil depth should be at least 30 cm deep, have at least 2% organic matter, and a pH that is slightly acid to neutral.

PRODUCTION AREA ENVIRONMENTAL REQUIREMENTS

Site Selection

In China, sites are selected within the daodi region with the appropriate soil, irrigation, and atmospheric conditions for growing *mùxiāng*. The site can be virgin soil, loamy soil with less than a 20-degree slope, table-land, or level fields. A layer of deep, loose, rich, and sandy soil is ideal. Do not use low-lying land where water can accumulate. Avoid continuous cropping; use only new land or a site that has not grown *mùxiāng* for at least 3 years. [Translator's Note: *Mùxiāng* is also grown in other regions of China but it is not daodi and the quality is considered to be markedly lower. This is probably because this plant is native to India and Pakistan; northwest Yunnan is the closest ecological niche related to *mùxiāng*'s native habitat.]

Soil Preparation

In December of the year prior to planting, the land is plowed to at least 25 cm deep and allowed to sit, exposed to the sun and weather, until about 10–15 days prior to sowing seeds. At that point, the land is tilled finely with the addition of 12000–24000 kg of decomposed manure, compost, or humus per acre. To this is added 120 kg per acre of standard NPK fertilizer. Finally, the site is harrowed so that the soil is broken into pieces no larger than 2 cm in diameter, and all weeds and any other plant material is either fully incorporated or removed. When growing on sloped land or a masa, trenches must be dug to assist with water drainage and preserve the land from washout. On flat farm land the trenches should be dug deeper to ensure proper drainage. Beds are built 25–30 cm high and 80–90 cm wide with the middle of the bed raised slightly to assist with water drainage. Drainage ditches must be dug around the sides on flat farm land to ensure that any excess water is drained from the land. In China, sites are selected within the daodi region with the appropriate soil, irrigation, and atmospheric conditions for growing *mùxiāng*. The site can be virgin soil, loamy soil with less than a 20-degree slope, table-land, or level fields. A layer of deep, loose, rich, and sandy soil is ideal. Do not use low-lying land where water can accumulate. Avoid continuous cropping; use only new land or a site that has not grown *mùxiāng* for at least 3 years. After beds are built, they are covered tightly with black agricultural plastic to warm the soil, prevent weeds, and help with production efficiency. Once the seedlings have developed the plastic can be removed.

SEED REQUIREMENTS

Growing for Seed

There are a significant number of varieties of *mùxiāng* and they commonly interbreed, therefore when growing *mùxiāng* for seed, the site should be at least 1 km from any other site growing *mùxiāng*. Spacing for plants should be 8000–10000 per acre. Seed should only be collected from healthy plants that are free from disease and have a strong appearance.

Seed Harvesting

Mùxiāng seeds mature from the middle of August through about early September. When the capitula (flower head) turns a yellow-tan color the seeds should be mature and ready for collection. Harvesting *mùxiāng* seeds should be done on a clear sunny day without wind. The flowering head is cut off with sufficient length of peduncle (stalk) to allow for it to be hung for 2–3 days in the sun. After this period the capitula are gently beaten with a stick or other appropriate tool to knock the remaining seeds out. The seeds are then winnowed from any foreign matter before being dried in the sun for 5–7 days. Seed moisture should be below 12% for proper storage.

Seed Quality Requirements

One-thousand seeds should weigh at least 20 g. Germination rate should be above 80%, no more than 15% foreign matter, and moisture content of at or under 12%.

DIRECT SEEDING

Pre-Sowing Seed Treatment

Seeds are generally soaked in a diluted (with water) fungicide for 12 hours, the seeds are then drained and allowed to dry in the sun prior to planting.

Sowing Seeds

Seeds are sown from April through mid-May. Seeds are sown at a rate of 4–6 kg per acre. Three to five seeds are placed in a 3–5 cm deep hole every 25–30 cm.

Thinning Seedlings

Seedlings are thinned twice, once when the plants have 4–5 true leaves, then again after they have at least 6 true leaves. Each hole should be left with 2–3 seedlings, which will grow together, for a total of 66,000–78,000 plants per acre.

RAISING TRANSPLANT SEEDLINGS

Sowing Seeds

Seeds are handled in the same manner as above, but planted more densely at a rate of 18–24 kg per acre.

Raising Seedlings Method

Beds are built 15–20 cm tall and 1.2 m wide. Seeds are cast evenly on to the beds, covered with a thin layer of soil (0.5–1.0 cm) then covered with a layer of dried pine needles (just enough to cover the soil) and finally watered.

Nursery Management

Soil must be kept moist. Weeding is done by hand. Once the seedlings begin to push against the pine needle mulch on the beds, the pine needles are carefully removed. Generally, seedlings are raised for one year before being transplanted.

Transplanting to Field

Seedlings can be planted either from late November through mid-December, after the leaves have withered and before the ground has frozen, or in the spring (April through early May) before the plant begins to sprout. When transplanting into beds, the beds should be 1.2 m wide and 30 cm tall. Three to four roots are placed in each hole 30 cm apart. Rows are built 30–35 cm tall and 60–70 cm wide; seedlings are planted every 25–30 cm.

FIELD MANAGEMENT

Cultivation and Weeding

Weeding is done three to four times per year, or as needed. Usually when the plants grow out in the second-year weeds are minimal. Weeding is done in June and July as needed. At the same time the beds or rows are cultivated to loosen the soil. Old leaves and weeds are removed in the autumn after the plants have withered.

Irrigation and Top-Dressing

In a long-term drought, *mùxiāng* is irrigated as needed. Generally, no watering is required. When entering the rainy season from June to September, it is necessary to maintain proper drainage to prevent flooding. Prior to the rainy season carefully check all drainage and repair any problems. Improperly drained water can cause significant crop loss. In the first year of growth, during mid-July, apply 75 kg of urea per acre to the area around the roots. In the second year, in mid-June, apply 120 kg of NPK fertilizer per acre.

Removing Flower Buds

In the second year during the months of May and June, when the plants begin to bolt, a clean sickle is used to cut off the flowering tops. This encourages root development.

PREVENTION AND TREATMENT OF DISEASE AND INSECT PESTS

Principles of Prevention and Treatment

Mùxiāng is not generally prone to disease and pest problems. When top-dressing, be cautious of excessive amounts of nitrogen. However, moderate increases in phosphorus and potash can be used. Carefully manage water drainage to avoid the accumulation of water on the site is very important. Pay attention to timely cultivation to loosen the soil, weeding, clearing the field of weeds, and watching carefully for diseased plants, removing them immediately followed by putting lime in the hole where the plant came from to eliminate pathogens still lingering in the soil.

HARVESTING

Harvest Season

Mùxiāng is grown for two years before harvesting. The plants do not flower in the first year. In the second year the seeds can be collected. However, as noted above, when growing plants for root harvest, the flowering tops are cut off. Choose a clear sunny day. Roots can be dug any time during the months of October and November as long as the above-ground portion has turned yellow and withered. The above-ground portion is then removed.

Harvesting Method

Roots are harvested by digging from the side of each plant, or a trench along a row, then they are carefully excavated. Once the root is removed, shake off any clinging soil before they are returned to the processing and drying location. Be sure to protect freshly harvested roots from frost.

ON-FARM PROCESSING

Grading

After roots are dug and most of the soil has been removed by shaking (*do not knock or beat the roots*), the roots are placed in a clean area (*do not wash with water*) and any weeds or other foreign matter is removed. Carefully appraise each root, discarding any roots that show signs of any disease or damage from the harvesting process.

Cutting into Sections

After the roots have been carefully selected, a knife is used to cut away fibrous roots and the fibrous head of the root. The root is then sliced into sections 10–15 cm long.

Drying

Once the roots have been cleaned and cut into sections, they are dried in the sun or in a drier. If a drier is used the temperature should be set between 50–60°C. Roots should be dried until they reach a moisture content below 14%.

Tumbling

Once the roots are dry, they are placed in a tumbler made with steel mesh and spun to remove any remaining fibrous roots, course skin, and soil. When the roots have turned a brownish-gray color they can be removed.

太行山射干

Leopard Lily

Belamcanda chinensis

DISTINGUISHING FEATURES

The dried rhizome of the daodi herb *tàihéngshān shègān* (*Belamcanda chinensis* (L.) DC.*), commonly known as *shègān* (射干) in China, is a member of the iris family (Iridaceae). Although this plant is often colloquially called a "lily" it is actually an iris native to eastern China, Japan, Korea, and eastern Russia. The plant has been cultivated extensively and its exact origin is unclear, but it can be found in many other parts of the world. The daodi location for cultivation of this herb is in the Taiheng mountain region, Ping Mountain, Wei and She counties, and the surrounding areas in Hebei province.

This medicinal is primarily used in Chinese medicine to treat severe sore throat. It is also used for phlegm-heat in the lung with coughing and wheezing. It has a very long history of use and can be found in formulas from the late Han period such as Belamcanda and Ephedra Decoction (Shegan Mahuang Tang) found in *Prescriptions from the Golden Cabinet* (*Jin Gui Yao Lüe*). The herb can also be used for abscesses and sores; however, it is less commonly used for this purpose.

Modern science has confirmed that *shègān* and some of its chemical constituents have the following pharmacological activities: anti-inflammatory, antibacterial, antioxidant, hepatoprotective, antitumor, and ichthyotoxic (toxic to fish).

* A paper was published in 2005 by Peter Goldblatt and David J. Mabberley in the journal *Novon*, based on molecular DNA research published in 2001 by Tillie, Chase, & Hall, arguing that *Belamcanda chinensis* be

formally renamed *Iris domestica*. Although many publications, including the *Pharmacopoeia of the People's Republic of China* (2015), still use the name *Belamcanda*, the *Flora of China* notes, "it might be better placed in *Iris*." There has been significant support for this by many other authors in the subsequent years since this publication.

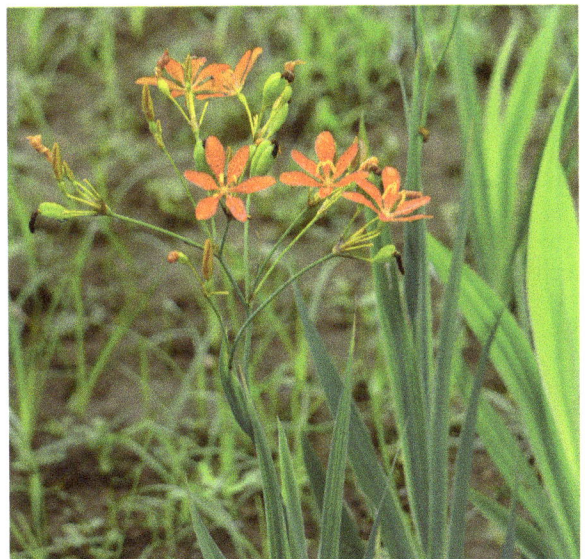

Contributing Authors

Xie Xiao-liang, Liu Ming, Hao Qing-xiu, Guo Lan-ping, Huang Lu-qi, Wen Chun-xiu, Liu Ling-di, Tian Wei, Liu Zhi-miao, Gu Dong-sheng

PRODUCTION SITE ECOLOGY

Elevation

Shègān is cultivated between 100–1000 m elevation.

Temperature

The average annual frost-free period is 200 days.

Illumination

Annual sunshine hours range from 1516–2016 hours and the sunshine percentage ranges from 34–46%.

Moisture

The average annual rainfall is 300–1200 mm with relative humidity of 35–65%.

Soil

A sandy soil with a pH from neutral to slightly alkaline is suitable. Low-laying land or saline-alkali soil should be avoided.

Topography

The site can be either sloping or level as long as it is not low-laying and has good drainage. North-facing slopes are not suitable.

Site Selection

Sandy soil with good drainage is best. The field should have proper drainage, good wind-flow, and irrigation.

Soil Preparation

Composted manure at a rate of 12,000–18,000 kg per acre should be applied. A super-phosphate fertilizer is applied at a rate of 150–180 kg per acre. After application of composted manure and super-phosphate, the site is plowed deeply and beds are built.

SOWING SEEDS & RAISING SEEDLINGS

Seed Quality and Pre-Treatment

According to the *Pharmacopoeia of the People's Republic of China* (2015) 1000 seeds must weigh more than 10 g and the germination rate should be better than 80%. One month prior to planting, soak seeds in water for one week (barely covering them), rinsing 3–4 times during this period. After each rinse it will be necessary to add, approximately, another 1/3 of the original amount of water to account for seed swelling. During the rinsing process, gently rub seeds between your hands to loosen the outer fruit layer, be sure to rinse after this process so that the water is clear during soaking. At the end of this first week, place the seeds in a wicker or other breathable container and cover with a cloth. Rinse water through this container 2–3 times per day so that bacteria and mold are not allowed to accumulate. When more than 60% of the seeds have sprouted, they may be planted. This treatment is for spring planting only and is NOT used when planting in the autumn season.

Raising Seedlings and Transplanting

Seeds planted for nursery seedlings may be planted at three different times of the year, in the spring in late March and early April, in early August, or in late autumn from early to mid-November. Furrows are dug with a hoe to 3 cm deep with rows 10–15 cm apart. Seeds are sown about every 8 cm within the furrow. Seedlings are transplanted when they have reached a height of approximately 20 cm. Choose a cloudy day and build rows 25 cm apart and place 1–2 plants every 4 cm within these rows; water thoroughly after transplanting. Transplants weighing between 60–84 kg will fill a single acre.

Direct Seeding

There is no special treatment needed for seeds when using this method. Seeds sown in the spring should sprout within 30–40 days. Seeds sown in August usually emerge within 25–30 days. Seeds sown in November sprout the following April. Furrows are dug in rows on beds 30 cm apart and 5–6 seeds are buried every 25 cm to a depth of 2 cm. A small amount of composted manure is often mixed thoroughly with the soil during this process. Water in thoroughly after sowing seed and do not allow to dry out. Seeds are sown at a rate of 15–18 kg per acre.

FIELD MANAGEMENT

Thinning and Final Singling of Seedlings

Initial thinning should be done early. All weak or diseased plants should be removed, selecting for strong healthy plants. Thinning is usually done twice, the first time when the plants are 6–8 cm tall and the second time when the plants reach approximately 10 cm tall; at this time, final singling is done leaving 1–2 plants in each hole. In large fields, singling and filling gaps is done at the same time. This should be done on a cloudy day or right before sunset. Gaps may be filled by transplanting from overcrowded holes or from seedlings raised in flats or beds separately. Each acre is planted with 72,000–90,000 plants.

Cultivation, Weeding, and Hilling

During the spring, weeds should be diligently removed and the soil loosened. Starting in June, the soil should not be disturbed but gently hilling soil around the base of the plant to prevent it from falling over is a common practice.

Irrigation and Water Drainage

When seedlings are young, it is important to maintain good and even moisture in the soil, the only exceptions to this are during thinning, singling, and filling in the gaps when the soil should be allowed to dry somewhat so that fields workers are not damaging the soil structure. If the land has any issues with poor drainage, these areas should be carefully monitored. Stagnate water is likely to cause significant damage to plants and lead to disease problems.

Top-Dressing

During the vigorous growth period in the second year, a NPK compound fertilizer is added at a rate of 180 kg per acre.

Removal of Flowers

Unless the plants are being used for seed production, the scape is pinched off during late July.

PREVENTION AND TREATMENT OF DISEASE AND INSECT PESTS

Principles of Prevention and Treatment

This plant is relatively easy to grow but because it is grown for its rhizome and because it takes three years from seed to harvest, diseases and pests can be challenging and potentially cause significant damage to the crop. Good drainage is critical to avoid most disease problems and careful monitoring of the crop is important for early detection of pests.

Rust (*Puccinia iridis*)

Prevention and Treatment

At the end of autumn any affected leaves that remain should be carefully removed from the field and properly disposed of to reduce the active disease-causing fungus in the field. Increase phosphorus to improve the health of the plant and increase disease resistance.

Leaf blight (*Alternaria sp.*)

Prevention and Treatment

After the autumn work is done, collect all twigs and leaves affected by the disease and get rid of these by whatever appropriate means so that the fungal disease can't survive the winter.

Bean Yellow Mosaic Virus (*Potyvirus sp.*)

Prevention and Treatment

Pre-treat seeds by soaking in a 10% solution of sodium phosphate for 20–30 minutes. Aphids can be a vector for this disease. As early as possible eliminate aphids. Be vigilant in finding infected plants and immediately remove and burn them.

Belemcanda Borer (*Oxytripia orbiculosa*)

Prevention and Treatment

During the evening, adults can be lured by lamps into traps. During late October the soil can be plowed to 20 cm to disturb the larvae and reduce the numbers of the insects that survive the winter. Removing buds and flowers can have a significant impact on the population of this insect. [Translator's Note: This species is only known to live in areas spanning from Europe to Asia, so North American growers are not likely to encounter it.]

Cutworms (*Agrotis ypsilon*)

Prevention and Treatment

Use a black light to lure adult cutworms to traps.

Grub (*Holotrichia* sp.)

Prevention and Treatment

Deep plowing and extensive harrowing are used to kill larvae and reduce the chances for those not killed to survive the winter. Black light can be used to lure adults into traps. Lights are deployed at 1 per 8–10 acres.

Biological Controls

To control larvae, apply *Bacillus popilliae* at a rate of 9 kg acre and *Beauveria brongniartii* at a rate of 2.0×109 spores per square meter. This treatment is applied to the soil near the plants.

HARVESTING

Harvest Season

When plants are started by direct seeding, rhizomes are generally harvested after three years. When seedlings are transplanted into the field, rhizomes are generally harvested after two years. Rhizomes should be harvested in October after leaves have withered.

Harvest Method

Chose a fine warm day to remove the withered leaves and flower stalks from the plants. Then, using a shovel, or other appropriate digging tool, dig the rhizomes and remove as much soil as possible by shaking before taking the entire bunch to another location for sun-drying. In commercial operations, *shègān* is commonly harvested by using a tractor with a rhizome digging attachment.

ON-FARM PROCESSING

Drying Method

There are two methods for drying and processing *shègān* on the farm. The first method is to remove all the fibrous roots by hand (hand tools such a sharp knife are needed) and dry completely in the sun or in a dryer. The second method is to use a dryer at a temperature of 50–80°C until all the fibrous roots are dry and brittle. At this point the roots are put into a drum and spun to brake off the dry fibrous roots. Finally, the remaining rhizomes are dried in the sun. The final product should have no more than 10% moisture.

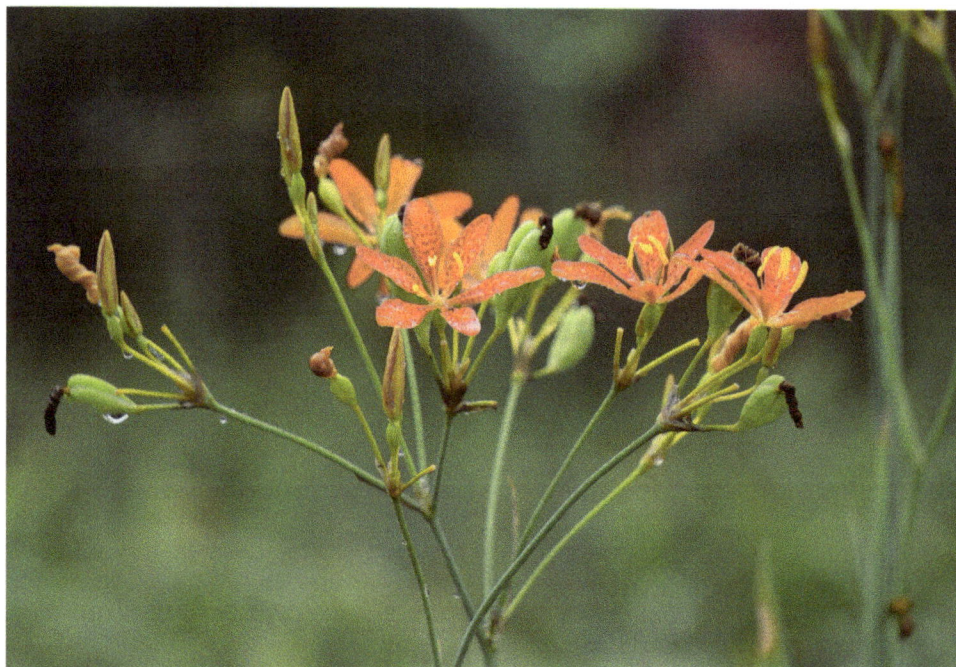

太行山柴胡

Bupleurum

Bupleurum chinensis & *B. scorzonerifolium*

The root of the daodi herb *tàihàngshān cháihú* (*Bupleurum chinensis* DC. and *B. scorzonerifolium* Willd.) commonly known as *cháihú* (柴胡) in China is a member of the carrot family (Apiaceae). The *Bupleurum* genus is large and complicated, with about 200 species found throughout the northern temperate areas, one disjunct species in South Africa, and one native species in western North America. Many species have recorded medicinal uses in China, and one species in Taiwan, however at least one species (*B. longiradiatum*) is known to be toxic. The genus is relatively easy to identify due to its simple and entire leaves, in a family that is well-known for difficultly to differentiate genera. However, species identification can be very tricky due to large morphological variation across regions. The daodi area for this medicinal is in the Taihang Mountain area in Xian county and the Yan Mountain Reserve, both in Hebei province.

In Chinese medicine *cháihú* is a very well-known herb with a long history. It is well-represented in many formulas, some dating back to the Han Dynasty. *Cháihú* is often used for fever but is most well-known for its ability to treat illnesses that are "half internal-half external." In some cases, this means that it is moving from the exterior to the interior, or it could mean that the illness is "stuck" and is not resolving, therefore the patient presents with symptoms of alternating sensations of heat and cold, stuffiness in the chest, headache, and possibly cough. This herb is also frequently used for its ability to course the liver qi, leading to the movement of qi and thus blood. Applications based on this action include the treat-ment of menstrual disharmonies such as irregular menstruation, painful menstruation, and a variety of premenstrual syndrome symptoms.

Modern science has studied this plant extensively and has shown pharmacological activities including sedative, antipyretic, analgesic, anti-inflammatory, immunomodulatory, hepatoprotective, antitussive, antifibrotic, and anticancer. Significant research has shown that this herb and its constituents have a strong anti-inflammatory action on the liver and can be used to treat a number of liver diseases. Recent research on the polysaccharide fraction of this herb showed strong antitumor action as well as an immune-potentiating action that suggests it could potentially be used for patients with liver cancer.

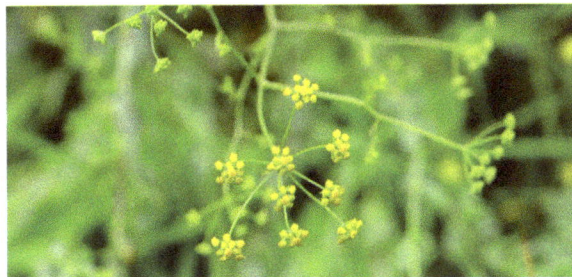

Contributing Authors

Zheng Yu-guang, Xie Xiao-liang, Guo Lan-ping, Huang Lu-qi, Hao Qing-xiu, Liu Ming, Hou Fang-jie, Wen Chun-xiu, Liu Ling-di, Gu Dong-sheng, Tian Wei

PRODUCTION SITE ECOLOGY

Elevation

Cháihú is cultivated between 260–1500 m elevation.

Temperature

The plant requires 181–204 frost free days.

Photo Period

Annual sunshine range requires 1998–2957 hours with daily sunshine percentage of 59%.

Rainfall

The average annual rainfall should be 331–1032 mm with a relative humidity of 35–45%.

Soil

A loose, humus rich, soil with pH in the 5.5–6.5 range is ideal.

Topography

A mountainous area with less than 15 degrees slope is ideal. If the field is sloped it should be facing either southeast or northwest to allow for proper drainage and wind-flow.

PRODUCTION AREA ENVIRONMENTAL REQUIREMENTS

Site Selection & Preparation

Select sandy soil with good water drainage. Add 3000 kg of organic fertilizer and 300 kg of compound NPK fertilizer per acre before tilling soil, then harrow finely.

SOWING SEEDS & RAISING SEEDLINGS

Sowing Seeds

Seeds should be full and plump from the previous year's harvest. Spring planting should be done during the months of March and April. Autumn planting is done during the month of November before the ground freezes. Space rows 20 cm apart and hoe a channel 1.0 cm deep. Distribute seeds evenly in the furrow, cover with soil and press gently. The site is seeded at a rate of 12–15 kg per acre.

FIELD MANAGEMENT

Cultivation and Weeding

While plants are young cultivation should be done regularly so that weeds are not allowed to become established and the soil is kept loose.

Irrigation and Water Drainage

While the plants are still young, do not allow the soil to become dry. Water after top-dressing applications. Be sure to maintain good drainage during heavy rains.

Top-dressing

During the month of July or August top-dress with diammonium phosphate at a rate of 180 kg per acre.

Removing Flowers

During the months of July and August, flowering stalks, which arise from the middle of the plant, should be pinched off to improve root production. Starting in the second year, the stalk can be allowed to grow until it can be easily cut with a sickle or other mechanical means. By allowing the flowering stalk to get to this height, plants can be handled in bulk, making the process more efficient.

PREVENTION AND TREATMENT OF DISEASE AND INSECT PESTS

Root Rot Disease (*Fusarium* sp.)

Prevention and Treatment

Water drainage is very important to prevent this disease. Ensure that water drains appropriately by choosing land with a mild slope and deep, sandy soil. Rational crop rotation and appropriate use of fertilizer is also important. Finally, timely removal of any diseased plants is important to avoid the spread of organisms that contribute to root rot.

Aphids (Aphidoidea)

Prevention and Treatment

Aphids are naturally attracted to the color yellow. Deploying "sticky yellow boards" or constructing areas with yellow painted boards will attract aphids to places where they can be killed. Deploy 180–240 boards per acre.

Biological Treatment

During the early stages when aphid populations are still low, the introduction of lady bugs can be very helpful. Other natural treatments such as 0.3% matrine or pyrethrins can also be used during the winged stage to kill aphids.

Black Cutworm (*Agrotis ypsilon*)

Prevention and Treatment

Prior to the time the adults lay their eggs, black lights can be used to lure them into traps. While the adults are active, traps can be set with a combination of sugar : alcohol : vinegar (1 : 0.5 : 2) put into trays and set at a height of 1 m. These traps are placed at a rate of 30–36 per acre.

Spot Blight (*Septoria lycopersici*)

Prevention and Treatment

Before the onset of winter, be sure to remove any diseased plant materials; these should be either burned or deeply buried. Also, pay close attention to proper field management, including cultivation and weeding, application of fertilizer and watering, and being sure that excess water during heavy rainfall drains from the field properly.

Yellow Swallowtail Butterfly (*Papilio machaon*)

Biological Controls

During the period when they are laying their eggs, or just after hatching, *Bacillus* (Bt) can be applied as directed by the manufacturer; Entobactenin (*Bacillus thuringiensis* var. *galleria*) can also be used.

HARVESTING

Harvest Season

Cháihú is harvested after 2–3 years of growth. *Cháihú* is harvested during the months of October and November around the time of the first frost when the leaves have begun to whither.

Harvesting Method

Small-scale harvesting is done by hand. The leaves and stems around the base of the stalk are removed just prior to digging. A digging fork or other appropriate tool can be used, being careful not to damage the roots. The root is dug, remaining soils are shaken free from the root, and the stalk is cut away before transporting to the drying and processing area. In large-scale farming, root excavators, attached to tractors, are used to dig roots.

ON-FARM PROCESSING

Drying Method

Cháihú is dried in the sun as a whole root. It should be spread out evenly is a sunny location and never piled-up. It is best to mix or flip the roots regularly during the drying process, while also inspecting them for the any mold, mildew, or other potential problems. Any diseased roots or foreign matter should be immediately removed.

Final Processing

When the roots have reached 70–80% dryness, and are still soft and pliable, cut off any remaining stem and remove the fibers at the top of the root, as well as any other impurities. Roots are then allowed to dry until they are below 10% moisture. Once they are dried to the desirable <10%, they are graded according to root diameter; 1) >0.5 cm, 2) 0.2–0.5 cm, 3) <0.2 cm. When *cháihú* is properly dried the root-bark is a light brown color and the inner woody portion is a yellow-white color.

河南红花

Safflower

Carthamus tinctorius

The dried flower of the daodi medicinal *Hénán hónghuā* (*Carthamus tinctorius* L.) is commonly known as *hónghuā* in China (红花 \ 红花), is a member of the aster family (Asteraceae). This plant is part of the *Carthamus* genus with about 47 species centered in Europe and Central Asia, however *hónghuā* is native to SW Asia and occasionally naturalizes in China. This is the same plant that produces safflower oil, commonly used in cooking. The flowers have also been found as an adulterant of saffron. Material produced in Henan province and the surrounding area is considered daodi.

Hónghuā is well-known for its ability to quicken the blood and eliminate blood stasis. It is primarily used in two areas of Chinese medicine. The first is to treat pain caused by a variety of diseases or trauma such as joint pain, pain due to traumatic injury, or pain and swelling due to sores and abscesses. The second area is gynecology, a use which goes back to Zhang Zhong-jing and the *Treaties on Cold Damage* (*Shanghan Zabing Lun*), where he used it for menstrual pain, lack of menstruation, and irregular menstruation. This herb can be used either internally or externally.

Modern science has found a wide array of compounds, primarily flavonoids, that are responsible for the pharmacological activities of *hónghuā*. Most likely due to its traditional use for pain and cardiovascular diseases, research has focused on these areas and the results have been very positive, showing its actions as an anticoagulant, antithrombotic, antifibrinolytic, and antioxidant. This has led to the development of a combination injection drug with *Salvia miltorrhiza* for the treatment of cardiovascular diseases. The plant has also shown neuroprotective, hepatoprotective , anti-inflammatory, and antitumor activities.

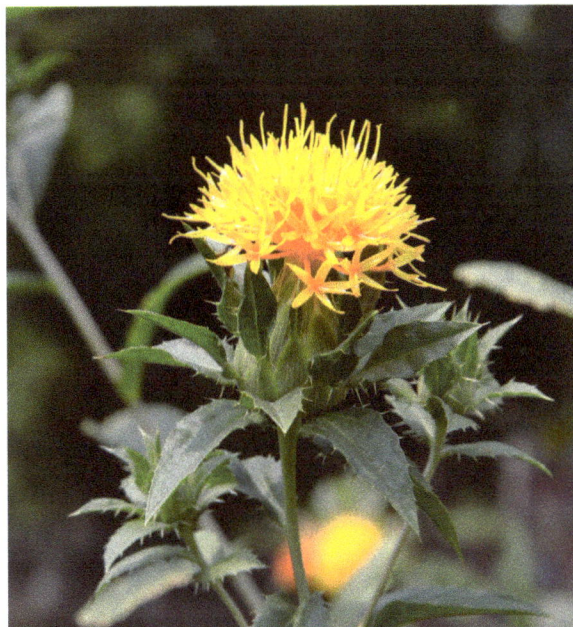

Contributing Authors

Huang Lu-qi, Guo Lan-ping, Zhang Yan, Zhao Dong-yue, Sun Hai-feng, Yang Guang, Kang Li-ping, Zhu Shou-dong, He Ya-li, Wang Ling, Wu Wei-xiao

PRODUCTION SITE ECOLOGY

Elevation

Hónghuā is cultivated between 100–1000 m elevation.

Temperature

The average annual temperature range should be between 8–12°C.

Rainfall

Annual average rainfall should be 150–300 mm, concentrated in the months of July–September.

Soil

Hónghuā can be cultivated in a range of soils including; chestnut soil, brown calcic soil, gray calcic soil, light carbonate brown soil, black humus-rich soil, and by using recovered land from pastures. The soil should be slightly alkaline (pH 8–9).

PRODUCTION AREA ENVIRONMENTAL REQUIREMENTS

Site Selection

Choose a site with good sun exposure that is hot and dry. The soil layer should be deep with moderate fertility. Well-draining sandy soil on a slight slope is best. There should not be significant rain during the flowering season. The best crops to have been grown on the site prior to growing *hónghuā* are potatoes, soybean, or corn; wheat or vegetables are also suitable.

Soil Preparation

Preparation begins in autumn before the first freeze; the soil should be plowed to at least 25 cm, and all plant matter from the previous year's cultivation can be integrated into the soil. The soil does not need to be harrowed. In spring, once the soil has thawed to 5–8 cm it can be shallowly tilled, however, the spring tilling is generally between 10–15 cm, after which it is harrowed smooth. During this time water drainage channels are dug or maintained to ensure the site drains properly. Prior to planting seeds, be sure the soil surface is soft.

Any areas where crust has formed must be broken up prior to planting seeds.

SOWING SEEDS & RAISING SEEDLINGS

Seed Quality Requirements

Seeds should be from the previous year's harvest, have no more than 5% foreign matter, and have a germination rate greater than 80%.

Seed Saving and Storage

Seeds should be collected only from healthy plants that are free of disease or pests. Seeds should be stored in a dry area at normal atmospheric temperature and with adequate air flow.

Sowing Seeds

Seeds may be sown from late March through mid-April; late planting is not suitable for this crop. Seeds are planted at a rate of 9–12 kg per acre for good quality seed and 12–15 kg per acre for lower quality seed. Seed can either be planted by hand or by machine. Seeds are planted 25–30 cm apart at a depth of 5–10 cm. Rows are spaced at 30–40 cm. Generally, seeds are planted 5–6 cm deep (Henan province), however, in very dry areas, seeds may be planted 8–10 cm deep (for example, Xinjiang province). Deep planting of seeds allows plant roots to penetrate the soil in excess of one meter deep to access water.

FIELD MANAGEMENT

Cultivation, Weeding, and Hilling-up

Hónghuā plant health is very much dependent on soil moisture and whether or not weeds are present. Cultivation should be done 2–3 times early in the season (April and May) to prevent weeds for getting a foothold. A hand hoe is most frequently employed for this process, however, weeds in close proximity of *hónghuā* should be pulled by hand. Care must be taken to not damage the roots of *hónghuā* during this process. During the final cultivation work, soil can be hilled-up around the plants to prevent them from falling over. Weeds should be removed from the site and composted or otherwise disposed of.

Irrigation and Water Drainage

If it is dry anytime during branching or during the bloom, the crop must be watered. Flood irrigation is most frequently used. Over-head watering during the flowering stage is not appropriate. Watering in the early morning or early evening is best. If there are thunderstorms or significant rains of any kind during the summer, care must be taken to avoid any pooling of stagnant water left in the field. Checking drainage during these times is strongly encouraged.

Pinching Flowers

The main stem is cut off when the plant has reached about 1 m in height and the plant has approximately 20 branches. After pinching flowers, plants are fertilized with 60 kg per acre of urea or 180 kg per acre of ammonium bicarbonate. However, today, due to increases in labor costs, this pruning process is rarely done.

PREVENTION AND TREATMENT OF DISEASE AND INSECT PESTS

Principles of Prevention and Treatment

Selection of varieties that are resistant to disease or insect damage can be an important strategy in reducing crop problems later. Careful monitoring of the crop for disease and pests is critical. Any problems should be immediately and appropriately resolved. Generally, diseased material is removed and burned. After the harvest the residual plant material is plowed deeply into the soil and the soil is allowed to be exposed to the sun in an effort to avoid further problems in the following year. Any plants that are damaged or diseased are removed from the field to avoid further problems. Keeping water drained from the site is critical, make sure that your site has properly draining soil, or the site can be drained with ditches. Any application of sprayed pesticides, even "organic" products, should be discontinued 30 days prior to the harvest of the flowers.

Rust (*Puccinia* sp.)

Prevention and Treatment

Sites on higher ground that are dry, or building tall beds are important to help avoid this disease. Keep the field clean and free of diseased material. Increasing organic fertilizer and phosphorus can be helpful. Foliar feeding with a 0.2–0.3% potassium dihydrogen phosphate solution can also help treat the problem, but early application is advised.

Safflower Aphids (*Uroleucon compositae*)

Prevention and Treatment

In the late autumn, tidy up the field paying attention to the stalks, branches, and leaves remaining in the field; deep plowing is the most common way to deal with this. Prior to the arrival of winter, tilling compost into the soil is recommended.

Soil-borne Insects

Prevention and Treatment

Plowing and harrowing, deep plowing, application of ample amounts of compost help to prevent cut worm, cricket, wire worm, grub, and mole cricket.

Biological Controls

During their adult stage, lights can be utilized to attract and trap the insects.

HARVESTING

Harvest Season

Hónghuā is an annual plant and is harvested in the first season.

As the flowering period for *hónghuā* is very short, it is critical to be well prepared for the harvest. This is especially important because the quality of *hónghuā* is dependent on timely harvest. Generally, *hónghuā* is harvested during the month of July. Within 2–3 days after bloom, the flowers are mature and ready for harvest. The best time for harvest is in the morning of the second day of bloom, once the morning dew has dried. The corolla should have begun to turn from yellow to red at the tips, the middle area is orange colored, and the edges of the receptacle (the structure below the flower) are beginning to turn yellow.

Harvest Method

Flower corollas are harvested by hand using the thumb and 2–3 fingers to grasp the corolla and pull straight up away from the plant to ensure the flowers do not break during harvest.

ON-FARM PROCESSING

Sorting

Immediately after harvest the flowers should be cleaned to remove any foreign material. Any damaged flowers or even slightly composted/rotten flowers should be rejected.

Drying Method

Flowers are spread out in a sunny or shady location on tarps or any appropriate clean surface no more than 7 cm deep (thinner if in the shade) and allowed to dry. Flowers should dry rather quickly; usually completed within a few hours. Generally, stirring of the flowers is not necessary, but if it is necessary it is best to refrain from doing so with one's bare hands, instead wearing cotton gloves is advised, or use a clean pole or other appropriate instrument. If there is a threat of rain, the flowers must be well-covered or brought inside. The flowers are properly dried when they turn to powder when rubbed between the thumb and forefinger; moisture may not exceed 13%.

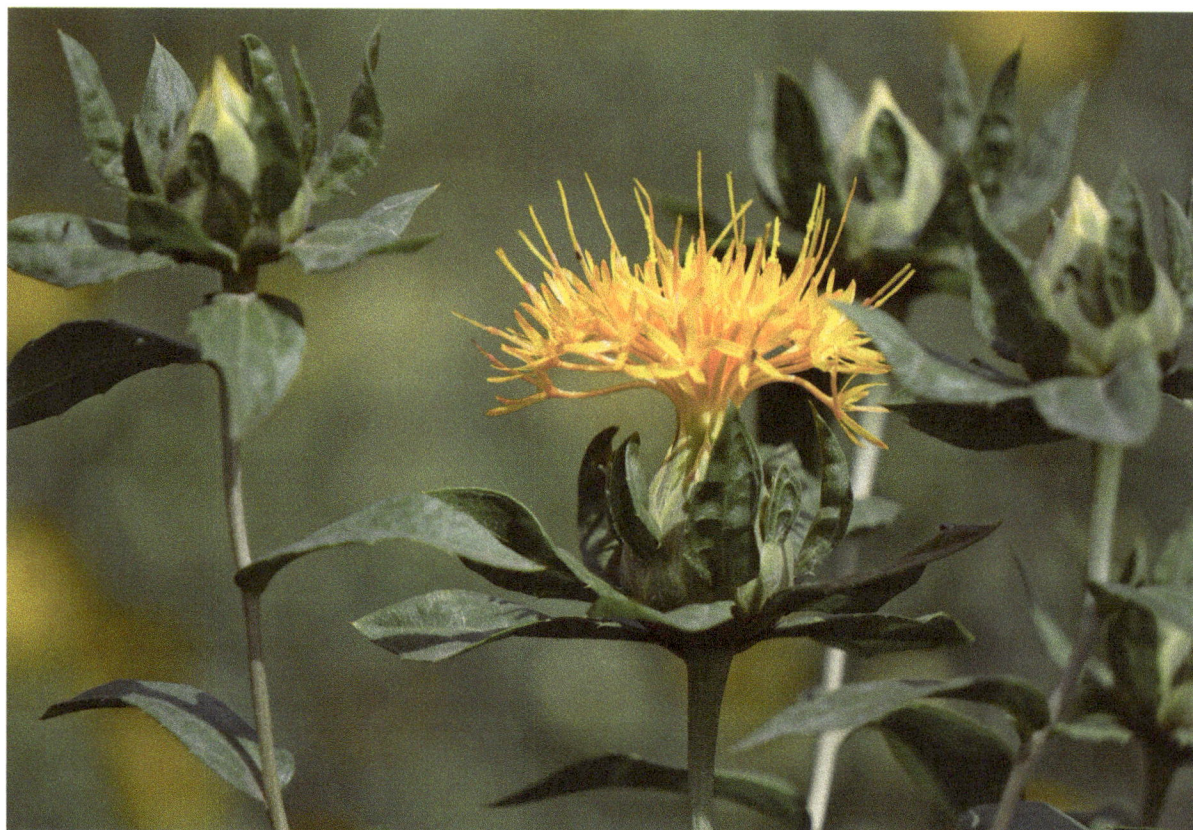

Flowering *hónghuā* at its peak waiting for harvest in Henan province, China.

祁菊花

Chrysanthemum

Chrysanthemum morifolium

The dried flower of *qí júhuā* (*Chrysanthemum morifolium* Ramat.), commonly known as *júhuā* (菊花), is a member of the sunflower family (Asteraceae). The genus identification is confused because of centuries of horticultural breeding. Although this species name has been widely accepted, it is not present in the Flora of China and it is possible that it is itself a cultivar since it is only propagated via root stock (not seed). It is a multi-branched woody perennial with whitish-pink to whitish yellow flowers. Daodi *júhuā* refers to the production of this herb is the area of Anguo in Hebei Province.

Traditionally this herb is categorized as a wind-heat-dissipating medicinal. It is commonly used for wind-heat attacking the exterior with symptoms of headache, red eyes, fever, etc. It is also well-known for clearing the liver and brightening the eyes. Because of this it is commonly drunk as a (steeped) tea in China, particularly in the summer and often with a bit of hard sugar (rock candy). It is an important herb for swollen and red eyes, especially due to liver and kidney depletion when the patient is seeing spots in their vision. However, it can be used for both vacuity and repletion patterns. Modern Chinese medicine doctors frequently suggest drinking this herb daily for patients with high blood pressure.

Most modern research has focused on the phenolic compounds found in the flowers. These compounds tend to peak around the time the flower is approximately 50% open. Many of these compounds have shown pharmacological activities such as anti-inflammatory, antioxidant, and even neuroprotectant. Some research also suggests an anti-diabetic activity partially via an anti-inflammatory action in adipose tissues which leads to increased adiponectin production, inducing the amelioration of insulin resistance and subsequently giving rise to a hypoglycemic effect. Some research of the polysaccharides suggests a positive shift in the microflora of the gut leading to benefit to those with ulcerative colitis.

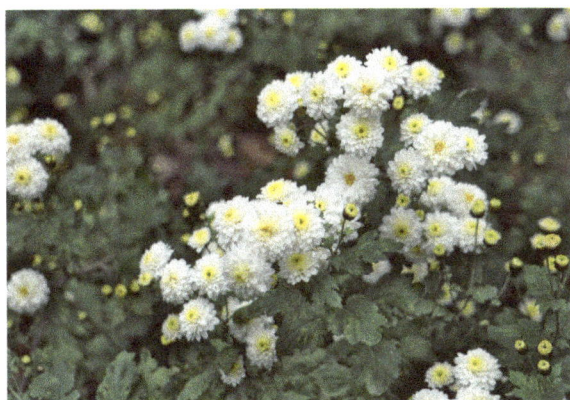

Contributing Authors

Wen Chun-xiu, Yang Tai-xin, Xie Xiao-liang, Guo Lan-ping, Huang Lu-qi, Hao Qing-xiu, Zheng Yu-guang, Liu Ming, Liu Ling-di, Jia Dong-sheng, Tian Wei

PRODUCTION SITE ECOLOGY

Elevation

Júhuā is cultivated at an elevation of 50–500 m.

Temperature

At least 197 frost free days. January is the coldest month with average temperatures below 3°C and July is the warmest month with average temperatures between 18–27°C.

Illumination

Average annual sunshine is between 2500–2757 hours. Sunshine percentage range is 35–70%.

Moisture

Average annual rainfall is 500–1000 mm with relative humidity of 34–55%.

Soil

A loose sandy-loam soil with a depth of at least 30 cm is ideal with soil pH in the 5.5–6.5 range.

Topography

Field can be either level or have a slope up to 15 degrees. If the field is sloped it should be facing either southeast or northwest to allow for proper drainage and wind-flow.

PROPAGATION

Propagation by Cuttings

During the months of April and May, when the plants have reached about 20 cm in height, choosing plants that are free from disease or insect pests, remove 12–15 cm of the stalk, discarding all but 1–2 leaves. Stems should be immediately sunk into a solution of naphthaleneacetic acid (NAA) (300 mg/L) to encourage root growth. Approximately 15 days after the emergence of new roots, plants may be transplanted. [Translator's Note: NAA is a synthetic rooting hormone in the auxin family. It is extremely common and although toxic to humans if ingested at high doses, it is generally considered safe.]

Propagation by Root Divisions

When planning root divisions flowering stalks should be cut off to allow the plant to put more energy into root growth. The following year, around April 15th, when the new growth has achieved 15–20 cm of vertical growth, sections of new white shoots that emerge from the main roots are dug and removed from the main root ball. Be careful to thoroughly check the plants for disease and insect pests, discarding any infected plants. These cuttings should then be planted as soon as possible.

TRANSPLANTING

Site Selection and Soil Preparation

Select rich and fertile soil that drains well; sandy-loam or clay-loam are both acceptable. Chose land that had grain (or other grass family plants) or a legume crop grown on it in previous years. This land should be plowed to 20–25 cm depth, turning in both the stubble from the previous year's harvest along with 12,000–15,000 kg per acre of composted manure or other organic compost. The field is then harrowed into 2 m wide beds.

Planting and Transplanting

During mid- to late April plants to be propagated by root division should be divided and transported immediately to the field for planting. Cuttings are transplanted from mid-May through mid-June. Planting or transplanting should be done on a cloudy day or after it has rained and the soil is moist and soft. Row spacing is 30 cm and plants are planted every 50 cm at a depth of 8–10 cm; one plant per hole, being sure that the entire root is covered by soil. When handling the cuttings, it is important not to damage the leaves and roots, being sure to maintain the integrity of the plants during the planting process. Pay attention to cuttings' size and plant so that sizes are evenly distributed in the field. Water thoroughly immediately after transplanting is complete.

FIELD MANAGEMENT

Checking Transplants & Filling Vacancies

After one week the field should be checked carefully for poorly developing or dying-dead transplants;

replacing them with new transplants to ensure proper spacing.

Cultivation and Weeding

Cultivation and weeding is generally done 3–4 times after planting. 1) about 2 weeks after transplanting; 2) twice during late July or early August; 3) when the plant is approaching its full growth. During the cultivation process soil can be hilled up around the plants to protect them from falling over. Cultivation must be done shallowly near the plants but more deeply between them, being careful not to damage the roots. Following a heavy rain, if there is hardening of the soils, this should be broken apart and loosened.

Top-Dressing

When plants begin to branch, urea is used at 120 kg per acre, when flower buds begin to form 60–75 kg per acre of superphosphate and 36–48 kg per acre of potassium sulfate is added. Fields should be watered immediately after top-dressing.

Irrigation and Water Drainage

It is inappropriate to water excessively within the first 30 days after transplanting, so be sure to maintain a reasonable moisture, neither too wet nor too dry; 40-60% soil moisture is ideal. After July watering should be done according to the needs of the plant when rainfall is insufficient. After watering, soil should be loosened to protect soil moisture.* During the rainy season when there is excessive rain, or accumulation of water in the fields, be sure to create appropriate drainage. [Translator's Note: The daodi region for this plant gets the vast majority of its rainfall from July through August. *Also, most of China's cultivated lands suffer from lack of good soil structure due to over-tilling and in some cases excessive use of fertilizers. Thus, crusting is common and "loosening the soil" is used to mediate crusting and keep soil moisture even.]

Pinching to Encourage Stem Development

When the plants have reached about 30 cm, choose a sunny day, and trim the main stems (1–2 cm). This is repeated every two to three weeks until the mid-July. At this point plants are left to develop with no further management.

PREVENTION AND TREATMENT OF DISEASE AND INSECT PESTS

Principles of Prevention and Treatment

Most of the diseases that affect *júhuā* are fungal in nature and are directly related to proper water drainage and airflow in the area. Therefore, it is critical to be mindful of these potential problems. Aphids can be a serious problem if not treated early, planting a companion crop that attracts predator species is encouraged.

Aphids (Aphidoidea)

Prevention and Treatment

Aphids are naturally attracted to the color yellow. Deploying "sticky yellow boards" or construction of areas with yellow painted boards (60×40 cm) will attract aphids where they can be killed. Apply oil to the surface of these boards so the aphids get stuck there, check to see when the board is coated with aphids, at which time the board can be scraped and more oil can be added. Boards are deployed at a rate of 180-240 per acre.

Biological Controls

Introduction of lady bugs early can be a very effective control of aphids. A 0.3% solution of matrine is diluted to a 0.1% concentration in water.

Damping Off Disease (*Rhizoctonia solani*)

Prevention and Treatment

Timely removal of affected plants. Crop rotation can also help to minimize this problem.

Verticillium Wilt (*Verticillium dahliae*)

Prevention and Treatment

When transplanting be sure to eliminate any diseased plants. During summer months, when rain is heavy, take care to drain water away from fields, not allowing it to accumulate. Use crop rotation. Take care to eliminate any infected plants immediately after discovering them.

Black Spot Disease
(*Diplocarpon rosae*)

Prevention and Treatment

Use a crop rotation of a grass family crop every 2 years, or as needed. Cut away infected leaves or plants and dispose of them away from the area as this will help slow the spread of this disease. [Translator's Note: Neem is known as an effective control of this fungal disease. However, there is not data to support its use on this crop.]

Chrysanthemum Gall Midge
(*Epirmgiu sp.*)

Prevention and Treatment

During the month of April any plants found to be infected with galls should be removed and disposed of, most commonly they are buried deeply.

HARVESTING

Harvest Season & Method

Flowers are harvested when they are 2/3 open during late October and early November before the first frost. Flowers are harvested on sunny days after the morning dew has dried. Flowers should be carefully snapped from the stem by hand, not cut.

ON-FARM PROCESSING

Drying Method

Flowers are dried below 45°C in a drier with good air circulation until 90% dry. At this time flowers are allowed to dry in the open air. Dried flowers may not exceed 15% moisture. [Translator's Note: Here, 90% dry does not refer to the total water content but rather when the ray and disc flowers have dried to 90% and the involucre appears dry on the outside, but the entire flower has a slightly soft feeling. If open air conditions do not allow outside drying, the temperature of the dryer should be lowered to 30°C and the drying completed. Do not over dry!]

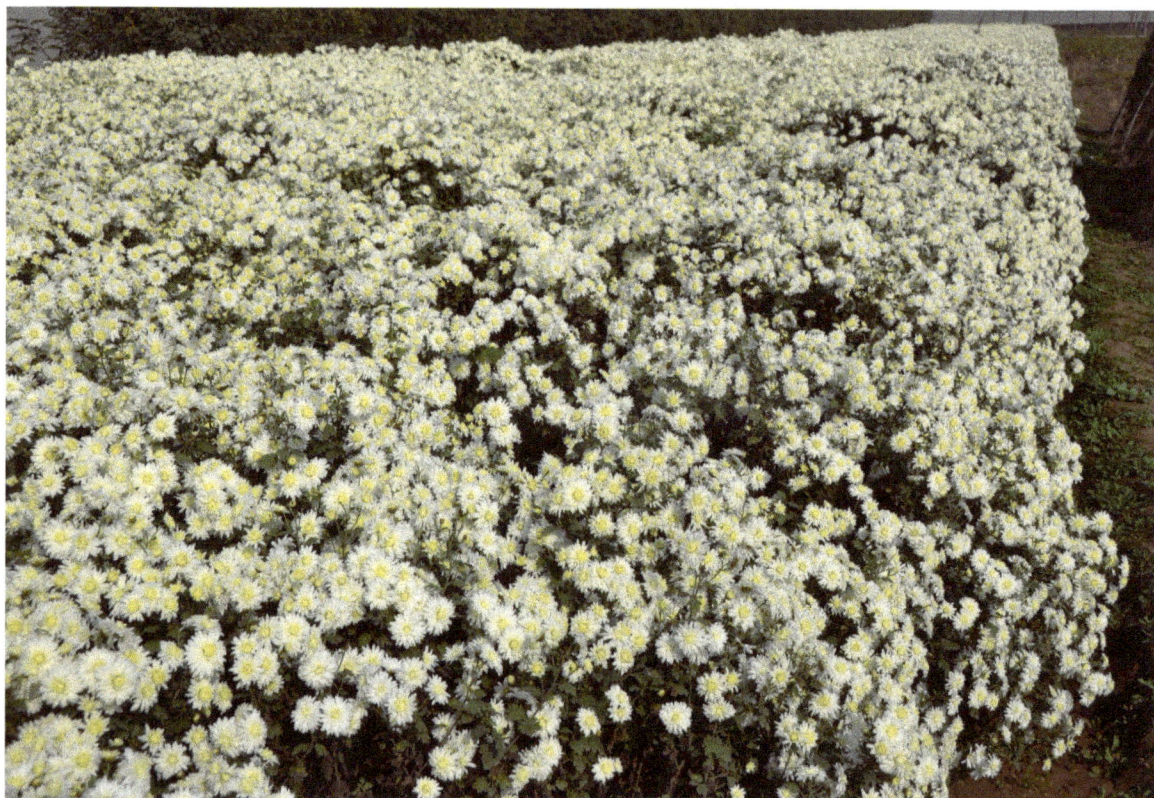

阿拉善肉苁蓉

Cistanche

Cistanche deserticola

DISTINGUISHING FEATURES

The dried, fleshy stem of the daodi herb *ālāshàn ròucōngróng* (*Cistanche deserticola* Y.C.Ma.), is a perennial parasitic plant known as *ròucōngróng* (肉苁蓉 \ 肉苁蓉) in China. It is a member of the broomrape family (Orobanchaceae) within the *Cistanche* genus. In the wild, the plant grows in the provinces of Inner Mongolia, Ningxia, Xinjiang, and Gansu, as well as in the country of Mongolia, in sandy locations from 200–1200 meters elevation. The daodi location for this medicinal is in A La Shan and the surrounding area of Inner Mongolia province.

This medicinal has been used for at least 2000 years and is a very important herb to supplement kidney yang and essence. Although it supplements kidney yang and is considered warm in nature, it is actually relatively neutral and does not cause over-heating or dryness, thus it can be used in cases where the patient also has kidney yin vacuity and essence depletion patterns. The herb is frequently used for older people with symptoms such as weakness and tightness of the muscles and tendons. It is commonly used in traditional Mongolian medicine as an anti-aging herb and is commonly used for elderly people with yang vacuity constipation.

There has been some very interesting research over the last few years about this holoparasitic plant. The pharmacological activities of the polysaccharides from this plant can modulate immune function and lipid balance, and has been shown to provide protection against aging, oxidative stress, and liver damage. Furthermore, new research suggests vul-nerable neurons can be protected by these compounds during ischemia stroke. Other research has shown that flavonoids from this plant exhibit neuroprotective actions.

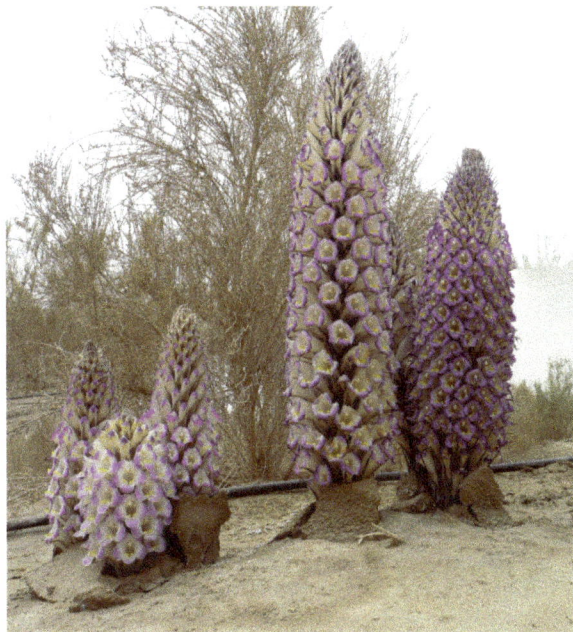

Contributing Authors

Li Min-hui, Zhang Chun-hong, Ha Si Ba Te Er, Wu Li-ji, Xu Jian-ping, Wang Jie

PRODUCTION SITE ECOLOGY

Elevation

Ròucōngróng is cultivated between 800–1400 m elevation.

Temperature

This herb requires a frost-free period of 120–180 days. The suitable annual average temperature 6–9°C. January is the coldest with temperatures of -14--3°C and July is the warmest with temperatures of 15–27°C.

Photo Period

Annual sunshine hours ranging from 3000–3700 hours with average daily sunshine of 70–73%.

Moisture

An average annual rainfall of 80–220 mm with an evaporation rate of 2900–3300 mm is typical. Soil moisture is generally very low at 2–3%. Suitable field water holding capacity should be around 50% and the area's average relative humidity should be 36–47%.

Soil

Sandy desert soil with neutral to slightly alkaline pH. Soils with high organic matter or clay content are not suitable for growing *ròucōngróng*.

Site Selection

Growing *ròucōngróng* requires abundant sunshine, minimal annual rainfall, good water drainage, and significant temperature difference between day and night. The water-table should be between 2–5 meters below the surface of a sand/sandy soil, which should be at least 1 meter deep. Growing within or surrounding a desert zone with neutral or slightly alkaline soils in best. Soils with salts between 2–3 g/kg are best and gray/brown or brown desert soils are acceptable. Heavy, hardpan, clay, and other similar soils are not suitable for growing *ròucōngróng*. Plants are grown at a density of 540–660 plants per acre. Host plants should be 2–3 years old, at least 1.5 meters tall, and be vigorous growers. *Haloxylon ammodendron* is the host of choice for cultivation.

SOWING SEEDS & RAISING SEEDLINGS

Seed Quality Requirements

Seeds stored under natural conditions can be 1 year or older when planted, seeds from wild plants are best. Germination should be above 85% and the material should have not more than 5% impurities.

Seed Collecting Requirements

Seeds should be collected from wild, healthy plants between the ages of 3 and 4 years; seeds may also come from cultivated sources. Plants grown for seed should be separated from plants grown for medicine by at least 200 meters to prevent accidental hybridization. Seeds are collected from late July through mid-August. The entire section of the plant that has flowers will eventually turn into a dense grouping of brown hard capsules full of seeds. One should take the capsules and rub them between your hands to remove seeds, which are then dried in the sun. Once the seeds have dried completely, they are winnowed from any foreign matter. Seeds should be full, plump, brown, and lustrous.

Pre-Sowing Treatment of Seeds

Seeds are mixed with sand and laid out in the sun for 20-30 days to bring them out of dormancy. Note that this assumes that seeds have been kept under natural conditions, which means that they are exposed to the same temperature fluctuations as their native habitat. If this has not been the case, seeds should undergo a similar warming and cooling environment for about 60 days to improve germination rates.

Sowing Seeds

Seeds can be planted any time between early April and late October. The best time to plant is during the months of May and June. The period from August through September is the next best time to plant. Select *Holoxylon ammodendron* trees between 2–3 years old and dig a wide hole 40–80 cm from the tree 50–70 cm deep, place clay or well composted manure in the hole (1–3 cm thick) and top it with a layer of sand (3–5 cm thick). Sprinkle 0.5–1 g of seeds on top of the sand and cover with 20–30 cm of sand, water until the entire hole is moist, then cover with a bit more sand and tamp down. Mark the area clearly.

FIELD MANAGEMENT

Management & Protection of the Host Tree

In the event of high winds or a sandstorm, the trees should be protected by adding extra sand around the tree or placing cut branches in the area to avoid excessive sand loss which could potentially expose the roots and damage the health of the tree. When growing seedlings, be sure to keep them moist; remove any other plants to avoid competition. Areas where trees are planted should be fenced to prevent domestic or other animals from damaging the trees.

Irrigation and Fertilization

When growing *ròucōngróng* it is best to keep human interference at a minimum; it is best to mimic nature. When the plant is less than 70 cm there is no need to water. However, in extremely dry weather, watering 1-2 times may be appropriate. In most cases fertilizer is not used, although it is occasionally applied close to harvest time; only composted manure is added in these cases.

Artificial Pollination

Ròucōngróng blooms in May. During the bloom, the plant can be covered with a bag or hand pollinated to improve pollination. These techniques have a significant positive impact on seed production.

PREVENTION AND TREATMENT OF DISEASE AND INSECT PESTS

Principles of Prevention and Treatment

Ròucōngróng is essentially free for diseases but insect and mammal pests are a threat. However, its host tree can develop disease, therefore careful monitoring of the host tree and treatment of any disease is critically important when growing this herb.

Powdery Mildew (*pathogen not identified*)

Prevention and Treatment

This is a significant threat to the host tree during the months of July and August. During the dry times, injecting a small amount of water into the sand close to the tree is a way to strengthen the tree and its resistance to disease. Keeping the soil loose and removing weeds will help to strengthen the tree. Do not over-water. Remove any diseased or dead plants to avoid infecting the other plants.

Root Rot of Host (*pathogen not identified*)

Prevention and Treatment

Preventative treatments are the same as powdery mildew (above). When planting the trees make sure the site drains water properly and loosen the soil if necessary.

Fly (*Delia platura*)

Prevention and Treatment

When *ròucōngróng* emerges from the sand to flower, the larvae of this insect can damage the tender stalk and drill into the stalk below the ground; this causes serious damage to the quality of the final product. However, there are currently no effective measures to avoid this other than traps to lure flies away from the plants, which may be moderately successful.

Grub (*Holotrichia sp.*)

Prevention and Treatment

Grubs during their larval stage are a serious pest that eat the stalk and roots or *ròucōngróng*. *Cynanchum hancockianum* (a milkweed family plant) is cut into 2 cm sections and dried in the sun. Then this plant is mixed with sand (1:3) and 300–500 g is added in and around the holes when planting *ròucōngróng*.

Great Gerbil (*Rhombomys opimus*)

Biological Controls

This animal is known to eat branches of the host tree and eat the *ròucōngróng*. Construct simple "houses" or dig holes and place water containers in the area to attract cats, weasels, foxes, etc. to the area to control these rodents. Building roosts for owls and hawks is also a good way to control these rodents.

Exterminating with Cement

Cook some rice, wheat flour, and corn flour over dry heat, add a little sesame oil, then mix in some dry cement. Take this mixture and place it areas where the rodent frequently travels or eats.

[Translator's Note: Although this rodent is native to China, the information above is included to help growers deal with other potential rodent pests.]

HARVESTING

Harvest Season

Ròucōngróng can be harvested anytime between 2–4 years of growth, but 3-year and older plants produce the best material. *Ròucōngróng* can be harvested in the late autumn or early spring, however the late autumn harvest produces the best quality medicinal material.

Harvest Method

It is common practice to use hand tools to harvest. Start just outside of the hole where the seed was planted and dig around that area. Carefully excavate around the base of the plant to avoid damaging it while removing the stem. Damage to the main plant could kill it, so careful removal is extremely important. Because *ròucōngróng* is a parasitic plant, careful removal of the medicinal material (stem) without disturbing the base of the plant may allow it to regrow, especially since there could be other, smaller or less obvious, stems that have already begun to grow. After harvest, use the same sand-soil to fill in the hole, press down, and mark the area for the future.

Cutting Away the Buried Flowering Head

During the process of harvesting, the flowering head of *ròucōngróng* that has yet to emerge from the sand can be cut away to focus the plant's energy on vegetative growth. This is done by finding the new growth that will become a flowering stalk and carefully holding the new growth while cutting the stalk 20 cm from the surface of the soil.

ON-FARM PROCESSING

Drying Method

Ròucōngróng is dried in the sun and the flowering-reproductive parts are removed, this is also known as the head of *ròucōngróng*. Once the head of *ròucōngróng* changes color either use boiling water to soften and remove the head, or use a knife to cut away the area that has changed color, then put in a clean area to dry in the sun. The herb should be frequently turned to avoid loss in quality. Drying is completed in the sun; moisture content should be below 10%. During sun drying, if there is rain or damp weather, the plants must be protected; do not allow the harvested plants to get moist during this process.

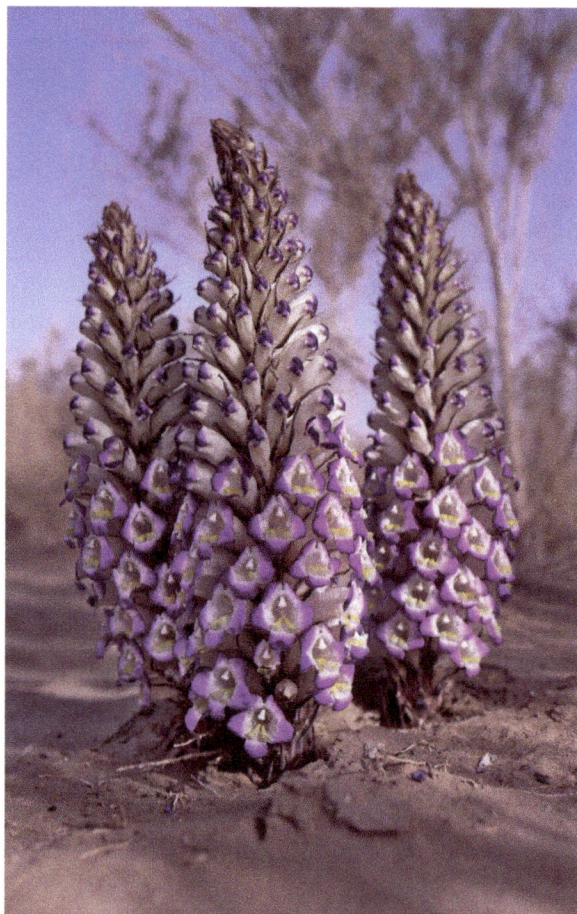

Flowering *ròucōngróng* at China Academy of Sciences Ecological Research Station in Xinjiang, China.

潞党参

Codonopsis

Codonopsis pilosula

DISTINGUISHING FEATURES

The herb *lù dǎngshēn* (*Codonopsis pilosula* (Franch.) Nannf.), commonly known as *dǎngshēn* (黨参 \ 党参) in China, is a member of the bellflower family (Campanulaceae). The genus is made up of about 40 species with more than half endemic to China. This species is common throughout much of China as well as Mongolia, Korea, and the far eastern area of Russia. The plant grows in forests, thickets, meadows, and forest margins between 900–3900 m elevation. Officially, the *Pharmacopoeia of the People's Republic of China* (2015) recognizes this species plus a variation, *Codonopsis tangshen*, however this monograph is specific to growing Codonopsis pilosula only. The daodi location for this herb is Changzhi and Jincheng cities, and the surrounding areas, in Shanxi province.

This medicinal plant became popular due to the extreme shortage of ginseng in the Shanxi region after excessive digging led to the extinction of wild ginseng in the region. Around the time of the late Ming and early Qing Dynasties (16th and early 17th centuries) *dǎngshēn* began to gain favor in the region as a substitute for ginseng, especially among those who could not afford the cost of real ginseng. This led to it becoming known as the "poor-man's ginseng" and it has since become a common substitute in formulas for ginseng. However, it is not a very good substitute for treating many medical conditions, and should be viewed as only a partial substitute for ginseng. *Dǎngshēn* is mostly used to supplement spleen and lung qi in Chinese medicine for conditions such as low appetite, diarrhea, lack of energy, and fullness due to spleen and\or lung qi vacuity.

Modern science has shown this and other plants in the genus have a variety of medicinal applications. *Dǎngshēn* has been shown to have the following pharmacological activities: anti-tumor, anti-diabetic, and anti-aging effects; protecting the gastric mucosa, stimulating the immune system; and protecting the nervous system.

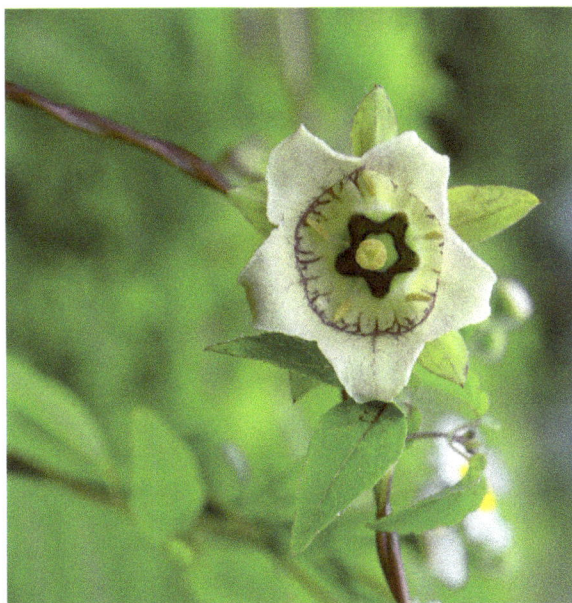

Contributing Authors

Gao Jian-ping, Cao Ling-ya, Sun Hai-feng, Zhao Guo-feng

PRODUCTION SITE ECOLOGY

Elevation

Dǎngshēn is grown between 1000–3200 m elevation.

Temperature

There should be between 157–182 frost-free days annually, and average annual temperatures should be between 5–11°C. The coldest month is January and the hottest month is July.

Photo Period

Annual sunshine hours should range from 1800–1900 hours, with 59% annual sunshine days.

Rainfall

Average annual rainfall should be 500–1000 mm.

Soil

A sandy soil that is primarily yellow with brown mixed in, or primarily red-yellow with brown mixed in, and a slightly alkaline pH is ideal. Soil should have a rich amount of trace elements including iron, copper, manganese, zinc, etc. These elements affect the color and luster of the exterior of *dǎngshēn*'s root, as well as efficacious chemical constituents found in the root.

Topography

The areas around the cities of Changzhi and Jincheng, in Shanxi province are the primary growing areas for *dǎngshēn*. Changzhi city is located in the southeast portion of Shanxi province (E113°01′, N35°50′). This area belongs to the moist continental monsoon climate at an elevation between 800–1500 m above sea level. Jincheng city is also in the southeast portion of Shanxi province (E113°01′, N35°50′), and has a continental monsoon climate at an elevation between 600–2000 m above sea level. Wild *dǎngshēn* grows in a wider elevation range, 1200–3200 m, and grows in semi-shaded habitats including forests, along forest edges, in thickets, and on mountain slopes with about 50% shade. Cultivation is mostly near the respective regions river headwaters with well-drained, loose, sandy, fertile soil.

PRODUCTION AREA ENVIRONMENTAL REQUIREMENTS

Site Selection

In order for the root system of *dǎngshēn* to penetrate the soil, it should be deep, loose, and drain well, with good fertility and abundant humus. Under these conditions the survival rate of transplants or field planted seeds will be very high and yield will be very good. *Dǎngshēn* growing areas have good quantities of complete nitrogen and quick-acting potassium; exchangeable magnesium is also in higher quantities than most soils. *Dǎngshēn*'s N, P, K, Ca, Mg, Fe, Mn, and Zn quantities are all very high. The plant has a tendency to assimilate excess Fe, Mn, and Zn, which helps to promote root growth.

Soil Preparation

Till soil in the autumn, to a depth of 20 cm, around the time of the first frost, to kill pathogenic fungi and bacteria, as well as pests and their eggs. This procedure also helps to reduce weeds. Before planting, break up clods, level soil, rake smooth, and dig ditches for drainage. Meticulous soil preparation is the key to high yields of *dǎngshēn*. The best choice is loose-sandy, but fertile soil, or fertile garden soil; an area that has no previous history of growing *dǎngshēn* and has few weeds and insect pests. Areas close to headwaters are the most ideal areas for its cultivation. The use of high-quality, thoroughly decomposed manure and/or compost is highly recommended. This material is spread on the field at a rate of 3000 kg per acre, then the soil is tilled deep to 40–50 cm. Deep tilling will loosen the soil and blend the fertilizer into the soil. Once soil is tilled, it can be harrowed and beds are built.

SOWING SEEDS & RAISING SEEDLINGS

Seed Quality Requirements

Seed purity >99%; <5% foreign matter; <10% moisture; >70% germination rate; free of insect pests. Seeds should be full and plump, brown, shiny, and free of contaminates. Seeds should be shiny, undamaged, and without mold or mildew. They should be from the previous year's harvest because fresh seeds sprout quickly and have a high germination rate, and they grow quickly with well distributed growth that is healthy and strong, making the crop easy to manage. Seeds stored at normal atmospheric temperatures for more than 8 months are not suitable for production (they have very low germination rates), and can be recognized because they will have lost their shininess and the color will not be as deep.

Saving Seed

Seeds are collected from the yellowed seed capsules of 2-year-old plants when the calyx has withered and dried. Seeds are a shiny, dark brown color when mature. When collecting seeds, the stem and capsule are removed together and transported to the drying area where they are spread out to dry in the sun for several days until the capsule opens. Use a board or stick to gently break open the capsule to free the seeds. Then the stem, which is still attached to the capsule, is held and gently tapped on the ground or other surface to free all the remaining seeds from the capsule. Finally, the seeds are garbled from the other plant material.

Seed Storage

Once seeds have been sifted and are free of foreign plant material, they are laid out in a fairly sunny location for 1-3 days until moisture content goes below 10%. Seeds are stored in a cotton bag in a dry shaded location with good air exchange and low temperatures (4–20°C). Do not use smoke-curing and keep the seeds dry.

Nursery Bed Selection and Preparation

Seedlings should be grown in moist, not wet, loose, fertile soil. *Dǎngshēn* seedlings do not like full sun. Seedlings prefer moist, shaded, and sloped areas. Do not choose dry, windy areas, or sunny, southern exposure slopes. Areas with little agriculture development or areas that at least have not had *dǎngshēn* or other related plants grown in the location for more than 3 years are best. Fertile soil that has undergone alternating freezing and thawing cycles makes for good quality soil and reduces insect pests and weeds. Before sowing seeds, break any hard surface that may exist on the soil, level the beds (1.2 m wide and 12–15 cm tall, with 25 cm deep trenches between the rows), remove stones, sticks, and sow seeds.

Sowing Seeds

Dǎngshēn seeds can be sown in the spring or autumn. Spring sowing is most often employed, from late February through early March, once the soil is no longer frozen. When sowing seeds in the spring it is best to do it early, do not sow late, early sown seeds allow for seedlings to get a tap-root deep into the soil early, this avoids damage from dryness and makes the plant stronger. Seeds sown in the autumn generally are left without any management, but it is important not to sow seeds too early and risk the seeds sprouting before the winter freeze, as this will have a negative impact on the second year of growth.

Seeds are very small, and one-thousand seeds must weigh ≥0.27 g. Due to their small size, it is important to pay attention to making sure that seeds are evenly distributed when sowing. In order to assist with even distribution, seeds can be mixed with sand or fine-grained soil at a ratio of 1:5. This mixture is scattered on the surface of the soil and covered by 0.5–1 cm of fine-grained soil. Seeds are sown at a rate of 12–18 kg per acre. Maintaining good soil moisture after sowing seeds is important and will benefit germination rate and survival of seedlings. After seeds are sown and raked in, mulch should be used to shade the area, pine branches, straw, or bean husks are most frequently used. Mulching is used to shade the area, but should neither be too thick nor too thin.

Raising Seedlings

Dǎngshēn seedlings are very tender and the mulch must be removed slowly. Once the plants emerge, a small amount of the mulch is removed to allow for about 15% sun exposure. Then, once the plants reach 3–5 cm tall, every 3–5 days more of the mulch is gradually removed until the plants reach 15 cm tall, when all the remaining mulch may be removed.

Seedling Bed Management

If a dry spell occurs when sowing seeds in spring, be sure to protect seedlings from excessive wind and do not allow soil to dry out. After there is approximately 60% germination, the seedling beds should be allowed to dry slightly before watering. If there is heavy rain, it is important to be sure to drain off excess water from the seedling beds. Once the seedlings have reached 5–7 cm tall, they should be thinned to a spacing of 2–3 cm apart; this should allow for 200 seedlings per square meter. During this time any weeds should be pulled; keeping the seedling beds well-weeded is key to strong sprouts.

FIELD MANAGEMENT

Transplanting

Seedlings are grown for one year prior to transplanting into the field. Roots grown in seedling beds should be between 0.3–0.4 cm thick, 15–18 cm long, evenly developed with few branches, the root color should be unmixed, must be without physical damage, and there are no signs of presence or damage due to insects. During late March and early April, after the ground has thawed, but prior to the grown buds sprouting, the one-year old seedlings are transplanted. Autumn transplanting can be performed during the first 2–3 weeks of October, after the plant's growth has halted and before the ground freezes.

Dăngshēn is planted in rows 22–25 cm apart. Trenches, which will form the rows, are dug 25–30 cm deep and plants are placed in the trenches every 8–10 cm. The tail of the root must be pointed straight down, never winding or crooked, and extend naturally downward into the trench. The trench should be filled and the top of the root covered with 2–3 cm of soil, which is then pressed firmly. Once plants have emerged from the soil, carefully inspect them, looking for roots that did not emerge. Any places that did not sprout can be replaced with roots that were kept in reserve. The best time to transplant to the field is on a cloudy day with cloud cover predicted for the following two days after transplanting. Water during periods of insufficient rain.

Cultivation and Weeding

Plants should emerge within 35–40 days after transplanting. Because weeds tend to grow faster, after 30 days weeds should be removed once by pulling. At this time the rows should be cultivated to loosen the soil and kill small weeds; this will also help to regulate soil temperature and maintain soil moisture, encourage root growth, and safeguard the health of the young plants; be very careful to avoid damaging the roots or budding plants. During the month of April gentle hoeing of the soil to loosen it and to kill small weeds should be performed. This

process should be repeated twice during the month of May, but at this time weeds should be killed via hoeing, not pulled as this could disturb the growing *dăngshēn*. Finally, this process is repeated once prior to the first frost.

IRRIGATION AND FERTILIZATION

Watering and Water Drainage

The daodi area for *dăngshēn* generally has abundant rain, so irrigation is not needed. After the start of the rainy season, it is important to dig trenches to drain off excess water. Excess water in the soil can easily cause root rot.

Top-Dressing

Growing daodi *dăngshēn* allows for two types of fertilizer: 1) organic thermal compost and 2) GAP approved chemical fertilizer. If using organic composting methods, the organic matter (animal manure) must be thoroughly rotted. Compost is generally applied during autumn at a rate of 3000 kg per acre. Thoroughly rotted seed compost is also applied at a rate of 3000 kg per acre. Top-dressing is done in the second year during the second half of May after the plants have reached a height of about 10 cm. This is done at the same time as the final bed cultivation and weeding session and is also applied at a rate of 3000 kg per acre.

Plant Management

Dăngshēn has a trailing vine that grows to indefinite heights. Once it is past the point of rapid growth, the most succulent 15 cm or so are cut off with an appropriate tool.

PREVENTION AND TREATMENT OF DISEASE AND INSECT PESTS

As long as basic prevention methods are used, cultivation of this plant comes with few pest or disease risks. Application of pesticides of any kind is not common practice. Continuous cropping is ill-advised, crop rotation for at least 1 year with a grass or pea family plant is considered best practice. Proper drainage of water during heavy rains is critical. Early weeding is critical. Removal of any insect eggs on leaves and elimination of the source of any insect pest is important. Any manure used must undergo high heat composting procedures.

HARVESTING

Harvest Season

Plants are grown for 2–3 years before harvest. Roots are harvested during the months of October and November.

Harvesting Method

Roots are dug from two sides and removed. Once removed from the soil, excess soil is gently removed, taking great care not to damage the root skin; the root is then placed in the sun to dry.

ON-FARM PROCESSING

Sun-Drying

After most of the soil is removed, roots are laid in the sun to dry for 1-2 days. Roots are flipped regularly so they dry evenly to 80% dryness.

Grading

Dǎngshēn roots are divided into three grades based on the diameter at the top of the root, below the crown; 1) more than 0.8 cm, 2) 0.6–0.7 cm, 3) 0.4–0.5 cm. Any roots with a diameter below 0.4 cm are considered substandard and not fit for use.

Washing

After preliminary sun-drying and grading, *dǎngshēn* roots are washed with water. Roots are soaked in water for 5–10 minutes, then a soft brush is used to remove the remaining soil, after which the roots are placed in the sun for drying.

Kneading

After the roots have dried 40-50%, hold the root crown tight with one hand, while the other hand smooths it from top to tail. Make sure the skin and woody parts stay together tightly and rub 8-10 times, then rub the root crown 8-10 times.

Make sure to avoid creating high temperatures with your hands, taking care not to rub too hard, otherwise the root skin will look like "female pig skin," which is considered low quality. Lay out in the sun for 1-2 days, then repeat. This process should be repeated 3-4 times.

Bundling

After the kneading process is completed and the roots are dry, make bundles of approximately 0.5 kg and tie together (in the middle) with cotton or other natural fiber. Finally, arrange the crowns neatly and use an elastic band to hold them in place.

Final Sun-Drying

After roots are bundled, the bundles are placed in the sun until dried to a moisture content of 10–13%.

川黄连

Chinese Coptis
Coptis chinensis

The dried root of the daodi medicinal *chuān huánglián* (*Coptis chinensis* Franch.) commonly known as *huánglián* (黄连 \ 黄連), is a member of the crowfoot family (Ranunculaceae). The *Coptis* genus is comprised of 15 species in East Asia and North America, six are present in China and five are endemic. This is a perennial forest dwelling herb, native throughout much of southern China, growing from 5–15 cm tall and found from 500–2000 m elevation. The daodi location this medicinal originates is in Sichuan province Emei mountian, Hongya county, and the surrounding area, Chongqing area, Shizhu county, Wu Mountain, Hubei province in Lichuan county, Shaanxi province in Zhenping county and the surrounding area.

Traditionally this herb is used to clear heat and dry dampness for treating conditions such as dysenteric diarrhea and bloody urination. It is an important herb for treating the qi aspect where it can clear heat and drain fire and treats mouth sores, toothache, and sores on the upper part of the body. It is also an important herb for stomach and heart heat, the latter of which can manifest in a number of psychological conditions such as anxiety, agitation, and delirious speech. The root is also used both internally and externally to clear heat and resolve toxin for sores, boils, and abscesses that are red, hot, and swollen.

There is a large body of research on this entire genus and some of the compounds found in it, particularly berberine. The herb is a well-known anti-inflammatory, antibacterial and, more recently, research suggests it can be used in the treatment of diabetes. Several variations of the primary alkaloid, berberine, are available as a single compound drug that is sold over-the-counter in China and other countries. It is primarily used for dysentery and other similar digestive disturbances from bacterial contamination of food and water, in fact it is popular among travelers as a easy-to-carry first-aid to take in case of "travelers diarrhea."

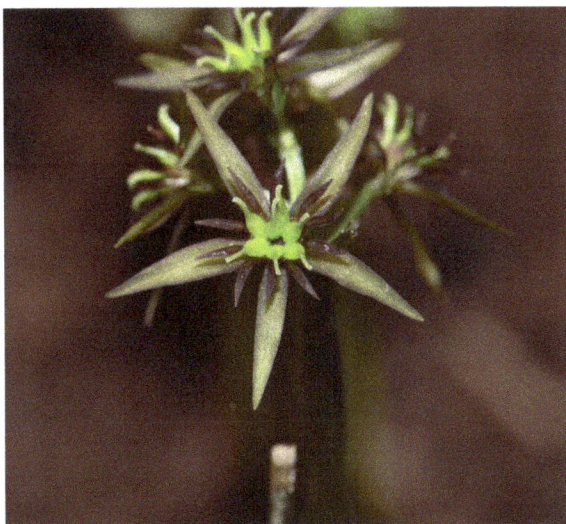

Contributing Authors

Song Liang-ke, Guo Lan-ping,
Zhao Man-qian, Tan Rui, Wang Yan

PRODUCTION SITE ECOLOGY

Elevation

Huánglián is cultivated between 1100–1800 m elevation.

Temperature

Average annual temperature ranges between 8–10°C. Annual frost-free days are 170–220. The hottest month of the year is July but it doesn't get hotter than 31°C and averages around 21°C. The coldest month is January, with the coldest temperatures dropping to -18°C but the average is around -3--4°C.

Photo Period

Average annual sunshine is between 1100–1400 hours. The strongest sun is in August around 6000 lx and the weakest sun is during October and November, which is between 1000–2000 lx. The rest of the year it ranges between 4000–6000 lx.

Moisture

Average annual rainfall is between is 1300–1600 mm. Humidity is usually between 80–90%.

Soil

A humus rich soil that is reddish-brown, grayish-brown, brown, or yellowish-brown with a pH between 5.0–6.5 is most suitable. A coarse sand or clay soil is unsuitable for growing *huánglián*.

Topography

Shady or morning sun mountainous areas with a slope under 20 degrees are most appropriate for growing *huánglián*.

PRODUCTION AREA ENVIRONMENTAL REQUIREMENTS

Site Selection

Sites with loose, thick, deep, rich humus soils are best. The area should easily drain and have good air flow. A virgin mixed forest location with nice brown or yellowish-brown soil is best. Continuous cropping should be avoided. Fields in cleared forest areas are sometimes used by growing *huánglián* for the first two years intercropped with corn.

Soil Preparation

Beds (1.6 m wide and 15–20 m long) are built on a slope and generally prepared across a slight ridge in the geography so that the bed can easily drain from the middle out. Pathways between the beds are 10 cm deep and 30 cm wide. However, at the lowest point where the beds are built, a larger drainage ditch is dug which is 30 cm deep and 40 cm wide. This allows for excellent water drainage so that water is not allowed to accumulate in heavy rain conditions.

SOWING SEEDS & RAISING SEEDLINGS

Seed Quality Requirements

Seeds that are fully ripe, plump, weigh a minimum of 1.3 g per 1000 seeds, germinate at a rate over 70%, and have no more than 10% foreign matter are considered good quality.

Saving and Storing Seed

Seeds may be harvested from plants starting at the end of the fourth year of growth. Seeds are collected when the seed capsules turn from green to yellow and begin to split open. Collected seeds are placed in a shady, cool area up to 3 cm thick. The seeds should be flipped 3 times per day. After 7–8 days when the seeds turn a khaki color they can be planted or stored. Seeds should be stored in a cellar on a bed of sand, then covered with 3 cm of pure sand or high-quality humus.

Preparation of Seedling Bed Area

A shady mountain slope with a less than 20% slope with at least 10 cm of high-quality, good draining, humus-rich soil with a pH of 5.0–6.5 is best. Soil is tilled to 20–25 cm deep and beds are prepared 130 cm wide and should not exceed 10 m in length, with 15 cm wide (10 cm deep) pathways in between. Well-composted cow or horse manure is applied at a rate of 30,000 kg per acre, it is mixed evenly with the top-soil and leveled. Then, another 3 cm of smoke-cured soil is added on top. A crop cover that allows 85–90% shade is put over the beds (80 cm high) to protect seeds and newly emerging seedlings. The illumination should be between 1500–4000 lx. [Translator's Note: Smoke cured soil is a technique used in mountainous, cold, and humid locations. The process is to burn grasses, fallen leaves, and/or other non-woody plant stalks to smoke or fumigate soil. This process tends to increase available nitrogen, phosphorus, and potassium; however, it can lower total nitrogen in the soil. Although this technique is common, it is not practiced by all growers.]

Sowing Seeds

Seeds are sown during the months of October and November at a rate of 15 kg per acre. Mix the seeds with fine humus-rich soil to assist with sowing, then broadcast the seeds evenly on the beds. Finally, the beds should be covered by a single layer of seed-free grass or straw.

Field Management of Seedlings

Once seedlings have produced one to two true leaves, they should be thinned to create rows approximately 1 cm apart. Beds should be weeded once after the plants produce their third true leaf. During the period of April and May, after the beds have been thinned, a nitrogen fertilizer is added at a rate of 48 kg per acre, or finely sieved composted manure at a rate of 6000 kg per acre. During the months of June and July a mixture of 150 kg of cake fertilizer and 780 kg of humus should be sifted together and added to the beds, acre by acre. During October and November, the final fertilization is applied; 900 kg per acre of powdered cow manure and 300 kg of cake fertilizer is applied. In the second year, after the snow has melted, manure or urea is applied once at the same rate as above. [Translator's Note: Cake fertilizer is produced from oil seeds that have already been pressed for their oil. Commonly used seeds include perilla seeds, hemp seeds, cotton seed, soy beans, etc.]

Pricking Seedlings for Transplanting

On a cloudy day, or after a rain, second year plants that are a minimum of 6 cm tall and have 4–6 true leaves can be pricked out for transplanting. The fine roots are trimmed to 2 cm and washed thoroughly with clean water, then plants are spread out from the rhizome to the leaves to form a fan shape. Note they should not be bundled, 100 plants form a single grouping for transportation. This arrangement is used to transport to the field for transplanting.

Transplanting

Transplanting can be done in the spring from mid- to late March, or in the autumn from late October through early November. Plants should be transplanted at 10×10 cm spacing, which works out to about 360,000 seedlings per acre. The soil should be firmly pressed around each plant after transplanting.

Building Shade Houses

Artificial shade is created by building shade houses two meters tall. Vertical beams are 10–15 cm in diameter and top beams are 10–12 cm in diameter; cross-members are 3–6 cm in diameter. This is covered with fronds of available tree branches (typically a local cedar is used - *Cryptomeria* sp. -, but anything that is local can be used). During the first year after transplanting, the light available should be 1500 lx, after this time, more and more light can be allowed to penetrate the shade house to mimic natural conditions.

FIELD MANAGEMENT

Filling in Gaps

Gaps in the beds due to death of seedlings can be filled in the autumn of the first year (after spring transplanting) or the spring of the following year.

Weeding

During the first through third years, weeding should be done 4–5 times annually. During the fourth and fifth year, 2–3 times should be sufficient. While weeding, it is advantageous to loosen the top-soil.

Hilling-up

During the spring of the second year, soil from the pathways is dug and placed between the plants, trying to get the soil in and around the plants as tightly as possible. During the autumn of the third year, after top-dressing, 1.5–3 cm of fine humus is applied to the top of each bed; this is repeated in the autumn of the fourth year with 3–5 cm of fine humus.

Fertilization

Two to three days after transplanting, a tea of manure (3600 kg) and water (6000 l) is sprayed on each acre. One month after transplanting, 7500 kg per acre of finely sieved composted cow manure is used as a top-dressing. During the spring of the second through the fourth year a combination of 6000 kg of composted manure and 300-600 kg of cake fertilizer is combined with 6000 L of water (per acre) and applied as a foliar feeding. In the autumn of these years, a 3 cm cover of well-composted manure or humus is applied at a rate of 7500-12000 kg per acre.

Water Drainage

Preventing Erosion: The upper and outside drainage ditches should be connected by ditches 30-45 cm wide and 25-30 cm deep.

The Side Drainage Ditches: Ditches vertical to the slope, should be 15 cm wide, 10 cm deep. Horizontal ditches should be 10 cm deep, 30 cm wide, and should be dug every 16–20 m along the slope.

Shade House Management

During the first three years, watch closely for any damage or loosening of joints. Repair any problems immediately. Be mindful of any areas where sunlight may be penetrating beyond recommended levels or where water may be dripping onto the bed. Any such issues should be repaired immediately. During the autumn of the fourth year or spring of the fifth year, the covering on the top of the shade house is removed to allow light penetration, this will strengthen the roots and help the rhizomes to grow larger.

Pinching Flowers

Plants should start to flower in their third year. With the exception of those plants used for collecting seeds, all flowering stalks should be pinched off when they reach 2 cm long.

PREVENTION AND TREATMENT OF DISEASE AND INSECT PESTS

Fundamental Prevention

Every year during the winter months be sure to clear excessive snow from the tops of the shade house. During March and April pay close attention to insect pests. April and May are the months to be concerned with root rot disease. Anthracnose disease is most likely to occur April through June. May to August is the most active time for diseases such as southern blight or powdery mildew. Measures such as maintaining the drainage system, repairing the shade house, adjusting the light penetration, and generally keeping a close eye on the growing area are strongly recommended. Timely weeding and removal of diseased plants is critical. During the months of September through December appropriate top-dressing, eliminating any signs of insect pests or potential origins of disease, while shoring up the shade house for winter are all important tasks.

Soil-borne Insects (*Holotrichia* sp. & Gryllotalpidae)

Prevention and Treatment

Because of the length of time it takes to bring *huánglián* to harvest, sites where *huánglián* is grown need to be used for 5–10 years, thus *Cryptomeria* sp. (or similar species) grow fast enough to offer ideal shade for growing *huánglián*. If using virgin soil, or soil that has been grown on before, all waste such as tree branches, fallen leaves, scraps from building the shade houses, etc. are burned and used to smoke the soil to reduce the risk of soil borne diseases and kill potential insect pests. Use thermal compost, do not use fresh or poorly composted manure or other material. Lights can be employed while insects are able to fly to attract and trap them.

Root Rot Disease (*Fusarium solani*)

Prevention and Treatment

Pay close attention to water drainage, immediately remove any plants that show signs of disease, add lime to the hole where the plant was removed.

Powdery Mildew (*Erysiphe aquilegiae*)

Prevention and Treatment

Pay close attention to ensure that the soil is draining properly. Check the shade house cover and adjust if needed, as increase in light penetration may help. Properly dispose of any accumulated withered stems and fallen leaves.

Anthracnose Disease (*Collectotrichum* sp.)

Prevention and Treatment

Do not allow the top of the shade house to become too open, keep the opening relatively small. Reinforce cultivation and water drainage.

HARVESTING

Harvest Season

Plants are harvested 4–5 year after they have been transplanted into the field. *Huánglián* is harvested from mid-September through November; this is the period when the rhizome has a lower water content. Harvesting can be on sunny or cloudy days but should not be done in the rain or when the ground is frozen.

Harvest Method

The shade house and any fallen leaves are cleared from the site 2–3 days prior to harvest. The soil around the plant is loosened with a digging fork and the entire plant is pulled free from the soil and shaken vigorously to eliminate soil and other plant matter that may be clinging to the root system. Scissors are used to cut away most of the fibrous roots, leaves, and the next year's bud. Do not wash with water.

ON-FARM PROCESSING

Drying on a Heated Brick Bed

Fresh *huánglián* rhizomes are spread evenly on a brick bed 30 cm thick, which is then heated for 40–60 minutes from below with a wood fire. When the soil still present on the rhizomes turns white, the pile is turned with a fork or rake. The pile is then turned in the same manner after another 60 minutes. After another 90 minutes, the pile is turned for a third time. After this period, as much soil and remaining fibrous roots as possible are removed. The rhizomes are then divided into two halves; one half is stacked on 1/3 of the heated brick bed, while the other half is spread across the other 2/3 of the brick bed. The second half, on the 2/3 of the brick, is then turned frequently and rather aggressively treated until nearly all the soil has fallen from the rhizomes, at which point it is dried. Then the other half is treated using the same method.

Alternate Method

Divide *huánglián* into three groups according to the size of the rhizomes (large, medium, small). Each group is dried as above, however rhizomes may be stacked 70–80 cm high on top of the heated brick bed. When the fibrous roots and petioles are burned crisp, the rhizomes are removed from the heat and laid on a mat in the sun to dry. Rhizomes are dry when water content reaches 10%. Once the rhizomes have dried, they are put into a cylinder cage (similar to a backyard compost turner), traditionally made with bamboo, but metal works well too. Carefully seal the cage door then spin the cylinder until all the soil and other material has fallen from the rhizomes.

Translator's Note: These techniques developed in the mountainous areas of Sichuan, China where access to electricity and other forms of power where not available and often far from production sites. Because of the distances farmers would need to travel with heavy fresh rhizomes that might develop mold or other rotting during transportation, these methods were essential, and still are in many places. However, the use of an herb dryer can be used and is used in some areas. When drying *huánglián*, temperatures between 45–50°C can be used. Final drying is accomplished when the rhizome is below 14% moisture.

Final Processing

Rhizomes are divided into two grades: large and small. At this time a final cleaning of soil, fibrous roots, leaf petioles, etc. is done before storage.

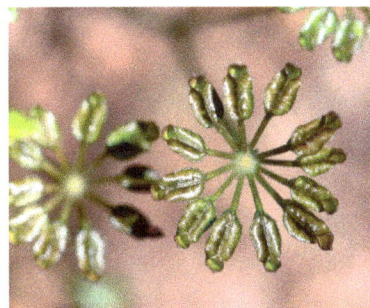

Huánglián seed capsules ripening in Sichuan, China.

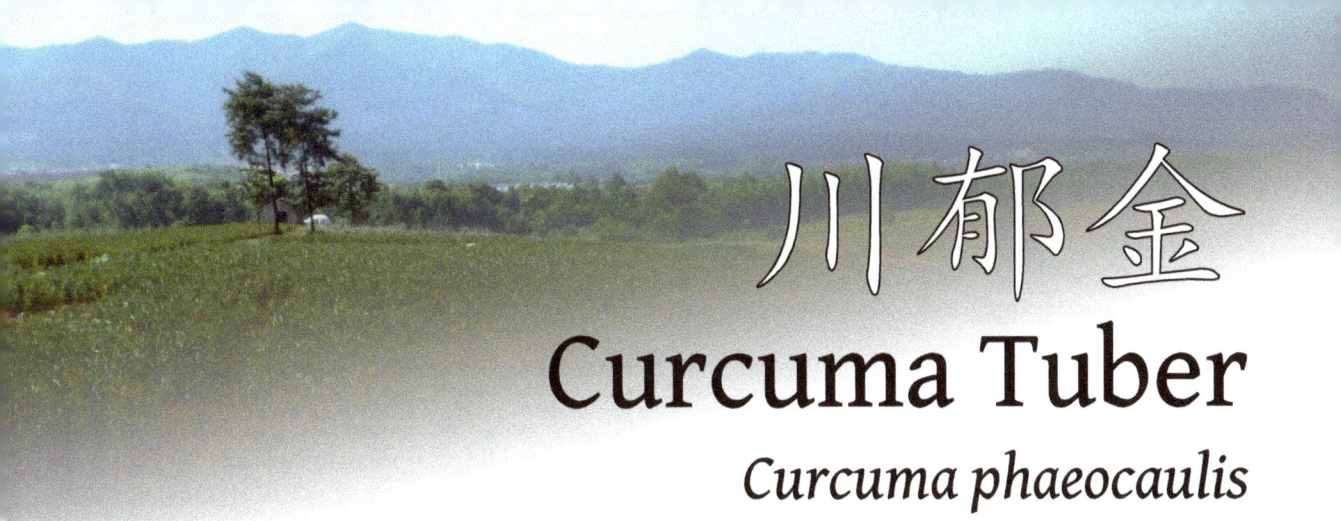

川郁金

Curcuma Tuber

Curcuma phaeocaulis

The dried root tuber of the daodi herb *chuānyùjīn* (*Curcuma phaeocaulis* Val.), known as *yùjīn* (鬱金 \ 郁金) in China, is a member of the ginger family (Zingiberaceae). The dried rhizome of this plant is known as *péngézhù* (蓬莪术) and is used as a different medicinal with different applications. While the native habitat for this species appears to be in Yunnan province, the daodi location for this medicinal is in Sichuan province throughout the river valleys of the Jinma river; along the banks and in nearby wet areas. These are the areas where *yùjīn* is most commonly grown and the material coming from these areas is considered daodi.

This herb is an important herb in traditional Chinese medicine. It has the function of quickening the blood and moving qi to resolve blood stasis and qi stagnation. However, it has a special quality among herbs with similar functions, it is cold and therefore is best used when treating a heat pathogen. The herb is primarily used for blood stasis and qi stagnation in the middle and lower burner and is frequently used for masses and accumulations in the abdomen. It is an important herb for treating menstrual pain with associated heat and is also used extensively for treating the heart. When treating heart conditions, it can enter the heart channel, cooling the blood and clearing the heart. This latter function is very important for diseases that have entered the construction and blood aspects. Finally, it is an essential herb for the treatment of gallbladder and liver diseases with heat, abdominal pain, scanty urination, blood in the urine, and yellowing of the skin.

Modern science has investigated this species, however identification can be very difficult; for this reason, most research must be taken with a grain of salt. The processed tuber of *C. phaeocaulis* is known for its effects on the cardiovascular and hepatic systems and research has proven some antitumor properties.

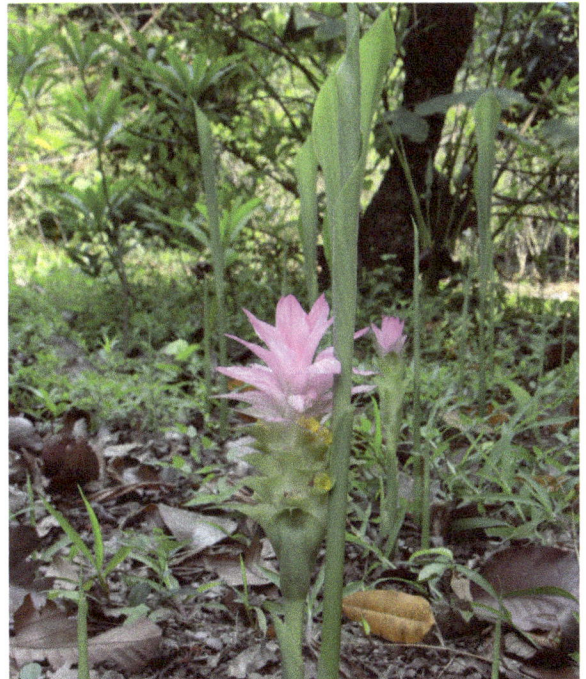

Contributing Authors

Yang Feng-qing, Zuo Hua-li, Li Feng

PRODUCTION SITE ECOLOGY

Elevation

Yùjīn is cultivated between 450–550 m elevation.

Temperature

Frost-free days must average about 290 days with an average annual temperature is between 15.8–16.2°C. The coldest month is January with an average temperature of 5.4–5.7°C. July is the hottest month with an average temperature of 25°C.

Photo Period

Average annual sunshine in the range of 1100–1200 hours is suitable.

Moisture

Suitable annual rainfall is 950–1000 mm with an average humidity of about 80%.

Soil

Alluvial soil or sandy-loam that is loose with a neutral to slightly acid pH is required.

Topography

A well-draining field in a river plain is ideal. Areas that mimic this environment can also be used, such as gentle sloping land near a river, beach areas along a river, etc.

PRODUCTION AREA ENVIRONMENTAL REQUIREMENTS

Site Selection

Sites free from pollution with a very good water source and good soil quality are critical. Sites should be far from main roads or highways, railroads, or any other potential source of pollution.

Soil Preparation

During late March and early April the site is covered with well-composted manure (quail manure is the best) at a rate of 30,000 kg per acre. After several days choose a sunny day and till the manure to a depth of 30–35 cm, then harrow smooth.

TAKING & RAISING RHIZOME CUTTINGS

Rhizome Cuttings Requirements

Rhizomes are dug around the time of the Winter Solstice and taken from mature plants that are free from disease or pests. Short, thick, plump, and healthy sections of rhizome with two to three buds are used to plant.

Rhizome Storage

Fibrous roots should be removed from the tuberous rhizomes, then the cuttings are placed on a muddy surface (outside) and stacked 30–35 cm tall (be sure to place root side of the rhizome facing down into the mud). The short stack is then covered with a layer of yellow sand, making sure to cover the entire pile. If the air temperature is expected to be below 5°C for more than a week, extra sand, a plastic tarp, or other means to protect the cuttings from potential frost damage should be used.

Planting Rhizomes

The rhizome cuttings are planted during early April. The rhizomes must be inspected for any sign of disease or insect damage; any damaged rhizomes are discarded. Holes are dug on the gentle slope 10–15 cm in diameter and 6–9 cm deep, plant 2–3 cuttings in each hole with the bud facing upward, then cover it with 3–6 cm of soil. Holes are dug 45–60 cm apart in single rows 50 cm apart. Do not plant too deep.

FIELD MANAGEMENT

Irrigation and Top-Dressing

During the months of July through September, when growth is vigorous, plants need extra water and should be irrigated unless natural precipitation is ample. Irrigation should be done early in the morning or around dusk, be careful not to cause erosion when watering. It is inappropriate to water after the month of October unless is it exceptionally dry, but do be careful not to let the soil become dry. At the same time, be sure that water is draining well after rain.

After all the sprouts have emerged, the initial top-dressing is done; heavy nitrogen is important at this time. Well-composted manure is applied at a rate of 9000–12,000 kg per acre, 60–75 kg per acre of super-phosphate is also applied at this time. During the month of June another 9000–12,000 kg per acre of well-composted manure is applied. Another application of calcium phosphate is sometimes added during July or August along with a mixture of composted manure, wood ash, and potassium dihydrogen phosphate (17:2:1), which is added at a rate of 12,000 kg per acre.

Cultivation and Weeding

This work is most frequently done concurrently with the addition of fertilizer. The first cultivation and weeding are generally done when the plants have reached 10–15 cm tall. This task is then done again sometime in late August or early September. If there is a need, this can be done at other times as well; do not allow weeds to compete with the herb for space.

PREVENTION AND TREATMENT OF DISEASE AND INSECT PESTS

Principles of Prevention and Treatment

Pests and diseases are not usually a serious threat to *yùjīn* cultivation. Using soils with poor water drainage or not maintaining the same can lead to some fungal diseases such as root rot, however this should not be a significant problem if the plant is given appropriate ecological conditions. There are few pest problems with this crop, but farmers should watch closely for the potential of grubs. Crop rotation is generally the best way to deal with any potential pests or diseases; improved fertilization strategies can prove useful for some diseases.

Leaf Spot (*pathogen not identified*)

Prevention and Treatment

Crop rotation is helpful. Keep the field clean and free of diseased material. Increasing organic fertilizer and increasing phosphorus can be helpful. Foliar feeding of a 0.2–0.3% potassium dihydrogen phosphate solution can also help treat the problem, but early application is advised.

Root Rot Disease (*Fusarium sp.*)

Prevention and Treatment

Do a crop rotation with a grass family plant for at least two years. Be sure that soil and seedlings are free of disease. Use of appropriate fertilizer application is very important. Increasing both organic compost and phosphorus is generally advised. Early removal of diseased plants with a lime application in holes is recommended to control this disease.

Soil-Borne Insects (grubs are most common)

Prevention and Treatment

Plowing and harrowing, deep plowing, and application of ample amounts of compost help guard against these problems. During their adult stage, lights can be utilized to attract and trap the insects.

HARVESTING

Harvest Season

Tubers are harvested at the end of the first season after planting. The optimal time to harvest is during mid- to late December, around the Winter Solstice. Harvest on a sunny day after the above ground portions of the plant have withered.

Harvest Method

Choose a fine sunny day, after the leaves have withered and remove the dead leaves and stems, most of these should be easily removed without the need for cutting; cut off any remaining above-ground portions of the plant. Using a digging fork or other appropriate tool, dig the below-ground portions, pulling up both the rhizome and the attached tubers. Be careful to dig deep enough when harvesting because you don't want to damage the root tubers or leave any behind. Be be careful not to damage the exterior of the root. In large commercial operations, tractor powered root diggers are employed for this operation. The entire root system is removed from the field intact. Wash the mud from the roots and rhizomes, then separate the root tubers from the rhizome and stack each separately.

ON-FARM PROCESSING

Sorting

Discard the old sections of rhizome that were used as cuttings the year before (this is called "old head"), remove fibrous roots, eliminate any foreign matter and wash away any mud. When separated, the rhizomes are called *péngézhù* and the root tubers are called *yùjīn*.

Steaming and Boiling

The *yùjīn* is put in a pot and the appropriate amount of clean water is added to cover the tubers, then they are boiled for at least two hours. The indications that the tuber has boiled long enough are as follows: when, after removing the largest tuber you can find in the pot, you press your fingernail into the tuber and there is no sound as your fingernail penetrates the interior of the tuber, or, when the color of the tuber has softened to a blanched-like color throughout. Once this has been achieved, strain the water out and dry them in the sun.

Drying Method

After the boiling process, the *yùjīn* must be dried in the sun, driers can't be used. While the tubers are drying in the sun, they should be flipped 1–2 times daily; at this time pay attention and remove any rotten or otherwise damaged tubers. If there is extended wet periods after harvest, wood ash are added to tubers (10:1) to help hasten drying and prevent rotting. Dried tubers should be stored at less than 15% moisture content.

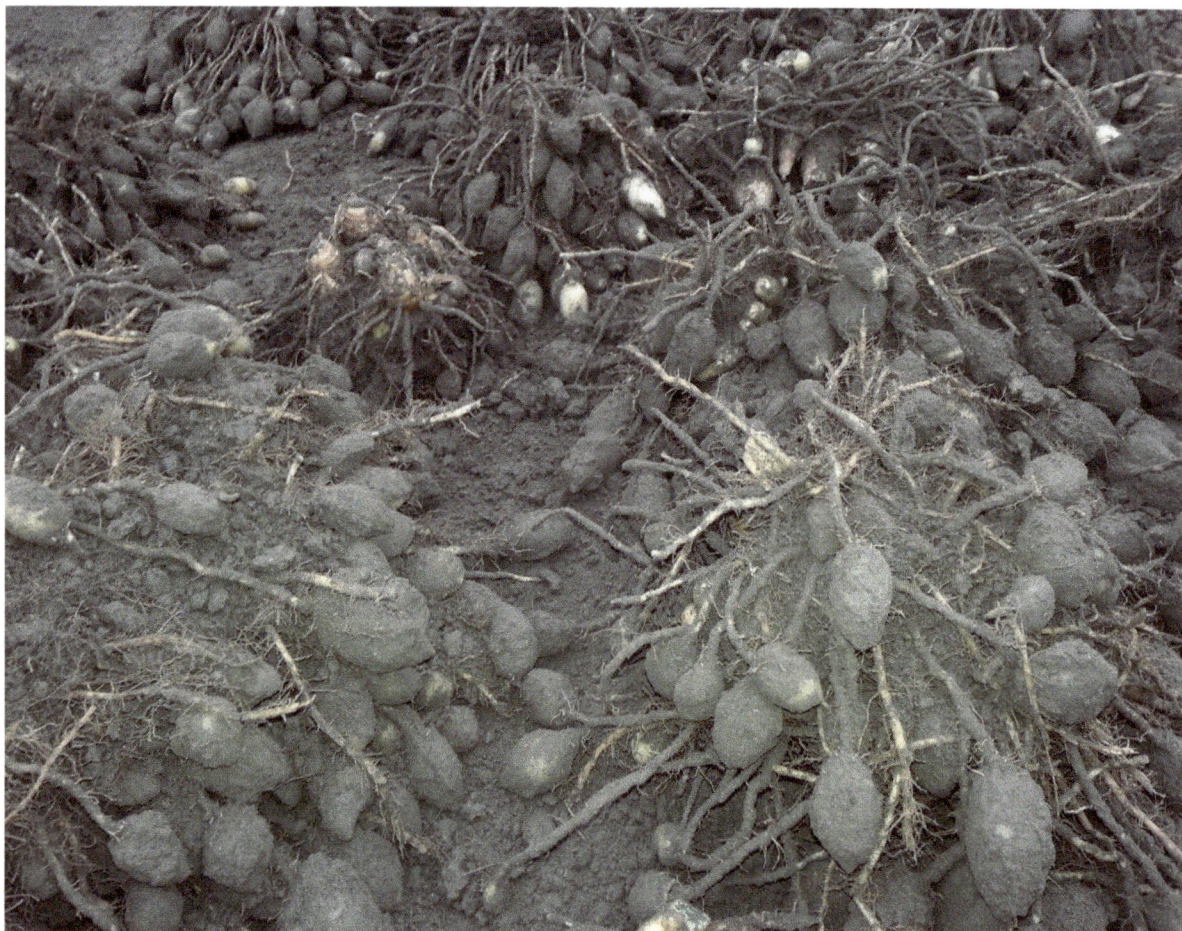

Freshly harvested *yùjīn* showing tubers still attached to main rhizome.

祁 瞿 麦

Dianthus

Dianthus superbus & D. chinensis

DISTINGUISHING FEATURES

The dried above-ground plant of the daodi herb *qí qúmài* (*Dianthus superbus* L. & *Dianthus chinensis* L.), commonly known as *qúmài* (瞿麦 \ 瞿麥) in China, is a member of the pink family (Caryophyllaceae). Although the official drug name for this plant is *qúmài*, the latter species, *D. chinensis* is often referred to as *shízhú* (石竹). These two species are common in most of China and the countries surrounding China, excluding the southern borders, growing in forest openings and margins, grassy hillsides, and meadows between 400–3700 m elevation. These species are also widely cultivated both in China and most of the world for their ornamental attractiveness. The daodi location for *qúmài* is around Anguo in Hebei province.

The use of *qúmài* is somewhat limited in Chinese medicine and is primarily known from the formula Ba Zhen San (八正散) used for urinary diseases. *Qúmài* disinhibits urine and frees strangury. It is a cold and bitter medicinal that is primarily used for painful urination associated with yellow urine with or without bleeding. It can be used for all types of damp-heat in the lower burner where disinhibiting the urine is the main treatment principle. The herb also quickens the blood and frees menstruation. However, it is rarely used for this application because it is not considered particularly strong.

The herb has been studied, elucidating many chemical components as well as a number of *in vitro* experiments using human cell lines as well as animal models. Using these models, *Dianthus* sp. has shown a number of pharmacological activities including, anti-inflammatory, antioxidant, antimicrobial, and anti-cancer actions. Research in animal models and human cell lines has shown ethanolic extracts may be useful to treat or prevent diabetic nephropathy.

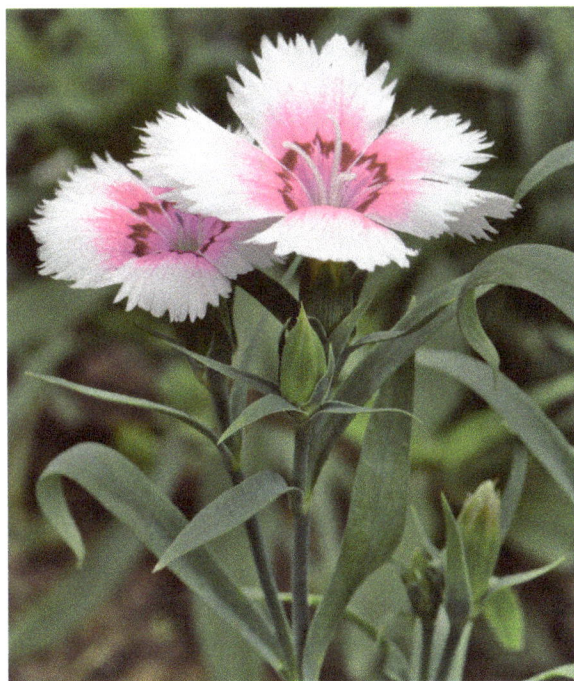

Contributing Authors

Liu Ling-di, Xie Xiao-liang, Liu Meng, Tian Wei Wen Chun-xiu, Zheng Yu-guang, Huang Lu-qi, Guo Lan-ping, Hao Qing-xiu, Jia Dong-sheng

85

PRODUCTION SITE ECOLOGY

Elevation

Qúmài is cultivated between 50–500 m elevation.

Temperature

At least 197 frost free days. January is the coldest month with average temperatures below 3°C and July is the hottest month with average temperatures between 18–27°C.

Photo Period

Average annual sunshine is between 2500–2757 hours. The average daily sunshine percentage range is 35–70%.

Moisture

An average annual rainfall of 500–1000 mm with a relative humidity of 34–55%.

Soil

A loose sandy soil with a depth of at least 30 cm is ideal with pH in the 5.5–6.5 range.

Topography

The field can be either level or have a slope up to 15 degrees. If the field is sloped it should be facing either southeast or northwest to allow for proper drainage and wind-flow.

Site Selection & Soil Preparation

Choose rich and fertile sandy soil that drains water well. Apply 12,000–18,000 kg of mature composted manure per acre, till deeply, harrow, and prepare beds for planting.

SOWING SEEDS & RAISING SEEDLINGS

Seed Quality Requirements

According to the *Pharmacopoeia of the People's Republic of China* (2015) seeds for *qúmài* (*D. superbus* and *D. chinensis*) should be thoroughly dried and mature.

Sowing Seeds

Seeds are sown in the second half of April. Prepare rows 20–25 cm apart and cut a furrow 1 cm deep. Plant seeds every 10 cm, cover with soil, and press down firmly. Seeds are sown at a rate of 9 kg per acre.

FIELD MANAGEMENT

Cultivation and Weeding

During the course of one-year, cultivation to kill weeds can be performed 2–3 times, or as needed. The first time is usually when the plants have reached 6–10 cm tall, after this it can be executed at appropriate times after watering or rain, or after top-dressing.

Irrigation and Water Drainage

Water requirements for *qúmài* are not high, but it should be watered if there are significant dry periods especially after sowing seeds or transplanting, and after top-dressing. During prolonged or excessive rains, be sure that water is draining from the field, do not allow soil to remain water-logged.

Top-Dressing

Each time after harvest, urea may be added at 120 kg per acre. Following application, the area should be raked to evenly distribute the fertilizer and help it to penetrate the soil, then water the entire field.

PREVENTION AND TREATMENT OF DISEASE AND INSECT PESTS

Principles of Prevention and Treatment

Qúmài rarely has disease problems. It has low water requirements but excessive water or water accumulation can lead to some problems.

Aphids (Aphidoidea)

Prevention and Treatment

Since this disease can be transferred via seed, it is critical to be sure your seed is free of the spores that cause this fungal disease. If improved varieties are available that resist this disease, and are appropriate for your area, this is the recommended course of action. Because this plant is a well-known host of crop pathogens, growing in a three-year rotation is recommended. Quickly eliminate any and all plants that show signs of disease before spores are released.

HARVESTING

Harvest Season

When seeds are planted in April, plants may be harvested in the first and subsequent years. Plants are harvested when approximately half the flowers have matured to seed and half are still blooming. When seeds are sowed in the spring, plants may be harvested twice, after which plants may be harvested 3 times in a single season.

Harvest Method

Choose a fine sunny day and harvest the entire plant by cutting close to the base, approximately 1–2 cm from the ground.

ON-FARM PROCESSING

Drying Method

Fresh *qúmài* cannot be piled, it must remain spread out to avoid mold and mildew. It should be spread out in a shady area with adequate air flow and turned regularly to avoid mold and mildew. Check carefully and dispose of any material showing any signs of mildew or rot. Dried *qúmài* should not exceed 12% moisture. [Translator's Note: Although *qúmài* is traditionally dried in the sun and now, as above, more commonly in the shade, modern drying systems can be used. If using a drying system, such as a forced air drier, the temperature should not exceed 45°C.]

Storage

After drying, the herb is minimally cut to allow for storage in bags. The herb should be kept out of the light and the storage area should not exceed 20°C or 65% humidity.

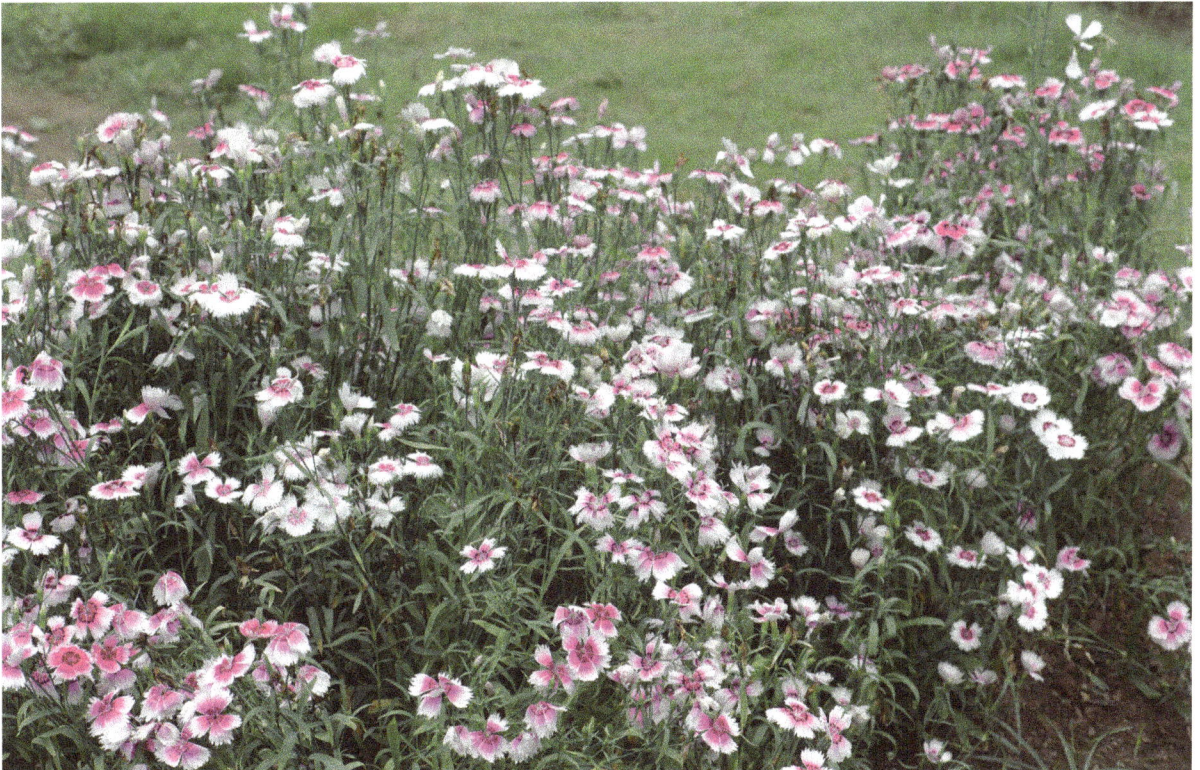

A stand of *qúmài* growing in the mountians of Hebei province, China.

怀山药
Chinese Yam Root
Dioscorea opposita

The dried root of the daodi herb *huái shānyao* (*Dioscorea opposita* Thunb.), which is commonly known as *shānyao* (山藥 \ 山药) in China, is a member of the yam family (Dioscoreaceae). The genus is large with over 600 species world-wide but only 52 in China. The daodi location for growing this medicinal is in Wen county and Meng county of Henan province.

[Translator's Note: The *Dioscorea* genus is large and it is a difficult genus to identify with many synonyms and misidentified species. While the original text and the *Pharmacopoeia of the People's Republic of China* (2015) continue to use this name, it is incorrect. The current name of this species is *Dioscorea polystachya* (Turcz.).]

This herb has a long history of use in Chinese medicine and is commonly consumed as a food. In Chinese medicine, *shānyao* is used to supplement qi and boost the yin of the spleen, lung, and kidney. The herb is used in a wide array of conditions including fatigue with loss of appetite and diarrhea, seminal emission, dribbling urine, and chronic cough among others. As a food it can be added to soups or porridge, sautéed, steamed, and mashed; it is sometimes used in dessert dishes as well.

Modern science has found that *shānyao* has anti-diabetic and antioxidant activities. In addition, studies have shown that consuming *shānyao* improves the bacterial composition of the intestine and may help to increase the ability of the gastrointestinal tract to absorb nutrients from food, thus making eating more efficient. These findings support some of the traditional applications.

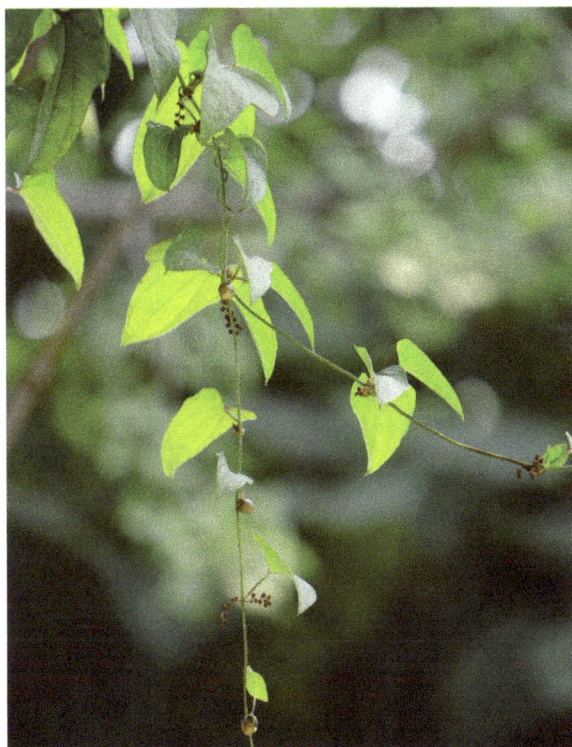

Contributing Authors

Gao Wen-yuan, Wang Ting-ting, Wang Hai-yang, Li Xia, Wang Juan

PRODUCTION SITE ECOLOGY

Elevation

Shānyao is cultivated between 150–300 m elevation.

Temperature

The average annual temperature is 14.1–14.9°C, with a frost-free period of 210 days. July is the hottest month and January is the coldest.

Moisture

The average annual rainfall is 550–700 mm.

Soil

The soil should be loam and\or sandy. The soil layer should be deep, loose, humus rich, and free of areas where the soil might stay wet for extended periods. Good water drainage and the ability to irrigate are necessary. Neutral to slightly acidic pH is suitable.

Site Selection

During *shānyao* rhizome development, it consumes significant nutrients. The growing site should be hilly or sloping with a deep, loose, rich soil layer. A sunny location (south-facing) with wind protection is ideal. Water must drain easily. A sandy\loam soil with a neutral to slightly acid pH is ideal. Low-laying areas, clay soil, and alkaline pH are not suitable for growing *shānyao*. Continuous cropping is a serious problem when growing *shānyao*, leading to significant disease and insect problems. Suitable crops to grow prior to *shānyao* include a grass or pea family species, or vegetables.

Soil Preparation

Shānyao can be grown on level fields or in raised beds. When using raised beds, they should be built after crop harvest but before the ground freezes. Generally, 18,000–24,000 kg of composted manure, 600 kg of cake fertilizer, and 300–900 kg of base fertilizer is applied per acre. The field is then watered and allowed to dry to the point where tilling will not damage the soil structure, then the fertilizer is tilled into the soil. After the beds are built or the soil leveled, an additional NPK fertilizer is applied at rate of 90 (N), 81 (P), 81 (K) kg per acre.

PROPAGATION & RAISING SEEDLINGS

Pre-Planting Preparation

There are two methods for growing this edible and medicinal rhizome. 1) Using the crowns of the rhizomes from the previous season, 2) using the aerial tubers, the latter is now considered the best method and is the most popular method used. About 15–20 days prior to planting out into the field, the aerial tubers are placed in moist sand (40–50% moisture content) while the temperature is maintained between 20–30°C. When more than 80% of the tubers have sprouted, they are carefully removed and the strongest, most healthy, tubers are chosen for planting in the field, the rest are discarded. In the daodi region, sprouted tubers are planted in the field from mid- to late April.

Sowing Aerial Tubers

Tubers should be planted when the soil temperature reaches 10–12°C for a period of three consecutive days. Trenches 3–4 cm deep and 20–30 cm apart are dug, sprouted aerial tubers are placed 10–12 cm apart in the trenches, then covered with soil and pressed firmly. Soil must be kept moist after planting. Sprouts should emerge from soil 15–20 days after planting. Rhizomes can be harvested in the first year, but aerial tubers are not produced until the second year.

Sowing Using Rhizome Crowns

During the period in mid- to late April when the soil temperature measured at 5 cm deep is above 10°C the crowns can be planted. Rhizome crowns are removed from the sand they have been stored in and dried in the sun for 5 days. The skin of these root crowns should be a grey color with some areas of green. Rhizomes are placed in a general antifungal for 15 minutes, then allowed to dry in the sun. Rhizome crowns are planted in trenches 8–10 cm deep at 15–20 cm intervals, in rows 40–60 cm apart, then covered with 6–8 cm of soil. When planting the crowns, they should all be facing in the same direction, this will allow for easier management as they begin to grow. Although this method is faster and easier, it can't be used for extended periods of time, after 4–5 years the quality of the roots begins to subside. For this reason, the aerial tubers should be used in regular rotation with the roots for propagation.

FIELD MANAGEMENT

Cultivation and Weeding

After the *shānyao* has sprouted, each time it rains or the fields are irrigated, the soil should be cultivated to loosen it. This process also keeps weeds in check; generally, this should be done 3 times. During the first cultivation process, when the plants have reached approximately 30 cm tall, a single post is erected close to the plant by pushing it about 3 cm deep into the soil, this will serve as part of a trellis that will be constructed later. Cultivation is done again between mid- and late June, and finally during late July or early August. Early cultivation must be done carefully so as to avoid damaging the young growing plants, later it is important to avoid breaking the vines of the plant.

Fertilization

The first fertilizer is applied just prior to the first cultivation. Nitrogen is applied at a rate of 42 kg per acre (or 90 kg of urea). Once the vines are growing vigorously another 54 kg of nitrogen (or 90 kg of urea) per acre are applied. Always water after fertilizer application. When the rhizome has grown large and the vines are filling up the field, a foliar feeding of 0.3% potassium dihydrogen phosphate can be applied 2–3 times.

Trellising

Bamboo is most frequently used; two stakes are added to the initial stake set during the first cultivation. Two bamboo stakes are added to create a teepee-like structure, directing the initial stake in a southerly position, which allows the vine to climb the first stake (planted next to it) toward the sun.

Irrigation and Water Drainage

Shānyao is drought resistant, but the highest yielding crop is well-watered. Generally, fields are irrigated after the first top-dressing or if there is a prolonged period without rain. If the soil has begun to show signs of crusting or excessive dryness, irrigation can be used 1–2 times until the soil is fully moistened. During the summer and autumn, if there are prolonged periods of more than one week with scorching heat and no rain, irrigate in the early morning to moisten the ground and cool the field temperature slightly. Usually *shānyao* is watered only once after mid-July. Do not allow the soil to become waterlogged. Make sure that water is properly drained during heavy rain.

Pruning

Generally, *shānyao* will only produce a single vine. However, if there is more than one vine growing out from the side, wait until they are about 7–8 cm long, then choose the most central and healthy sprout, pruning away the others. There is one variety that frequently gives birth to multiple sprouts, but the same procedure should be used so that the plant will not consume too much of the soil nutrition and impede proper air-flow through the crop, which can be a problem leading to disease.

COLLECTION & STORAGE OF AERIAL BULBS AND RHIZOME CROWNS

Collecting Aerial Bulbs & Rhizome Crowns

Generally, *shānyao* is grown from aerial bulbs, which take two years of growth to form. At the end of the first year the rhizome crown is well formed. When autumn turns to winter, late October to early November, the rhizome crowns are dug from the ground. Choose crowns with green sprouts, that are plump, thick, healthy, and free of any disease or insect damage. Cut the rhizome about 15–20 cm from the crown (this should weight 40–60 g) then place in an area with good airflow and dry for about one week (this can also be done outside in the sun but care must be taken not to allow the rhizome to freeze). After the cut wound has dried, the rhizome crowns are stored indoors over the winter (see below for details).

Over-Wintering Aerial Bulbs

Aerial bulbs are harvested in late October when the leaves have begun to turn yellow. Select the largest, roundest bulbs that are devoid of any damage, including insects or diseases. After picking, mix with moist sand and store in a cellar. Around early April, the aerial bulbs can be removed from the cellar and placed in the sun for one day to dry, then are immediately planted.

Over-Wintering Rhizome Crowns

About one week after cutting the rhizome from the crowns, when the wound has healed, the crowns are stored in coarse sand, such as river sand. There are two methods for storing rhizome crowns. The first is indoors where the ambient temperature will range between 0–8°C over the winter. Using this indoor method, dry sand is first piled with any size footprint 15 cm thick, then a single layer of the *shānyao* rhizome crowns are laid on the sand. This is then covered with another layer of sand (15 cm) and then another layer of *shānyao* is added. This can be continued until the pile has reached 80–100 cm tall. Finally, the top layer of sand is added and the entire pile is covered with a 15–20 cm thick layer of hay. Using the outdoor method, a trench is dug 24 cm deep and just wide enough for the crowns to be placed inside. The root crowns are placed standing erect with the crown up. The trench is back filled and left until spring when the root crowns are dug and transplanted into the field.

PREVENTION AND TREATMENT OF DISEASE AND INSECT PESTS

Principles of Prevention and Treatment

Shānyao is generally not particularly disease prone. Most diseases are associated with poor drainage or poor air-flow through the field. Therefore, choice of site and soil and draining excess water in heavy rain events is extremely important. The only major pest is nematodes, which can be treated as above, keeping diverse soil ecology is the best preventative measure.

Anthracnose (*Colletotrichum gloeosporioides*)

Prevention and Treatment

Crop rotation every three years with a grass family plant or any vegetable from the mustard family is good practice to prevent or treat this disease.

White Rust Disease (*Albugo* sp.)

Prevention and Treatment

This disease is usually associated with soggy soil conditions. Be sure that the soil is never too wet or stays wet for extended periods of time. Dig drainage ditches if necessary. Cover cropping with a grass family plant is sometimes necessary.

Brown Spot Disease (*Cylindrosporium dioscoreae*)

Prevention and Treatment

Covercrop with a grass family or a mustard family vegetable for three or more years.

Nematodes (*Pratylenchus coffeae*)

Prevention and Treatment

Cover crop with a grass family plant for at least three years.

Biological Controls

Active spores of Paecilomyces lilacinus, 200 million spores/g, 1200–2400 g per acre. This is applied to the area around the root, then again after one week.

HARVESTING

Harvest Season

In field situations, rhizomes can be harvested at the end of the first year; remember that plants should be given 140–160 days to mature. Rhizomes are generally harvested during the first 2–3 weeks of November.

Harvest Method

Either by hand or with a trench digging machine, dig a trench about 20 cm from where the roots were planted. This trench should be 80–100 cm deep and about 40 cm wide. Then, from the trench the soil is carefully dug away to expose the shānyao root, being careful not to damage it.

ON-FARM PROCESSING

Soaking, Washing, and Peeling Skin

Rhizomes are first soaked in potable water for 30 minutes. Then clean water is used to wash the roots clean of any soil. After the roots are washed, a special knife is used to remove the skin. When using this knife, it should be sharp, using even, gentle strokes to remove the skin, removing as little as possible of the rhizome flesh but making sure to remove all the skin. Roots are then piled into baskets. [Translator's Note: This special knife is similar to a vegetable peeler. However, it is more durable than a vegetable peeler; more like a farm tool than a kitchen tool. It is also slightly curved so that it peels more skin and less flesh from the rhizome. This process is very time consuming and to date has not been automated.]

A second method, used when rhizomes have a lot of rootlets, is as follows. After the rhizomes have dried to the point where the outside is hard, but the inside is still soft, the roots are soaked in water for 1–2 days. The rootlets are then rubbed off by hand or, if necessary, with a knife. Some rootlets may be difficult to remove, in which case a second stage is used. In this second stage the rhizomes are allowed to dry for about half a day before spinning the rhizomes between the hands to remove the rest of the rootlets. At this time the crown is also cut away. After this process is completed, the rhizomes are placed in the sun to dry, as before, and left until they are completely dried. Sulfur is very frequently used as a preservative to avoid oxidation of the naturally white rhizome in the processing of *shānyao*. If you choose to use it, do not exceed 400 mg/kg.

Drying Method

Rhizomes are dried in the sun by spreading them out evenly in a single layer. Avoid stacking.

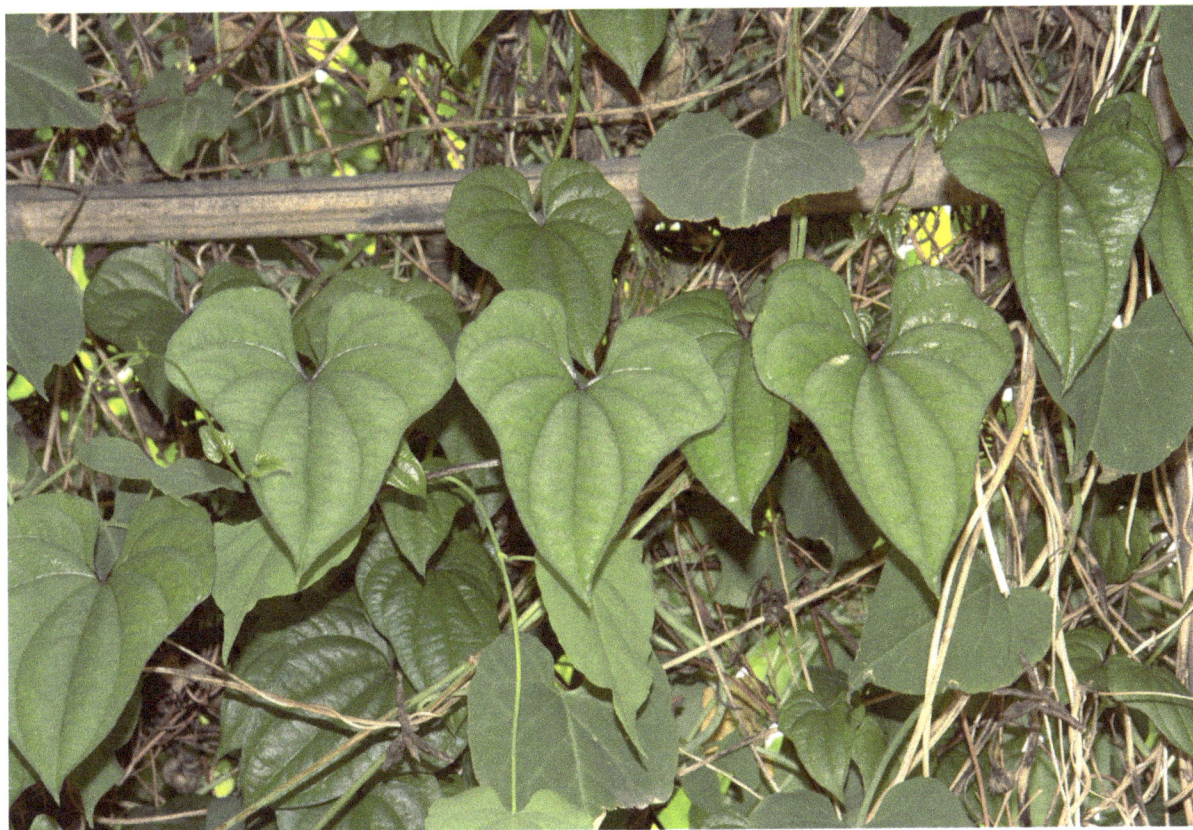

Leaves of *shānyao* hang on the fence at our farm in Beijing, China.

巫山淫羊藿

Epimedium Leaf

Epimedium wushanense

The dried leaf of the daodi herb *wūshān yínyánghuò* (*Epimedium wushanense* T.S.Ying), commonly known as *yínyánghuò* (淫羊藿) in China, is a member of the barberry family (Berberidaceae). The genus *Epimedium* is made up of about 50 species from China to Europe, but 40 of those species are endemic to China. This species' native habitat is in Chongqing, Guangxi, Guizhou, Hubei, and Sichuan provinces in forests and thickets between 300–1700 m elevation. The *Pharmacopoeia of the People's Republic of China* (2015) lists the species in this monograph separately from the monograph simply called *yínyánghuò*, which has four different species listed as being acceptable for use. However, the clinical applications for all five species are the same. The daodi location for this plant is in Lei Mountain county, Xiuwen County, and Longli county in Guizhou province.

This medicinal plant, or other members of this genus, has been used in China for at least 2000 years. It is sometimes called "horny goat weed" based on a rough translation of the Chinese name and has become popular in some Western countries in recent years owing to its action to enhance men's ability to achieve and maintain erection. It is traditionally used to supplement the liver and kidney yang for yang insufficiency leading to impotence, sore lower back and knees, fatigue, and coldness in the joints and muscles. It has also been used for asthma, high blood pressure, and menopausal symptoms.

Modern science has shown this herb has applications that include aphrodisiac, anti-osteoporosis, anticancer, antioxidant, anti-fatigue, anti-aging, anti-inflammatory, and antiviral functions. There has been significant research on its anti-osteoporosis activity and research suggests a promising therapy in the future, parti-cularly for women.

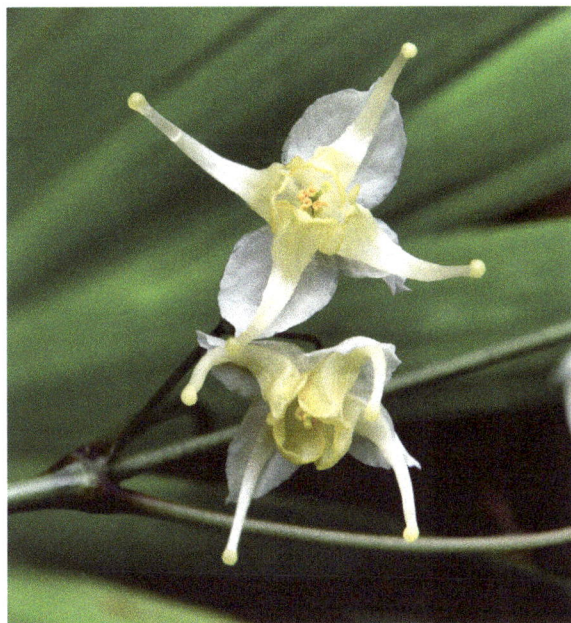

Contributing Authors

He Shun-zhi, Yang Xiang-bo,
Wei Shang-hua, Zhou Ning, He Yong,
Wang Da-min, Hu Ding-lan

PRODUCTION SITE ECOLOGY

Elevation

Yínyánghuò is cultivated between 300–1700 m elevation.

Temperature

The average annual temperature should be about 12°C. The average temperature in January should be about 2.9°C with more than 270 frost-free days a year.

Photo Period

Annual average sunlight should be between 1200–1500 hours.

Moisture

Average annual rainfall should be about 1000 mm and an average relative humidity of 70-90%.

Soil

Loam and sandy loam with a large amount of humus and organic matter (>2.5%) are needed, this protects moisture and nutrition in the soil. Soil pH should be between 4.5–6.

Topography

A north, northeast, or northwest slope is suitable.

Site Selection

When growing using a woods-grown method, the mountain slope should be between 25–50° with about 70% shade under a mixed forest canopy. If there is no forest canopy, shade houses must be built. Fruit trees and grapes are not appropriate shading for *yínyánghuò*. However, shading with *Perilla*, corn, and other crops can be done. Open fields are not suitable.

Soil Preparation

Wild simulated *yínyánghuò* is grown on forested mountain slopes by first removing shrubs and other small plants; beds are prepared 40–80 cm wide between the trees. Using standardized cultivation, the soil is tilled at least 30 cm deep with 12,000–18,000 kg per acre of well-composted manure (straw and other plant material may be included) or a founda-

tional fertilizer at a rate of 300–600 kg per acre, or 1800–3000 kg per acre of organic fertilizer. This is tilled in deeply (30–35 cm) then harrowed fine. Beds are prepared 1.5 m wide (beds 40–80 cm wide are some-times used if necessary due to land conditions) and 25 cm tall with 25 cm paths between beds; site conditions will determine the length of the bed. The entire field should have a drainage ditch 40 cm wide and 40 cm deep to avoid accumulation of rain or irrigation water.

SOWING SEEDS & RAISING SEEDLINGS

Seed Quality Requirements

Seeds should be from the current year's harvest. Germination rate should be above 70% and the seeds should contain no more than 5% foreign matter.

Nursery Bed Selection and Preparation

The nursery must have a good source of clean water for irrigation, fertile sandy loam soil, level topography, and be well drained. The area should be tilled more than 30 cm deep, tilling in 2500 kg of well-rotted compost per acre, then it is harrowed and any rocks, sticks, etc. are removed. Beds are built 1.5 m wide and pathways are dug 30 cm wide and 20 cm deep. There should be approximately 70% shade, which is usually achieved by using shade cloth.

Sowing Seeds

Seeds are sown from mid-December through early January. Seeding is done at a rate of 18–30 kg per acre by mixing the very small seeds with fine sand then scattering on the beds. After the seeds are sown, use a rake to spread the seeds evenly, then cover with about 1 cm of soil. Finally, the bed is mulched with a layer of straw or other appropriate mulch to preserve soil moisture. Do not allow the soil to dry out; water as necessary prior to and during the germination period.

Managing Seedling Area

After seeds are sown, carefully observe seed beds, checking soil moisture and potential seedlings every two to three days. After seedlings have emerged, carefully remove any weeds by hand. While weeding, soil can be hilled up (approximately 2 cm) around any seedlings.

TRANSPLANTING

Pricking Seedlings Out for Transplanting

Seedlings should be transplanted as soon after taking them from the seedling beds as possible. From the time they are dug out to the time they are transplanted, they should be kept out of the sun and wind and not allowed to dry out. A hand pick axe or other tool can be used to carefully dig the seedling out from the soil. The fibrous roots should be trimmed to about 4 cm in length and any unhealthy plants should be rejected. Seedlings can be bunched in groups of 50 for transportation to the field for transplanting.

Transplanting into the Field

When the seedlings are at least 1.5 years old they can be transplanted. Transplanting can be done in the autumn or spring (before March). Transplanting is best done the day after a rain or on a cloudy day. When planting in intensive field plots, plants are planted in holes every 30×30 cm, digging deep enough to allow for the roots to be placed straight down (about 4–5 cm); only the sprouting part of the plant must be above the soil. Seedlings are planted at about 32,000–60,000 seedlings per acre. Seedlings should be watered immediately after transplanting, do not use flood irrigation, avoid over-watering the site. When planting in a forest using a "woods-grown" technique, plants should be planted in holes every 45×45 cm. When planting in this fashion, 1680 sqare meters per acre is considered the average area available to cultivate, in this case 7200 plants per acre can be planted.

FIELD MANAGEMENT

Cultivation and Weeding

It is important to keep beds weeded. Generally, beds are weeded once between late May and early June. When using the "woods-grown" method, larger tools such as a sickle may be employed to cut back larger or more woody plants growing with the *yínyánghuò*. This should be done once during the year when these plants are at their most vigorous growth.

Irrigation and Top-Dressing

Irrigation must be used if there are extended periods of dry weather, do not allow the young plants

to dry out. Before watering, 240 kg of urea per acre is applied. If there is standing water after a rain or irrigation, this water must be drained and not allowed to sit accumulated. Generally, "woods-grown" *yínyánghuò* does not need to be irrigated or fertilized.

PREVENTION AND TREATMENT OF DISEASE AND INSECT PESTS

Principles of Prevention and Treatment

Yínyánghuò grown in a wood's grown environment is relatively disease and pest free. While some issues are noted above, they mostly are related to improper management, primarily due to excessive moisture in the area because of poor drainage or lack of good airflow. Pests should be easily controlled when there are good ecological conditions.

Leaf Brown Spot (*Macrophoma* sp.)

Prevention and Treatment

Remove diseased plants in a timely fashion and dispose of them properly. Manage sources of potential diseases. [Translator's note: This genus of fungi is the cause of a number of know diseases in apples, guava, boxwood, and other plants. An important preventative measure is to improve airflow through the cultivation area. Therefore, if this or a similar fungal disease is present a key action is to remove any barriers to good air circulation throughout the planting area.]

Rust (*Puccinia* sp.)

Prevention and Treatment

Keep the site clean and clear. Eliminate any sources where the disease may be harbored or latent.

Locusts (Locustoidea sp.)

Prevention and Treatment

If only a small number of grasshoppers is observed, then they can be left alone and control methods should not be applied. In the autumn and spring, cut back any grasses or other weeds around the site where eggs could have been laid. Allow these to dry in the sun and\or allow to freeze. Protect or encourage natural enemies such as sparrows, frogs, etc.

HARVESTING

Harvest Season

For both woods grown and field planted, harvest may begin two years after planting. After this initial harvest, leaves may be collected once per year. Harvest of leaves can happen any time from June - October.

Harvest Method

A sickle or similar tool is used to cut off the leaves above ground level including the petioles, which are bound together in small bundles and collected in large baskets for transportation.

ON-FARM PROCESSING

Drying Method

After untying the bundles made in the field, remove any weeds or foreign matter, including pedioles. Leaves can be open-air-dried, either in the direct sun or in a shaded area.

Baling and Storage

Using a baler, leaves are pressed into bales for transportation. Bales should be 50 kg with four 2 cm ties per bale. Bales are then fitted with a burlap bag for shipping. Generally, bales are not stacked higher than 5 layers and there should be about 30 cm between stacks to allow for good air circulation. The air temperature should not exceed 25°C and the humidity should not exceed 60%.

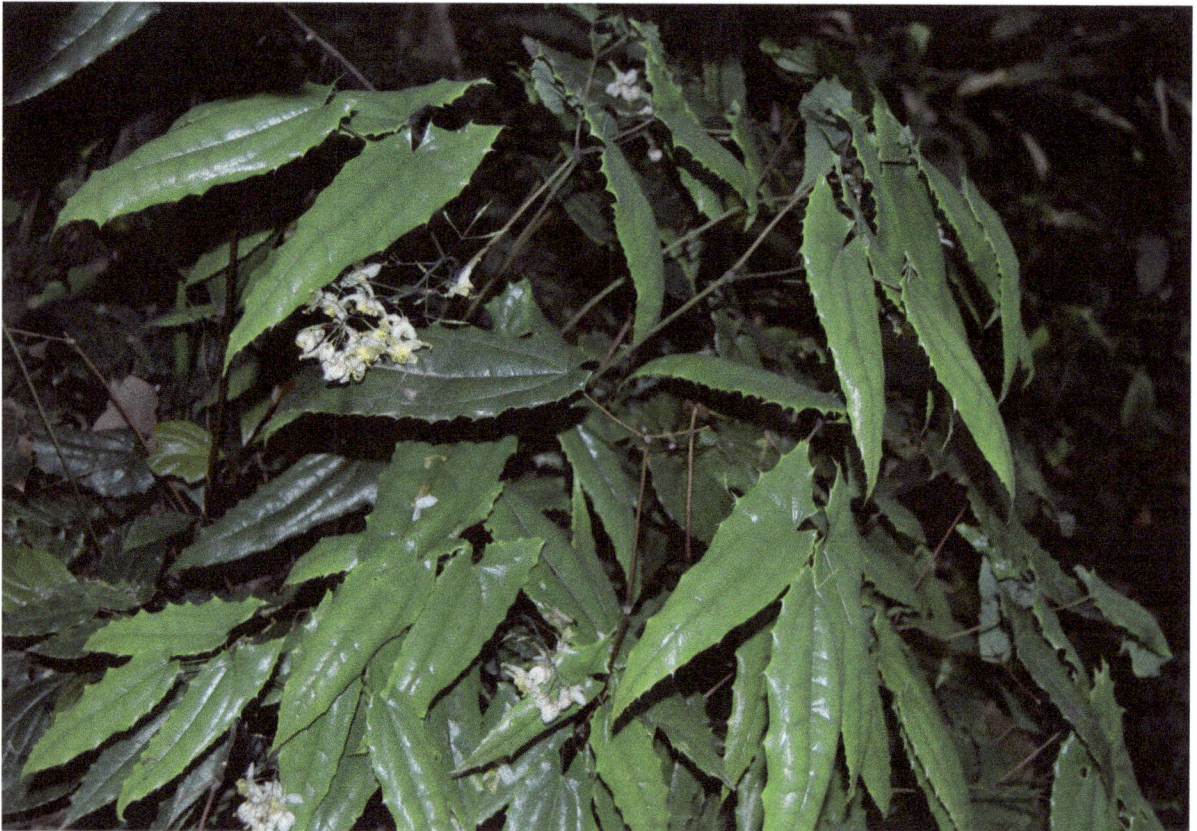

Wild *wūshān yínyánghuò* in Guizhou province, China.

太行山连翘

Forsythia

Forsythia suspensa

DISTINGUISHING FEATURES

The dried seed capsule of the daodi herb *tàihàngshān liánqiáo* (*Forsythia suspensa* Thunb.), commonly known in China as *liánqiáo* (连翘 \ 連翹), is a member of the olive family (Oleaceae). The *Forsythia* genus is small with only about 11 species, but more than half (six) are found in China. The shrub is common in thickets or grassy areas on slopes, valleys, and gullies between 300–2200 m elevation throughout much of central China. The shrub is a common ornamental widely valued for its yellow flowers, which appear before the plant's leaves in the very early spring. Material produced in the Taihengshan region, She county in Hebei Province is considered the daodi medicinal.

Although *liánqiáo* has been in use for at least 2000 years, other than a few formulas, one of which is found in the Shang Han Lun, it did not become prominent in the formulary literature until the Qing dynasty with the development of Warm Disease Theory. This herb is commonly classified as a clear heat and resolve toxin herb but it also has the function of coursing and dissipating wind-heat from the exterior. Therefore, while it can be used for all four aspects (defense, qi, construction, and blood) it is most effective for treating the defense aspect, especially when combined with *jīnyínhuā* (*Lonicera japonica*). This combination is also very important for treating boils and abscesses due to heat-toxin as well as summer-heat with diarrhea.

The pharmacological activities of this herb have been studied extensively. It has a wide range of anti-inflammatory activity from many different compounds, particularly flavonoids and phenylethanoid glycosides. Some of these compounds have proven to have hepatoprotective, antiviral, and neuroprotective, amongst other activities. The herb is antioxidant, which has led to research exploring the potential for beneficial activities in the treatment of diabetes and high cholesterol with some initial positive results in animal models. Studies show the herb has antibacterial, antiviral, and anticancer actions, as well as a number of other pharmacological activities.

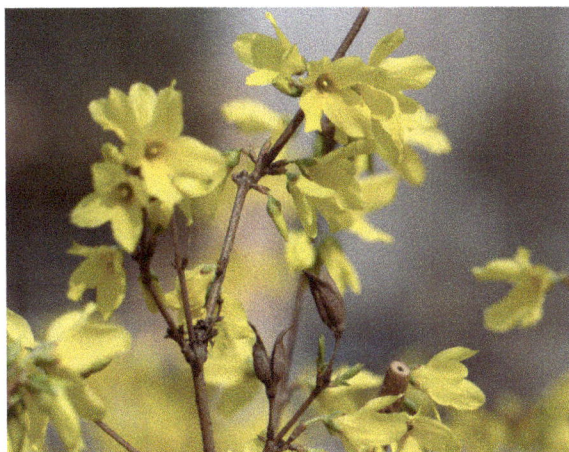

Contributing Authors

Zheng Yu-guang, Xie Xiao-liang, Guo Lan-ping, Huang Lu-qi, Hao Qing-xiu, Liu Ming, Song Jun-nuo, Wen Chun-xiu, Liu Ling-di, Gu Dong-sheng, Tian Wei

PRODUCTION SITE ECOLOGY

Elevation

Liánqiáo is cultivated between 300–2200 m elevation.

Temperature

A frost free period of at least 196 days is required. The coldest month is January with average low temperatures below 3°C and the warmest month is July with average temperatures between 18–27°C.

Photo Period

Average annual sunshine ranges from 1916–3216 hours. Daily sunshine ranges from 38–49%.

Moisture

Average annual rainfall is 300–800 mm and annual humidity ranges between 35–55%.

Soil

Soil quality is not overly important, average soil will do. Soil can be between slightly acid and slightly alkaline and still produce good product.

Topography

Mountain slopes with dense shrubs and thick undergrowth, in forests or in thickly covered grass areas, or mountain valleys, gullies, and open forests are all suitable for growing *liánqiáo*.

PRODUCTION AREA ENVIRONMENTAL REQUIREMENTS

Land Preparation Prior to Planting

Liánqiáo is a common wild plant growing between 600–1600 m elevation on mountain slopes and in forests. Cultivation is most suitable between 200–800 m elevation on craggy terrain in the mountains. Choose loose, sandy, deep, and fertile soil with a more or less neutral pH. Terraced land will help to control the growing environment, particularly when it comes to water. Composted manure is added prior to planting at a rate of 120–180 kg per acre.

TAKING CUTTINGS & MANAGEMENT

Seed Selection

According to the *Pharmacopoeia of the People's Republic of China* (2015) seeds for *F. suspensa* is the original source for the herb *liánqiáo*. However, propogation from cuttings is almost always used rather than planting seeds.

Taking Cuttings

During the month of June, 15 cm cuttings are taken from the new growth of 3–4-year-old plants. When taking cutting, the cut should be made 0.5–1 cm below a stem bud, the cut is made flat, not at an angle. If the nodes are spread far apart leaving two leaves is sufficient, but if the nodes are close together 3–4 leaves may be left on the stem.

SPECIAL ATTENTION

Liánqiáo naturally has two types of flowers, 1: Styles approximately 2X as long as stamens, 2: Styles approximately ½ as long as stamens. It is important to note this prior to taking cuttings because these two types must be relatively evenly mixed when planting out to the field. Research has shown that when pollen from flowers with the long-type styles gives pollen to the flower with the short-type styles, the reproduction rate is approximately 80%. When the opposite is true, the reproduction rate is approximately 50%. However, when flowers from the same type give pollen to each other the rate of reproduction is between 3–34%.

Bed Preparation for Cuttings

Dig a ditch 40 cm deep and 1–1.3 m wide. Within the ditch, place plastic planting bags (20 cm deep × 10 cm wide) within the ditch and fill with soil. [Translator's Note: Plastic planting bags are commonly used in China. The primary reason for using this method here is for future sale of the new starts. For ecological reasons, fabric is strongly suggested as a replacement for plastic.]

Managing Cuttings

Cutting are dipped in a solution of ABT #1 rooting powder with a concentration of 100 mg/ml for 10 seconds. Cuttings are then placed in the planting bags at a depth of approximately 4 cm before covering the entire ditch with soil, and finally watering in the cuttings. Rows are then covered with a temporary poly-tunnel, approximately 1 m tall, to protect them from external weather conditions and keeping the soil consistently moist. The poly-tunnel is left sealed for up to four weeks before opening, at which time there should be signs of growth from the cuttings; check to make sure they are rooting. Once they have good root growth the poly-tunnel can be removed, this should occur within 5 weeks. [Translator's Note: ABT is a plant growth regulator developed in China for woody species application. It is widely used in China and other countries and generally considered safe.]

Transplanting

Rows are 2 m apart and *liánqiáo* starts are planted 1.5 m apart from each other.

FIELD MANAGEMENT

Cultivation and Weeding

After final selection of transplants, be sure to cultivate and manage weeds in a timely fashion.

Irrigation and Top-Dressing

Always water after top-dressing; water once when the plants begin to flower. Prior to maturity, when the plants are setting fruits, top-dress with diammonium phosphate at a rate of 0.2 kg per bush. Once mature and setting fruit, apply 0.3 kg per bush.

Flowering Season Treatment

Spray boron while the plant is in bloom to increase the proportion of fruits produced. A solution of boron-sucrose-water (1 g : 400 g : 10 L) is made and sprayed to evenly cover the plants.

Pruning

During the winter after saplings reach a height of about 1 meter, after the leaves have dropped, cut the top off at about 70–80 cm tall. In the summer, after the fruits have been picked and growth is vigorous, select 3–4 main branches going in different directions from the leader and remove the other branches. Likewise, in the winter, any branches that run crosswise, are weak and small, or are diseased, should be removed. After the plants have been bearing flowers and fruit for several years, the main branches should be trimmed short by 2/3.

PREVENTION AND TREATMENT OF DISEASE AND INSECT PESTS

Principles of Prevention and Treatment

Liánqiáo has very few diseases or pest problems. Cuttings can succumb to several different fungal disease, but once the plant is mature there are no know serious diseases that cause loss of the production of kill the plant. There are a few pest problems, but they are generally easily managed.

Snail (Fruticicolidae)

Agricultural Controls

Snails are most active in the evening, early morning, and on cloudy days. Search out snails on the plants and kill them, or use branches, weeds, or waste vegetables. to lure them out and kill them. Clear the area of weeds and stones, which offer places for snails to rest and hide. Scatter lime to reduce populations. A 10 cm strip of lime can be spread around the edges of fields to prevent snails from entering the planted area. Turning the soil can help to kill young snails before they develop a shell.

Coleoptera Beatle (*not identified*)

Agricultural Controls

Be sure to identify the larvae and pupa before it becomes a beetle and destroy as many as possible.

HARVESTING

Life-Span

Liánqiáo is a perennial shrub, it flowers every year and produces fruit, with proper management 7–8 years into its life it will begin to produce a significant crop and continue for many years.

Harvest Season

Green fruits (*qīngqiáo*) are harvested from July to September; mature fruits (*lǎoqiáo*) in October.

Harvest Method

For efficient harvesting of the green fruits, entire branches may be cut from the plant, being sure not to do serious damage to the plant, then transport to another area for further processing.

ON-FARM PROCESSING

Drying Method

Green fruits are subjected to a steam bath for 15 minutes or boiled in water (amount of water should be four times the fruits weight by volume) for 10 minutes. [Translator's Note: Research has shown that two of the main active chemicals in *liánqiáo* (phillyrin & forsythiaside A) can be as much as five-times higher in the fruits when the boiling method is used. Therefore, this method is increasingly common in production of this medicinal.]

Drying Method

After steaming the water content of fruits is relatively high, so it is important to move the steamed fruits into an area where they can be dried in the sun in a timely manner. Each day the fruits should be raked or moved so that they will dry evenly. During these turning times, take notice of any mold, mildew, or other disease and quickly remove and discard affected material. Post-steamed fruits can also be oven dried at a temperature not to exceed 60°C. Dried *liánqiáo* should not exceed 10% moisture content. [Translator's Note: Although sun drying is the traditional method and still commonly used today, the use of dryers is recommended to avoid mold and mildew.]

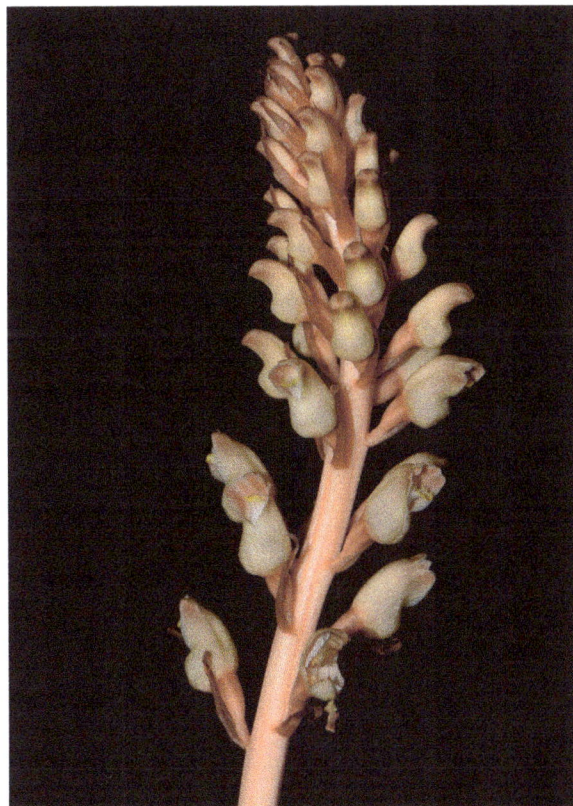

昭 通 天 麻
Gastrodia
Gastrodia elata

The dried stem tuber of this daodi herb *zhāotōng tiānmá* (*Gastrodia elata* Bl.), known as *tiānmá* (天麻) in China, is a member of the orchid family (Ochidaceae). The genus has about 20 species from India to Australia with nine species endemic to China. This species grows widely in sparse and open forests, and forest margins from northeast India through most of China and into far eastern Russia and Japan. It grows at elevations between 400–3200 m. The daodi locations for this medicinal are the areas near Zhaotong city, Yiliang County (including Zhenxiong, Yanjin, Yong-shan, Weixin, Daguan, and Suijiang counties), and the Zhaoyang region in Yunnan province.

Traditional use of this plant spans at least 2000 years, exclusively from wild sources, but the discovery of symbiotic fungi in the late 1990s allowed for commercial cultivation. The plant is used to settle wind stirring internally and stop spasms. Because it is neutral it can be used for both vacuity and repletion patterns when combined with the appropriate herbs. It is also commonly used in pediatrics for chronic fright wind, i.e. infantile convulsions, and is considered a very important herb for this disease. It is also used to calm the liver and subdue rising yang with symptoms of spasm, headache, etc.

Modern science has found many pharmacological activities including sedative, anti-epileptic, anti-anxiety, anticonvulsive, antidepressant, neuroprotective, anti-oxidative, hypotensive, anti-inflammatory, and antipsychotic. It has also been shown to treat vertigo and improve memory loss.

Contributing Authors

Liu Da-hui, Wang Li, Guo Lan-ping, Yang Ye, Zhang Zhi-hui, Fang Yan, Wang Jia-jin, Li Peng-zhang, Cui Xiu-ming, Xu Nuo, Shi Ya-nuo, Zuo Zhi-tian

PRODUCTION SITE ECOLOGY

Elevation

Tiānmá is cultivated between 1400–2300 m elevation.

Temperature

Annual mean temperature 7.9–12.5°C; the coldest month is January with an average temperature of -0.9–2.5°C; the hottest month is July with an average temperature of 15.2–21.5°C; the climate is relatively cool for the latitude.

Moisture

Annual average rainfall 972–1125 mm. Relative humidity ranges between 70–90%; it is often foggy in the area; snow and frost are common in the winter.

Soil

Yellow-sandy soil is most common, occasionally yellow-brown soil is used, soil structure is a loose soil, which maintains temperature and moisture well. This loose soil allows for optimum air penetration and good drainage. Soil pH should be in the range of 5.0–6.5. The topsoil layer should be at least 30 cm deep. The soil should be able to maintain approximately a 50% moisture level year-round.

Topography

Suitable areas should have slopes between 5–30 degrees. In cool mountainous regions, such as the Zhaotong ecosystem, the southern slope is preferred for growing *tiānmá*. In lower elevation areas either grow *tiānmá* on the north side of the slope or grow in areas that are under the cover of the forest canopy. In middle elevation areas choose locations with approximately half sun and half shade.

Site Selection

Sites should be either virgin forests or planted forests, abandoned land or grasslands are rarely used and not recommended. The area should be consistently humid, with relatively frequent fog, summer rain, and winter snow. Generally, bracken ferns are common in areas where the orchid can be cultivated successfully, so one can look for these when selecting a site. Other than noted above, the

soils should be rich in humus, very fertile, and drain-off water well but still be able to maintain approximately a 50% moisture content. Continuous cropping is problematic and should be avoided; land is usually allowed to rest at least five years before growing *tiānmá* on it again.

Soil Preparation

Growing *tiānmá* does not have significant soil preparation requirements. Small shrubs and trees along with other plants are removed from the area to facilitate ease of working in the area. Large rocks are removed but the soil is not plowed or tilled. Steep slopes are generally terraced and other work can be done to ensure that water can drain properly from the site. Level areas with high rainfall are not suitable for growing *tiānmá* because water accumulation is very detrimental for the growth of this medicinal. The site should be well protected from excessive downpours and strong winds therefore forested areas are best.

SOWING SEEDS & RAISING SEEDLINGS

Selecting Seeds

Seeds should be harvested from full seed pods lacking black spots that appear to be healthy and strong, have no physical damage or any sign of insect damage, and arise from an ovoid or broad-ovoid stem tuber. A single stem should produce seed pods that weigh 100–300 grams, which helps to ensure healthy plants with many flowers.

Raising *Tiānmá* for Seeds

Choose a location that is conveniently managed, is protected from heavy winds, has shade, and is isolated from other crops as much as possible. Currently, most breeding is done either indoors or in greenhouses. These rooms need sufficient control of temperature, moisture, wind, and have appropriate lighting.

Planting Tubers for
Indoor Cultivation for Seed

Tiānmá is started from February through April. Deep trays are filled with 10 cm of soil and tubers are placed in the tray (terminal bud facing up), separated by 3–4 cm (2–3 fingers width), then covered with 5–8 cm of soil.

Management

Temperature should be kept between 18–22°C with humidity between 76–85%. In order for *tiānmá* to bolt, scattered light is necessary, avoid direct or bright sunlight. Bolting *tiānmá* is generally staked to prevent it from falling over. Aphids and black-spot disease are common issues that need to be carefully watched for and immediately managed if they arise. During the flowering period, some flowers and buds must be removed. This is done be excising the bottom 3–4 flowers\buds and then the top 3–5 flowers. This prevents the plant from using excessive energy to produce seeds on all the flowers and concentrates that energy so that aborted flowers are rare. Large capsules should be left to ripen while smaller ones should be removed.

Artificial Pollination

Tiānmá is naturally pollinated by insects (entomophilous) but most modern cultivation requires human assistance to pollinate flowers. The optimal period to pollinate flowers starts one day prior to the flower opening and continues until the third day a flower is open. Pollination should be done either in the morning before 10 am or in the afternoon after 4 pm. Avoid pollinating flowers during the middle of the day when the temperature is high and humidity is low. Flowers are held firmly so that they open slightly allowing the pistil and stigma to show themselves. Using a needle or other appropriate tool, pollen is taken from the pistil and applied to the stigma, being careful not to damage the stigma with the tool. When performing this task, it is important to spread pollen from one flower to as many other flowers as possible to help avoid inbreeding.

Seed Collection

Seeds of *tiānmá* mature within a capsule. Approximately 16–25 days after pollination capsules begin to mature from the bottom to the top. The capsule goes from hard to soft and at the same time changes from deep black to a lighter black color with white lines delineating the sections of the capsule. When the capsule reaches this color, they are ready to be harvested for seed. Once seeds have reached this stage, they are cut off the stem directly into a container and protected from being dispersed in the wind. [Translator's Note: Seeds of *tiānmá* are extremely small, dust-like, and can easily blow away with the faintest wind. It is extremely important to safeguard them from

any wind.] Harvested seeds should be planted immediately, or, if this is not possible, they may be stored under refrigeration at 5°C.

Seed Quality Requirement

One-thousand seeds should weight more than 0.0005 g. Seeds should have at least a 20% germination rate with no less than 35% of seedlings reaching maturity. Seeds should have no more than 2% foreign matter.

GROWING SEEDLINGS FROM SEEDS

Pre-Treatment

Seeds should be planted from June through August. However, they first must be exposed to a fungal symbiont. This fungus is generally purchased in 500 ml bag. These packages are torn open and the fungi is left in the package. The seeds are then put into this bag, pouring them out directly from the capsule, and discarding the capsule. Four to five capsules can be treated with a single 500 ml bag. Seeds are kept out of the light, in the bag with the fungi, at room temperature for 3–5 days.

SPECIAL ATTENTION

Fungi isolated from seeds that have been found to assist in germination include species from the genus *Mycena*, including, *M. osmundicola*, *M. orchicola*, *M. dendrobii*, and *M. anoectochila*.

Materials Preparation

Wood from broad-leaf trees (oak, wild cherry, birch, etc.) with a diameter of 4–8 cm is cut into 12–15 cm long pieces. Smaller branches 1–2 cm in diameter are cut into 8–10 cm pieces. Dry leaves from members of Fagaceae (oak, beech, chestnut, etc.) are soaked in water for one day before planting; they are removed from the water and used directly. Fresh leaves can also be used, but these do not need to be soaked.

Fungal Bed Inoculation

A rectangular pit is dug (60×40×30). Do not allow the subsoil to dry out, if it does it must be watered to keep it moist. The materials, as prepared above, are spaced at intervals of 2–3 cm. Place 5–6 segments of wood, previously inoculated with honey mushroom fungus, at the ends and the middle of the segments (each bed uses one 500 ml bottle). On the prepared fungi beds, spread one bag of previously combined seed and fungi in one even layer and mix with tree leaves, using one bag for four pits. Spread leaves, branches and twigs on top of the fungi-leaf mixture. Place a 2–3 cm thick layer of leaves on top of that (fresh or dry). First cover with new soil, which has been taken from a field or anywhere locally, then cover completely with fungal material, finally cover with approximately 10 cm of soil.

FIELD MANAGEMENT—SEEDLINGS

Temperature Control

If the temperature drops below 0°C on the surface of the bed during the winter season, the beds should be covered by more leaves or another layer of soil to protect the temperature inside the bed. If the temperature on the surface of the bed rises above 30°C during the summer, the bed should be covered with leaves or other plant material to cool down the bed.

Moisture Management

Checking the beds regularly is important to ensure that water does not accumulate in or around the bed, and also to make sure that the surface of the beds has not eroded. If either of these problems occurs, they must be rectified immediately. If there has been water accumulation, the inside of the bed should be ventilated to ensure anaerobic growth does not bloom. If the soil on top of the beds dries out during summer, the soil should be moistened evenly and kept moist.

Protective Fencing

If the beds are accessible by either animals or people, it is advised to fence the area to avoid trampling.

COLLECTING SEEDLINGS

Collection Time and Method

Seedlings are collected from the end of November of the second year through March of the third year. Carefully remove the soil and upper layers of the beds to expose the seedlings. Wearing gloves, carefully pluck the seedlings from the bed, and sort according to ranking, then store in a cool, shady, well ventilated area. Because plants grow at different rates and sizes, and these different sizes can have a significant impact on the resultant medicinal materials, it is very important that they are divided and the different grades are planted together. The grades are, for an individual stem tuber: superior grade (> 250 g), grade I (200–250 g), grade II (150–200), grade III (100–150 g), grade IV (< 100 g).

FIELD CULTIVATION—SEEDLINGS

Building the Fungal Bed

Beds are dug from April through June. Beds should be dug in accordance to the terrain, digging the bed along the slope at a length of 60–80 cm, 40–50 cm wide, and 20–30 cm deep. The bottom should be dug in line with the slope at an angle of 5–15° to assist in drainage. Based on the terrain, dig 1200–1500 beds per acre with 50–100 cm between each bed.

Fungal Material Selection

Wood to be used for the fungal materials can be a mixture of long-acting and fast-acting types of wood. The most important factor when considering the species of wood are their hardness, which determines how quickly the honey mushroom (*Armillaria mellea*) will colonize and consume the wood (softer *and* fast-acting), or more slowly acting woods which will last for an extended period of time (harder *and* long-acting). The wood needs to be 5–10 cm thick, and can be split in half or quartered if it's thicker than 10 cm in diameter. [Translator's Note: These materials will hereafter be referred to as "fungal wood."]

Processing and Placing the Fungal Wood

Cut the fungal wood into sections 12 cm or 20 cm long; make sections of the same lengths as much possible. The ratio of long-acting wood to fast-acting wood should be 6:4. Use a combination of thin and thick fungal wood when placing it out for cultivation. Put a layer of soft fresh soil at the bottom of beds. Place 2–3 pieces horizontally on the steep slope direction of the slope (wood stick should be in parallel with equal-height rope, 3 pieces 12 cm long and 2 pieces 20 cm long). Make 5–10 vertical rows (decide number of rows according to the diameter of the fungal wood), and make sure it occupies all the space. On the gentle slope, 3–5 pieces of fungal wood should be placed vertically (the wood should be placed vertical to the equal-height rope, 5 pieces of 12 cm long ones, 3 pieces of 20 cm long ones), 4–6 rows should be placed horizontally (number of rows to be decided by the diameter of fungal wood), place until all the space is used. There should be 2–3 cm of space between every two pieces of wood. No space should be left between fungal wood and bottom soil, and so one should fill the space with soil after all the wood has been placed. Place 5–6 segments of wood, previously inoculated with honey mushroom fungus, at the ends and the middle of the segments (use one 750 ml bottle for each bed), and then spread a layer of small fresh tree twigs and leaves no bigger than 5 cm long and 2 cm thick on the fungus. First cover with new soil to cover completely the fungi, using about 3–5 cm of soil. After this, the entire area is covered with 5–10 cm of soil, using thicker covering for drier areas. Covering should be equal across the entire area. In areas that have more moisture, the covering can be on the thinner side and should be formed with a ridge in the middle, sloping out toward the edge to allow water to flow away from the center. Once the bed is covered with soil, tree leaves are used to cover the entire bed (~1 cm) to preserve soil moisture and protect the soil from the sun.

SPECIAL ATTENTION

Selected species of "long-acting" and "fast-acting" wood. While some of these species are available outside of China some are not. This is meant as a guide to allow growers to choose local wood that is as close as possible to these species.
Long-acting woods include:
Japanese blue oak (*Quercus glauca*), Chinese cork oak (*Q. variabilis*), saw tooth oak (*Q. acutissima*), Chinese chestnut (*Castanea mollissima*), sequin chestnut (*C. sequinii*), long petiol beech (*Fagus longipetiolata*), wedding cake tree (*Cornus controversum*), Sichuan cherry (*Prunus szechuanica*), autumn olive (*Elaeagnus umbellate*), and winter fruit poplar (*Populus purdumii*). Slow-acting woods include: Chinese alder (*Alnus cremastogyne*), Nepalese alder (*A. nepalensis*), western Chinese birch (*Betula alnoides*), Chinese red birch (*Betula albosinensis*), common apple (*Malus pumila*), Chinese catalpa (*Catalpa ovata*), and Korean mountain ash (*Sorbus alnifolia*).

Fungal Bed Management

If the temperature rises above 30°C during the summer, the bed should be covered with leaves (3–5 cm) to help lower the temperature. If it is dry during the summer months and the soil dries out, watering should be done to the point where soil can be formed into a ball in one's hand but breaks apart easily when it drops on the ground (40–60% moisture). When it rains, be sure that water is draining sufficiently and repair any eroding soil from the tops of the beds. Do not allow weeds to accumulate on top of the beds or in the drainage ditches. If there is any risk of domestic animals entering the area, be sure to properly fence the site. Domestic animal intrusion can cause significant damage to a *tiānmá* growing site.

FIELD CULTIVATION

Cultivation Season & Seedling Selection

Tiānmá can be planted from December of the same year through March of the following year, after establishing the honey mushroom fungus on the wood. When growing seedlings, they are classified into two categories, seeds that were harvested in one year and planted the following spring are considered first year "white head *tiānmá*"* and seeds planted in the autumn are considered second year "white head *tiānmá*." White head *tiānmá* should be between 5–25 g each and free of mechanical damage, have normal and healthy outward appearance and color (fresh pale yellow), be free from disease, and without any pests or pest damage.

* White head *tiānmá* refers to root tubers that are about the length of a thumb or pinky finger. These plants do not have obvious buds and should be grown together according to when they were planted, and not combined during transplanting.

Cultivation Method

Planting should only be done on a dry sunny day. Do not plant in the rain, freezing weather, or snow. Do not use hybrid fungal material. Dig the surface soil of the fungal bed away to expose the inoculated logs. The white head *tiānmá* is between the ends of the cut surfaces of two pieces of fungal wood. These white head *tiānmá* have two distinct ends. One end has a round scar (generally called the "bellybutton") and the other end has the bud that will sprout and eventually flower. At the edges of the bed, a single white head *tiānmá* is put at the cut-off surface of fungal wood, the "bellybutton" of white head *tiānmá* should be close to the cut-off end and the sprout should face up. After placing the white head *tiānmá*, place 3–5 fungal materials that nurture fungus (fresh small sticks, 2–5 cm thick, 4–5 cm long, cut surfaces should be sliced on the bias, not flat cut, to expose more surface area), and then cover with 3–5 cm of fresh soil, followed with 5–10 cm of cover soil (the cover soil can be thicker if the area is dry, make surface even; make surface soil thinner if in a humid region and make the surface into a turtle shell shape to facilitate draining). Finally, add a layer of tree leaves (~1 cm) is added to protect the beds from the sunlight and to help maintain the moisture of the soil.

FIELD MANAGEMENT

Temperature Regulation

In the late winter (February and March), if the temperature drops below 0°C fallen leaves and or soil should be added to the beds to preserve the temperature. During the summer if the temperature rises above 30°C fallen leaves are added to the beds to protect from high temperatures.

Water Management

During the rainy season (July-September) closely monitor the site, making sure all drainage ditches are functioning well; do not allow water to accumulate.

Weeding and Covering Beds

Starting in early to mid-April and through late July, weeding is done regularly and pulled weeds are simply added to the bed to cover and protect it in addition to adding organic matter.

PREVENTION AND TREATMENT OF DISEASE AND INSECT PESTS

Principles of Prevention and Treatment

Any discovery of disease or pests should be taken very seriously, spread of diseases can cause significant damage in short periods of time. Creating and maintaining an environment as close as possible to the native habitat of *tiānmá* reduces the risk of disease.

Stem Rot (pathogen not identified)

Prevention and Treatment

Select undeveloped land, do not continuously grow on the same land for more than 5 years. Make sure water is drained properly. Be sure that the fungal strain used is pure and free from other strains. Only the honey mushroom (*Armillaria mellea*) should be used. Add more of the honey mushroom spores to the beds. Be sure to only use freshly cut wood. Do not use dry dead wood. The size of the beds is very important, making them larger or more shallow will likely cause problems. Maintaining the bed's moisture is very important. If the bed gets too moist remove some of the covering from the top to help it dry out or remove it completely if necessary. Make sure that air is flowing well through the site and that water is drained properly. Water if necessary. If there is an incursion of another fungi, the covering of the bed can be removed and the sun allowed to penetrate for 2-3 days in an effort to kill the other fungi. If this is unsuccessful, the bed and its wood must be abandoned and cannot be used for cultivation of *tiānmá*. Only use the strongest and healthiest starts, never use any that appear diseased or weak.

Honey Mushroom Fungal Pathogens

Prevention and Treatment

Choose sandy humus soil with good water drainage. Be sure to check drainage ditches during periods of rain so that water is not allowed to accumulate.

Mole Cricket (Gryllotalpidae)

Prevention and Treatment

The use of black lights to lure and kill the crickets is an effective measure.

Grub (*Holotrichia* sp.)

Prevention and Treatment

During bed building, pay close attention and if these pests are found they should be killed. Black lights are used to lure and trap the grubs.

HARVESTING

Harvest Season

Tiānmá is harvested in November of the first year through March of the second year after transplanting.

Harvest Method

First a shovel is used to unearth the beds, then the roots are removed by hand, being very careful not to damage them.

Post-harvest Bed Management

After *tiānmá* is harvested the beds should be cleaned-up by carefully going through and looking for any intrusion by other fungi besides the honey mushroom fungi, discarding any found. Also, the status of the wood must be checked. If it has rotted too much than it should be discarded and replaced with new wood.

Transporting to Processing Area

If processing is not done on-site immediately, the fresh roots must be transported to a well-ventilated area with well-ventilated containers such as baskets, and kept at a temperature that does not exceed 10°C. The tuber of *tiānmá* can be stored up to one week in this manner.

ON-FARM PROCESSING

Grading

Initial grading of fresh *tiānmá* is done to facilitate processing and the final grading process. The fresh root has three grades which are based on weight: grade 1: more than 150 g; grade 2: 75–150 g; grade 3: less than 75 g or root that have been damaged.

Cleaning

After grading, a pressure washer is used to remove all the soil still stuck to the root; use a soft brush to carefully assist in this process. During this process do not remove scales, scrape the root skin, or remove the bud. Roots that have been cleaned cannot be left for extended periods and cannot be left over-night before being steamed.

Steam Processing

As soon as the cleaned *tiānmá* arrives in the steaming facility it must be processed immediately. Root tubers are placed in stainless steel baskets and placed in a steaming machine. Starting from the time the temperature of the water reaches 100°C the root tubers are left to steam according to their weight. Larger than 250 grams: 35–40 minutes; 200–250 grams: 30–35 minutes; 150–200 grams: 20–25 minutes; 100–150 grams: 15–20 minutes. The steaming process should not penetrate so deeply that it reaches the center of the tuber; this will produce sub-par final product. After steaming the roots are laid out on screens to dry in the air.

Drying

High Heat Drying: Roots are first put into the drier for 3–4 hours at 40–50°C. The temperature is then raised to 55–60°C and the roots are roasted for 12–18 hours until the outer portions of the root show tiny wrinkles. The roots are then packaged or piled to allow the moisture from the middle of the root to move to the exterior, then the roots are subjected to the 55–60°C drying process again for 12 hours. At the end of this period the roots should be properly dried.

Low Heat Drying: After steaming and initial drying, root tubers are dried at 45–50°C for 24–48 hours until the root tuber is 50–60% dry. The root tubers are then packaged or piled to allow the moisture from the middle of the root to move to the exterior, then they are dried again until the exterior begins to harden. This process is repeated regularly until the root tuber is dry, which takes 10–15 days. Properly dried, the root tuber should not exceed 15% moisture.

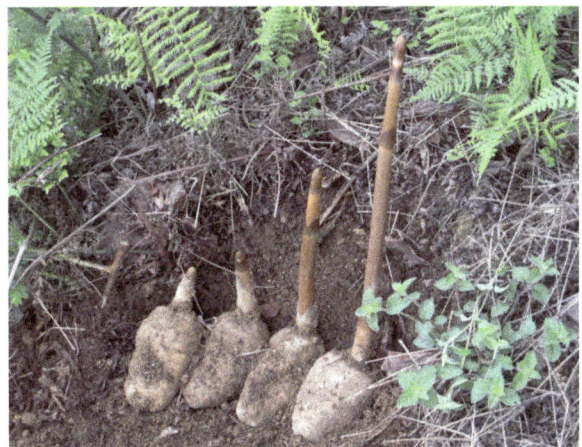

Four stages of flowering stem growth of *tiānmá*.

滇龙胆

Yunnan Gentian

Gentiana rigescens

DISTINGUISHING FEATURES

The dried root of the daodi herb *diān lóngdǎn* (*Gentiana rigescens* Franch.), known as *lóngdǎn* (龍膽 \ 龙胆) in China, is a member of the gentian family (Gentianaceae). The large genus has about 360 species and approximately two-thirds of those are native to China. This species grows in southwest China and Myanmar on grassy slopes, and in valleys, scrub, and forests that are between 1100-3000 m in elevation. The daodi location for this medicinal is Lincangyun and Yongde counties, Linxiang region, and Honghezhou in Honghe county (and the surrounding region) in Yunnan province.

This herb, or related species, have been used in China for at least 2000 years. The herb clears heat and dries dampness and is primarily used for liver and gallbladder damp-heat patterns with diarrhea, constipation, headaches, loss of appetite, etc. The herb drains fire and is a key herb for liver fire ascending with headaches, red and painful eyes, dizziness, and related signs.

According to the *Pharmacopeia of the People's Republic of China* (2015), there are 4 species of *Gentiana* recognized as the medicinal *lóngdǎn* including: *G. manshurica* (条叶龙胆), *G. scabra* (龙胆), *G. trifolia* (三花龙胆), and the species in this monograph. However, the content of gentiopicroside, an iridoid glycoside, in the species in this monograph is only about half of the other three species. Scientific investigation of this plant supports most of the traditional uses, showing hepatoprotective, anti-inflammatory, and antioxidant actions. The plant is abundant in iridoid glycosides, which give it its characteristic bitter taste. The iridoid glycoside, noted above, which can be has high as 4.5% of the total dry root and serves as the standard marker used for quality control.

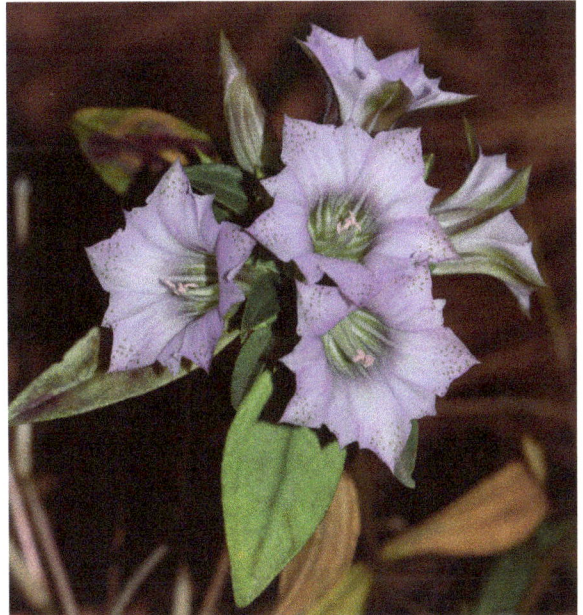

Contributing Authors

Zheng Yu-guang, Xie Xiao-liang, Guo Lan-ping, Huang Lu-qi, Hao Qing-xiu, Liu Ming, Song Jun-nuo, Wen Chun-xiu, Liu Ling-di, Gu Dong-sheng, Tian Wei

PRODUCTION SITE ECOLOGY

Elevation

Lóngdǎn is cultivated between 1700–2500 m elevation.

Temperature

Average annual temperature ranges between 7–21°C.

Photo Period

Sunlight is sufficient, but short. [Translator's Note: *Lóngdǎn* prefers cool areas with limited direct sunlight. However, while it is found in forests, it prefers open areas where the sun is mostly obstructed by daily cloud cover, the plant will not thrive in conditions where the sun is consistently bright.]

Moisture

Average annual rainfall is between 800–1400 mm and average humidity is 60%.

Soil

Red and yellow soils are most frequently used, but others could also be appropriate. Soils should be loose but hold water fairly well. Soils that are rich in humus or sandy are considered best. Soil should be between pH 5.0–6.5 for best results. A deep soil layer extending down to more than 30 cm is important.

Topography

Sites should have no more than a 30-degree slope.

PRODUCTION AREA ENVIRONMENTAL REQUIREMENTS

Site Selection

In China, sites are generally chosen because they either have or did have this plant growing on them as part of the native ecology. A headwaters area with a gentle slope is preferred, where the soil layer is deep and loose with a slightly acid pH. The area should be moist but with good drainage and the soil should be rich and fertile. Daytime sun is generally in the morning before clouds build up. Virgin soil is best. Continuous cropping is not recommended.

Soil Preparation

The site is plowed in the late autumn or early spring to a depth of 25–30 cm and any large clods of soil are broken up while other vegetation is removed from the land. The land is then often treated with a general fungicide before plowing again and harrowing. This process is thought to kill many of the potential underground pests (insects) and disease organisms (mostly fungi). [Translator's Note: Fungicidal treatment of the soil is somewhat common when growing some herbs in China. This is not an ecologically sound practice and is not recommended. This information has been retained here as a warning to those who may attempt to grow this herb because cultivation without this treatment is reportedly quite challenging.]

SOWING SEEDS & RAISING SEEDLINGS

Seed Quality Requirements

The weight of 1000 seeds should exceed 0.015 g with a water content of less than 12%, a germination rate above 30%, and foreign matter should not exceed 40%.

Pre-Sowing Process

Seeds should be soaked (often in a fungicide solution) for 12 hours then allowed to dry in the sun prior to sowing.

Sowing Seeds

Seeds are sown from late May through mid-June, this timing should be adjusted based on potential heavy rainfall, i.e. don't sow seeds if a heavy rainfall is predicted in the near future. Seeds are sown at a rate of 0.75–1.80 kg per acre. [Translator's Note: Research has shown that seeds sprout best between 23–25°C. Although this temperature is rarely if ever reached in the plant's daodi location, the takeaway here is that sowing prior to forecasted high temperatures is advised to increase germination rate.]

If there has not been recent rain, the site should be watered prior to sowing seeds. Seeds are combined with 5–10 times their volume of a fine sand and mixed thoroughly. The seeds (and sand) are then broadcasted on the site. It is best to broadcast each area twice to ensure even distribution of seedlings. Interplanting with foxtail grass (*Setaria viridis*) is strongly recommended. This is done at the same time the *lóngdǎn* seeds are planted at a rate of 9–15 kg per acre. The use of this grass helps to create shade for the small seedlings and to preserve moisture in the soil.

FIELD MANAGEMENT

Weeding

Once weeds and the foxtail grass reach a height of approximately 30 cm, they can be mowed short once between October and December. The mowing height is determined by the growth of the *lóngdǎn*; it should be cut just above the tallest plants allowing them to access sunlight. Weeding is done twice in the second year between the months of July and December depending on the needs of the site. In the third year, weeding is done according to the needs presented.

Fertilizer Application

During the months of June and July an application of NPK is applied at a rate of 60–75 kg per acre. During the third year, before the bloom, the same fertilizer is applied at a rate of 120 kg per acre.

SEED COLLECTION

Seed Collection Requirements

Plants must be at least three years old before seeds are collected. Seeds should only be collected from plants that are healthy and free from disease. The best plants to collect from are those with a tall, thick, and robust stem.

Seed Collection Time

Generally, seeds are ripe during the months of November and December. Seeds should be collected on a sunny day when there is no significant wind and no fog. When the capsule stretches out, the seeds should be khaki color, this is the best time to harvest.

Seed Collection Method

The entire capsule should be held while it is cut off and placed in a bucket or other similar non-porous container. The seeds and capsules are placed in an area with good air flow where they can dry in the sun. After 2–3 days the capsules are lightly beaten with a stick or other appropriate tool; the seeds should easily fall out of the capsule. All foreign matter should be winnowed away and the seeds should be left to dry in the sun for another 5–7 days until the seed water content is below 10%.

PREVENTION AND TREATMENT OF DISEASE AND INSECT PESTS

Principles of Prevention and Treatment

When growing *lóngdǎn* the standards of agriculture must be maintained, including keeping the site clean and free from disease, crop rotation, appropriate plant spacing, and maintaining the site in accordance with the surrounding ecosystem. These will all help to ensure minimal disease problems. By encouraging the natural ecosystem and all its diversity, diseases will be minimized and strong growth and development will be encouraged. Staying within this scope will discourage disease and minimize economic loss.

Clean Growing Site

Soil-borne diseases will survive the winter so that in the second year they can infect the young plants as they emerge. Therefore, it is important that the field is cleared of any diseased plant material each year after the harvest and disposed of properly.

Crop Rotation

After harvesting *lóngdǎn* a cover crop of a grass family plant or pea family plant is grown to help avoid any diseases from getting well established. Other plants such as tobacco are planted to reduce potential problems with nematodes. Some plants, such as spinach and cilantro encourage nematode eggs to hatch early. These plants attract nematodes and thus lure them away from the *lóngdǎn* crop. At harvest time these plants are pulled up by their roots and disposed of properly (usually burned) to reduce populations of nematodes. Other plants such as marigold, which are known to reduce pathogenic nematodes, are also grown on sites.

Proper Plant Spacing

One of the most significant disease problems when growing *lóngdǎn* is pathogenic fungi. When humidity and rainfall are highest, pathogenic fungi are most prevalent. Plants must be spaced so that there is sufficient free flow of air and light can penetrate, which will reduce the risk of pathogenic fungi infecting the crop.

Imitating Environmental Conditions

Wild *lóngdǎn* has very few disease problems and sometimes no diseases at all because *lóngdǎn*'s surroundings have a diverse community of plants that seem to offer a protective environment. After the development of large-scale cultivation efforts, fungal and other diseases became pervasive. After careful study, we know that keeping a diversity of native plants growing in proximity has proven to help prevent these problems. *Lóngdǎn* is also interplanted in tea plantations, which has proved to be very effective. Another major pathogen is anthracnose, which is significantly lessened with the use of the above techniques. These techniques also preserve the environment, reduce costs, and improve the quality of the resulting medicinal material.

HARVESTING

Harvest Season

The root of *lóngdǎn* is harvested after three years of growth. It is best to harvest *lóngdǎn* in November. Plants grown for seeds are best reserved until January when seeds are collected.

Harvest Method

Wait for a sunny day and dig the root and rhizome system from at least two directions. Take care to avoid damaging the root system; do not snap off roots when digging. After digging the root and rhizome, carefully remove soil and place in a basket or other appropriate vessel for carrying.

ON-FARM PROCESSING

Initial Processing

After bringing in the material the leaves are cut off, leaving 0.5–2 cm of the stem connected to the roots.

Sun-Drying and Removing Excess Soil

After removing the leaves, roots are placed in a shaded area (about 50% sunlight) and allowed to dry to about 50% moisture content (roots should remain flexible). Then roots should be rubbed between your hands to loosen and remove remaining dirt and any other foreign matter.

Bundling

Once roots are dried to about 50% moisture and have been processed as noted above, roots are tied in bundles of about 40–60 grams. Roots are dried in the shade in this manner at a temperature between 18–25°C; avoid direct sun. Good quality roots should have irregular nodes and the top should have a woody stock tapering to a finer root-tip. The exterior should be reddish-brown with extensive longitudinal wrinkles. The root should be firm and brittle. When snapping the root, the interior should have a yellow center (heart wood). Finished product should be very bitter, free of leaf or stem material, and without other impurities or mildew. Final dried material should not have more than 9% moisture.

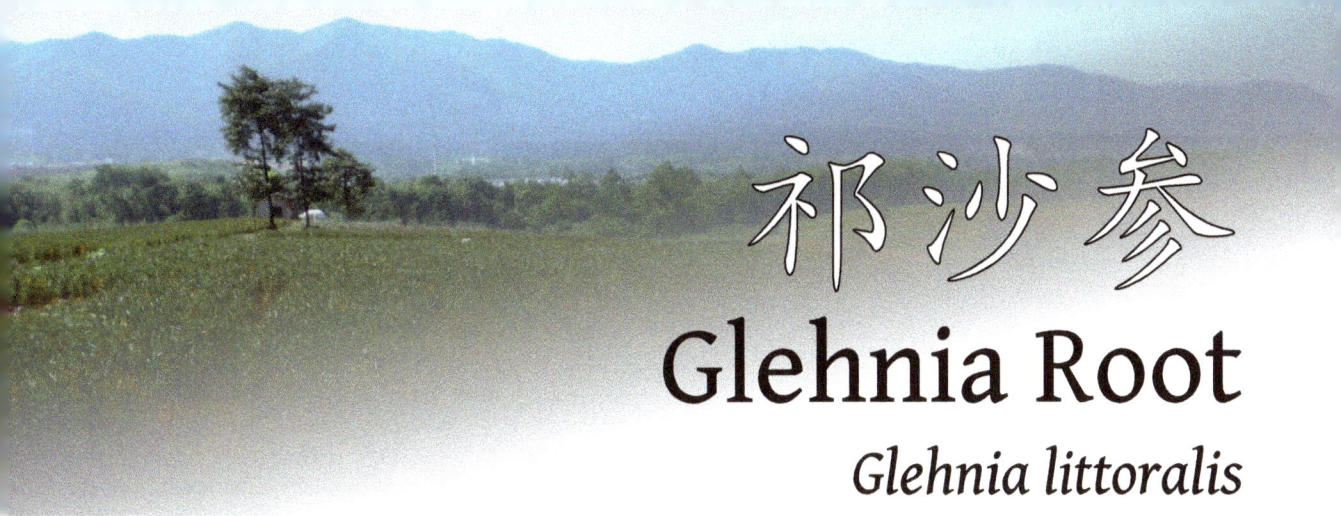

祁沙参
Glehnia Root
Glehnia littoralis

DISTINGUISHING FEATURES

The dried root of the daodi herb *qí shāshēn* (*Glehnia littoralis* Fr. Schmidtex Miq.), which is commonly known as either *běishāshēn* (北沙参 \ 北沙参) or simply *shāshēn* (沙参 \ 沙参) in China. The "*běi*" here means "north" and is a way to differentiate this herb from a botanically unrelated herb which is sometimes simply called *shāshēn*, creating confusion, but which is most often referred to as *nánshāshēn*; because "*nán*" means "south" in Chinese. *Běishāshēn* is member of the carrot family (Apiaceae). The *Glehnia* genus is a monotypic genus, but does have a subspecies, *Glehnia littoralis* ssp. *leiocarpa*. The species skirts the Pacific rim from China (Qingdao province), north into Russia and down through Alaska along the West Coast of North America; the subspecies has been recorded as far south as the San Francisco area. The plant is listed as endangered in China. The daodi location for this herb is in Hebei province in the area of Anguo city, which is also the site of one of the most important herb markets in the country.

Although the herb name *shāshēn* has been used for about 1500 years for other medicinal plants, this medicinal is a relatively recent addition to the Chinese materia medica, first appearing in the Ming Dyansty text *Materia Medica of Collected Statements* (1624). In Chinese medicine this herb is used to supplement lung and stomach yin, clear lung heat, moisten the lung, and is frequently used for various dry cough syndromes. The root is also commonly used in Chinese cooking, usually in soups or porridge.

There is limited modern research on this plant, however research has shown that the root of this plant has antibacterial, antifungal, antioxidant, and anti-inflammatory activity. Recent research suggests it may promote neurogenesis.

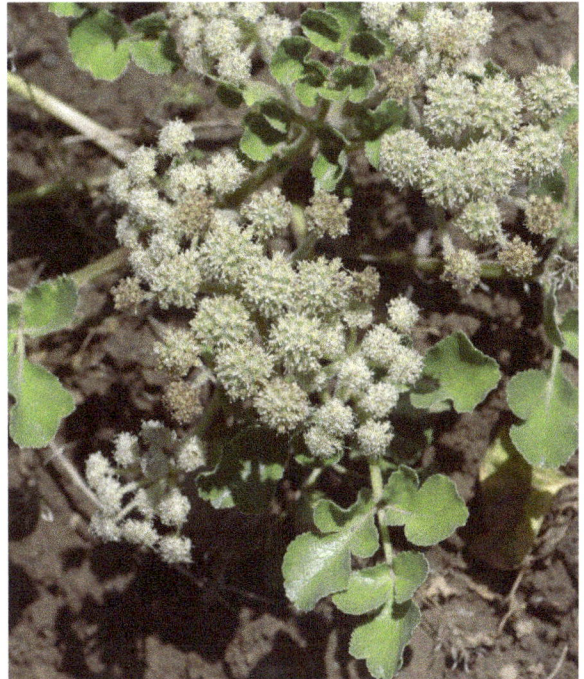

Contributing Authors

Liu Ming, Wen Chun-xiu,
Xie Xiao-liang, Huang Lu-qi,
Hao Qing-xiu, Guo Lan-ping, Liu Ling-di,
Bo Jian-ying, Gu Dong-sheng, Tian Wei

PRODUCTION SITE ECOLOGY

Elevation

Shāshēn is cultivated between 50–500 m elevation.

Temperature

An average annual temperature of 12.4°C with a minimum of 197 frost free days are required.

Photo Period

Annual sunshine 2500–2757 hours and a sunshine percentage range of 35–70%.

Moisture

Average annual rainfall 500–800 mm with a relative humidity of 34–55%.

Soil

A loose sandy soil with a depth of at least 30 cm is ideal and pH in the 5.5–6.5 range. Clay soils are not appropriate for this herb.

Topography

Both level and sloped land can be used, but good air circulation and water drainage are both important. A source of irrigation may be necessary.

Site Selection and Soil Preparation

A site should have at least a plough depth of sandy soil, but deeper is better. Add 3000 kg NPK and 360 kg composite fertilizer per acre. Till in deeply and harrow finely.

SOWING SEEDS & RAISING SEEDLINGS

Seed Quality Requirements

According to the *Pharmacopoeia of the People's Republic of China* (2015) seeds for *Glehnia littoralis* of the Apiaceae family are the original source for the herb *shāshēn* in Chinese medicine. Seeds should not be stored for longer than one year and should ideally be plump and not excessively flat with a feeling as though they are empty inside.

Seed Pre-Treatment

After the start of winter, seeds are soaked in clean water for 5–6 days, after the water is strained away, seeds are mixed with sand until the ratio of seeds to sand is 1:3 (i.e. add 3x as much sand). The seed-sand mixture is buried in a hole 40 cm deep, with the sand-seed layer about 30 cm thick. The following spring, when the ground has thawed, the mixture is removed and planted. For autumn planting, seeds are soaked in 40°C water for 8–12 hours, then allowed to dry slightly in the sun before sowing. [Translator's note: This method was developed traditionally to simulate over-wintering and to protect the seeds from damage from freezing. While this method is valid, the same could also be accomplished if the seed was stored (with the moist sand) under refrigeration for the same period of time.]

Sowing Seeds

Spring planting is done during the month of March; autumn planting is done between late October and early November. In prepared beds, furrows are dug 1.5–2.0 cm deep, 25 cm apart. Seeds are sown evenly in the furrow and covered slightly with soil, then gently pressed by hand or with a roller. Seeding rate is 30–36 kg of seed per acre.

FIELD MANAGEMENT

Thinning and Final Singling of Seedlings

When seedlings have reached 4–6 cm tall they are thinned to 4–5 cm apart. If there are places where there are larger gaps, robust seedlings can be removed from other beds to fill in the holes; this should be done on a cloudy day or at the end of the afternoon, just before sunset.

Cultivation and Weeding

Pull any weeds during the thinning process. When cultivating with a hoe or other tool, loosen the soil shallowly the first time, after this the soil can be loosened more deeply. After watering or rain, cultivate to eliminate weeds and keep soil loose.

Irrigation and Water Drainage

Water after transplanting and top-dressing. Watering before harvest should be done only when needed. Because *shāshēn* root easily rots in poorly drained soils or locations where water has accumulated, any excessive water from rain or irrigation should be immediately drained.

Top-Dressing

During the second half of June, plants should be top-dressed with NPK compound fertilizer at a rate of 300 kg per acre.

PREVENTION AND TREATMENT OF DISEASE AND INSECT PESTS

Principles of Prevention and Treatment

Diseases and pests can be problematic when growing this herb. Proper water drainage is critical to help keep the plant healthy and avoid root rot diseases. Aphids can be a major problem; early identification of this pest will help significantly with control. Boring insects and grubs can easily go undetected unless vigilant monitoring of the crop is done.

Rust Disease (*Puccinia phellopteri*)

Prevention and Treatment

Increase phosphorus and potash fertilizer. Improve control of water drainage during the rainy season or heavy rain periods so that the field does not remain soggy for any extended periods of time.

Root Rot (*Fusarium sp.*)

Prevention and Treatment

Rotate with a grass family crop every 3–5 years. Consider potential over use of fertilizer, particularly nitrogen, while also increasing phosphorus and potash. Identify and remove any diseased plants.

Boring Insect (*Epinotia loucautha*)

Prevention and Treatment

Adults can be lured to a trap using lights. When borers are present, any seedlings found* during harvest should be buried at least 20 cm deep. During harvest petioles should be inspected for chrysalis and larva, any found should also be buried as least 20 cm deep. (*Seedlings can sometime arise from seeds dropped by the current crop. These plants are likely to harbor borers and so should be buried when these pests are present.)

Aphids (*Aphidoidea*)

Prevention and Treatment

Aphids are naturally attracted to the color yellow. Deploying "sticky yellow boards" or construction of areas with yellow painted boards (60×40 cm) will attract aphids where they can be killed. Vegetable oil can be applied to the surface of these boards so the aphids get stuck there. Periodically check to see when the board is coated with aphids, at which time the board can be scraped and more oil can be added. Every acre should have about 180 boards.

Biological Controls

Introduction of lady bugs early can be a very effective control for aphids. A 0.3% concentration of matrine diluted to a 0.1–0.167% solution; or natural pyrethrins diluted to a 0.01% solution; sprayed according to the manufacturer's instructions.

Grubs (*Holotrichia sp.*)

Prevention and Treatment

Prior to winter and subsequent transplanting, plow deep (perhaps several times) to destroy the insect.

Biological Controls

Use *Bacillus popilliae* and *Beauveria bassiana* as non-toxic spray controls. *B. popilliae* is applied at 9 kg per acre; *B. bassiana* is applied at 2.0x109 spores per square meter.

HARVESTING

Harvest Season

Shāshēn roots are generally harvested at the end of October of the first year of growth, after the plant has withered.

Harvest Method

Choose a sunny day with good weather. Digging should begin from the radius created by the first areal leaf (30–40 cm) to safely excavate the root without damage. The root should be shaken to remove any loose soil.

ON-FARM PROCESSING

Root Bark Removal

Immediately after harvest, when the roots are fresh, they are put into boiling water for 6–8 seconds. Make sure they are continuously moving within the boiling water. Once they are removed from the water and cool enough to handle, the root bark is promptly removed by hand.

Drying Method

After removal of the root bark, roots are spread out in a cool shady area with good air circulation for drying. During the drying period, roots should be turned 1–2 times per day to avoid potential mold or mildew formation. Roots are considered dry when they reach 10% moisture. Roots with any sign of mold, mildew, or rot of any kind must be discarded. Forced air drying can also be employed. When using this technique the drier temperature should be between 50–55°C.

梁外甘草

Chinese Licorice
Glycyrrhiza uralensis

DISTINGUISHING FEATURES

The root of this medicinal plant, *liángwèi gāncǎo* (*Glycyrrhiza uralensis* Fisch.), is commonly known as gāncǎo (甘草) in China and is a member of the pea family (Leguminaceae). *Glycyrrhiza* is a genus represented by about 20 species in Europe, Asia, Australia, North America and South America. While this monograph only covers a single species, there are three official species in the *Pharmacopoeia of the People's Republic of China* (2015) including *G. glabra*, which is the officially-designated species in many other pharmacopoeias, particularly in Western countries. Licorice (*G. glabra*) is the source of licorice candy.

The herb has long been used in many systems of traditional medicine. Its use in China dates back at least 2000 years and it is one of the most commonly used plants in clinical practice. It is frequently used as a harmonizing herb when combined with other herbs in formulas. However, it has its own unique actions, which are to supplement the spleen and stomach qi, moisten the lung, clear heat, counter or reduce toxicity of other herbs, and supplement heart qi. It is commonly used for a wide range of ailments including poor digestion, stomach heat, cough, dry throat, anxiety and stress, and many more ailments.

Modern science has studied this plant extensively and the list of actions and indications that have been shown or proven through scientific research is extensive. Some of the pharmacological activities identified include gastroprotective, hepatoprotective, neuroprotective, cardioprotective, antiviral, anti-microbial, antidiabetic, antiasthma, anticancer activities, and immunomodulatory. Moreover, the traditional uses noted above are but a small selection of the many medicinal uses and herbal combinations for *gāncǎo* that have been recorded in the traditional literature. Unlike most other medicinals, it is commonly used in both formulas that supplement and nourish as well as those directed at infections and inflammatory processes.

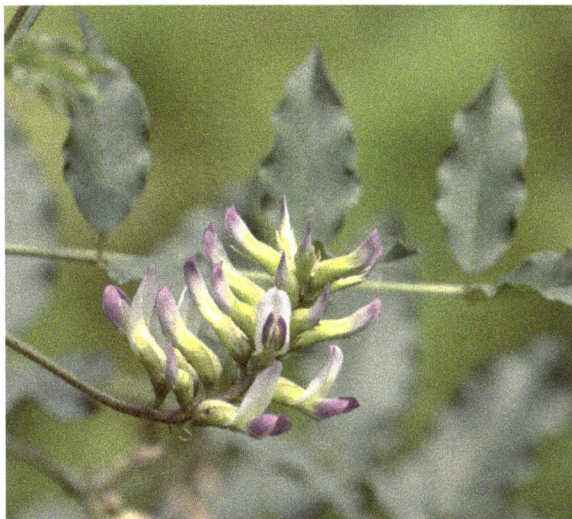

Contributing Authors

Wang Wen-quan, Wei Sheng-li, Hou Jun-ling, Huang Ming-jin, Yu Fu-lai, Liu Ying

PRODUCTION SITE ECOLOGY

Elevation

Gāncǎo is cultivated between 1000–1500 m elevation.

Temperature

An average annual temperature of 6–8°C; January average temperature between -14--8°C, and July average temperatures between 22–24°C.

Rainfall

An average annual rainfall of 150–300 mm, mostly coming from July through September.

Soil

Suitable soil types include: chestnut, brown, sierozem, light-carbonate brown, black soil, or saline desert meadow soil. Soil should be alkaline, between pH 8–9.

SOWING SEEDS & RAISING SEEDLINGS

Seed Quality Requirement

Seeds should be free of impurities, and one should discard damaged seeds, or seeds that are not plump and full (>20%). A germination rate between 65–75% is acceptable, 1000 seeds should not weigh less than 9 g, and water content should not exceed 10%.

Collection and Post-Collection Methods

Gāncǎo seeds are collected from mid-August through mid-September by removing branches with ripe pods. Seeds should be collected with the seeds inside the pods when they change from green to black-green color. Branches that are healthy and strong, free from disease or insect pests should be chosen from each plant for harvesting. Remove the entire branch and transport to an area where the branches and pods can dry completely in the sun, if there is any threat of rain be sure to protect the material from the rain. Spread evenly across the area to dry, once dry use a stone or other appropriate tool to roll over the dried material to free the seeds from the pods. Remove the stems from the area and winnow the seeds from the remaining plant material. Be sure seeds are properly dried, if not leave them in the sun they are very dry.

Seed Storage

Seeds should be saved in a well ventilated, cool, dark, dry area indoors. Containers should be airtight to protect seeds from insect pests.

Selection of Seedling Area

The area should be level and smooth, with deep soil layers, good fertility, a deep water table, and sandy soil. Excess water from irrigation should be easily drained away and the soil should be around pH 8.

Soil Preparation

In the autumn prior to sowing seeds (mid- to late October), plow the soil deeply to cultivate it and disturb over-wintering insect pests; 18,000 kg per acre of well composted manure is first spread on the land and plowed into the soil. At the end of October and beginning of November irrigate and allow the water to freeze to preserve soil moisture. Prior to sowing seeds (late April to early May) deeply plow soil (30–45 cm), harrow the beds once and rake smooth, this improves the germination rate and protects the seedlings. Beds are built to dimensions of 10×30 m, irrigated with a sprinkler, and every 30 cm a small mound is built extending the length of the bed so the area can be flood irrigated.

Pre-Sowing Seed Processing

Seeds are put into a rice polishing machine or similar processing to scarify them prior to sowing; this process is essential. Seeds can be processed this way until they appear yellow-white. The critical moment is when the size of the seeds has lost its uniformity. Immediately sieve the seeds to separate them away from the remains of the seed coating and broken seeds. If there are seeds that have not been fully processed, continue until they have all been processed. Fully processed seeds are then placed in 40°C water to soak for 2–4 hours. After this period the seeds are rinsed clean of all viscus liquids and are ready for sowing.

Sowing Seeds Timing and Method

Seeds are sown in late April and early May, when the average daytime temperature has risen above

5°C. Diammonium phosphate is spread on the land at a rate of 90 kg per acre prior to sowing seeds.

When done by hand, 3–4 cm deep rows are dug every 20 cm, seeds are scattered in the small trench and covered with 1–3 cm. In geographical areas where dust storms are possible, the thickest covering is suggested. Seeds are often sown mechanically in large production areas.

Management of Seedling Beds

Seedlings are top-dressed once or twice, both soil application and foliar feeding are acceptable. Irrigating after top-dressing is important. Generally, weeding is performed twice during the growing season. Cultivation can be done when seedlings reach about 10 cm tall, loosening the soil to a depth of 3 cm.

TRANSPLANTING

Preparing the Soil

Either level or sloped land can be used, however a tree windbreak is important, along with an irrigation canal (for flood irrigation). Plow deeply in the autumn of the year prior to transplanting, harrow smooth, and prepare canals. Prepare the beds in the area according the needs of the land. A layer of thermal manure compost is spread evenly on the surface of the bed and raked or harrowed in evenly. Finally, the beds are irrigated.

Digging Seedlings

Starting the day before transplanting, dig a deep trench along the side of each bed, deep enough that the entire seedling root can be removed in its entirety. The root should be at least 30 cm long; do not cut the root. Seedlings are examined, discarding diseased or weak plants, then they are bound in bundles of 100–200 plants for ease of handling and transport to the field. Protect seedlings from drying out through exposure to heat or sun during digging and transporting. Before transplanting, examine seedlings again to ensure they are all healthy and free of any signs of disease or physical damage.

Transplanting Timing and Method

Transplanting and sowing seeds are done at the same time. Growing *gāncǎo* can be done on both level and slopped areas. On level fields a 10 cm trench is dug and roots are laid flat in the trench every 10–15 cm, covered with soil, then that soil is pressed firmly. On slopped fields a 20 cm trench is dug and the roots are laid in the trench with the head of the root staying about 2 cm below the level of the soil. Roots are planted every 10–15 cm within the row, roots are covered with soil, then firmly depressed. Generally, *gāncǎo* is planted in rows 25–30 cm apart with 10–15 cm spacing; approximately 12,000 plants are planted per acre.

Measures taken after transplanting to protect the seedling: The most importing measure is not to allow the plants to dry out. As soon as the soil begins to dry at the surface, the area should be watered to allow the water to penetrate. This is especially true when transplanting in the autumn.

FIELD MANAGEMENT

Cultivation and Weeding

Generally, cultivation and weeding is done 3 times per year. The first time is in late May. Again, when the plants have reached a height of approximately 30 cm cultivation and weeding is combined with fertilization. Finally, around mid-July when the plants have reached approximately 40 cm, cultivation and weeding are done for the third and final time. Always weed in a timely fashion.

Irrigation and Top-Dressing

Flood irrigation or sprinklers may be used, and they both work well for this plant.

When growing *gāncǎo* do not water too frequently; three times annually is generally considered enough. About 10 days after transplanting assess the soil moisture content, and, depending on conditions, the fields can be watered again once. In late June top-dressing followed by watering is performed once. After this, depending on rain and other weather factors, a final watering is done along with a final top-dressing of fertilizer; there is no set time for this, it is entirely weather dependent.

Gāncǎo is fertilized once or twice during the season by top-dressing, depending on the conditions of the soil it is planted in; if the soil condition is good, once is sufficient.

PREVENTION AND TREATMENT OF DISEASE AND INSECT PESTS

Principles of Prevention and Treatment

Growing *gāncǎo* in China has specific challenges that may not pose a problem for growers in other countries. Specifically, the Gancao Cochineal is native to China and is not likely to be present in other regions. However, other potential pathogens or pests could exist that are not addressed here.

Rust (*Uromyces glycyrrhizae*)

Prevention and Treatment

During autumn any and all diseased plants should be removed and burned. Always be careful to removed weeds, drain excess water, and be sure that there is good air flow and light penetration in the fields.

Powdery Mildew (*Oidium sp.*)

Prevention and Treatment

Immediately remove any diseased plants. Use appropriate spacing when transplanting into the field (*do not plant too close*). Use organic fertilizer, paying attention to nitrogen, phosphorus, and potassium; using suitable methods to increase the amounts of trace nutrients in the soil. Do not use excess nitrogen. Be sure to use a grass family cover crop.

Brown Spot Disease (*Cercospora astragalis*)

Prevention and Treatment

Remove all above-ground portions of the plant during the autumn, including all fallen leaves and dispose of them properly.

Leaf Bettles (*Diorhbda tarsalis*)

Prevention and Treatment

Improve field management, irrigate during winter, and remove withered and fallen leaves.

Gancao Cochineal (*Porphyrophora sophorae*)

Prevention and Treatment

Timely clearing of leaves and other withered herbaceous matter surrounding fields.

HARVESTING

Growing Period Before Harvest

Gāncǎo is harvested after at least 4 years of growth.

Harvest Season

Gāncǎo is harvested both in the spring and autumn, however spring harvested roots are considered the highest quality.

Standard for Assessing When to Harvest

When the root and rhizome have reached a diameter of 0.5 cm and a length of 20 cm, this is generally an indication that it is large enough for harvest. However, assessment of the chemistry is usually done on large farms to ensure quality, particularly assays for glycyrrhizin (>2.0%) and liquiritin (>0.5%). When these standards are met, there is no need to grade the roots by size.

Harvesting Method

Prior to digging, the above ground portions are cut away with an appropriate tool. Then, along either side of the plant a 45–50 cm deep trench is dug. When the root and rhizome are removed from the soil, any remaining above ground portions are cut away, any chunks of soil attached are removed, and the material is laid in the sun to dry. On large tracts of land, a plow is used by plowing on one side of the bed approximately 40 cm deep. The roots are removed with hand tools. Specialized plows are sometimes employed to dig the roots and rhizomes.

Special Precautions

When digging roots try to avoid the following: damaging the root skin and washing the roots with water. Soil should be removed by other means, not with water.

ON-FARM PROCESSING

Initial Processing and Drying

The area used for drying should be spacious, clean, and sunny. Roots are first carefully inspected to separate any foreign matter and soil. Using a sharp knife any herbaceous portions left at the crown of the root should be cut away. All thin fibrous or lateral roots are removed and discarded. The roots are then carefully examined for damage due to cold, insects, or other pathogens; any roots that show any sign of damage should be discarded.

Preparing Roots for Classification

Using a sharp knife or clippers, remove and discard thin fibrous roots and the root-heads, along with any remaining soil or foreign matter. All root sections that are damaged or diseased should also be cut away and discarded.

Classification

"Twig *gāncǎo*" is processed by removing all of the heads and thin-fibrous lateral rootlets, and is then divided by size. This is the material seen most commonly on the market.

"Ungraded *gāncǎo*" material is the same as the above, but has not been divided by size.

"Hairy *gāncǎo*" has not been processed as above, or all the parts are mixed together.

Drying

Roots are lined up according to their shape so that they dry evenly. They are dried in the sun, or in a drying house. When drying, roots should be placed on a wooden or similar platform. Do not lay roots directly on the ground. Be sure to protect them from rain or morning dew. Dried roots should not exceed 12% moisture.

大别山百合

Lily Bulb
Lilium lancifolium

DISTINGUISHING FEATURES

The daodi herb *dàbiéshān bǎihé* (*Lilium lancifolium* Thunb.), commonly known as *bǎihé* (百合) in China, is a member of the lily family (Liliaceae), a family famous the world over for its beautiful and fragrant flowers often sold in flowers shops. The genus is very large and found throughout much of the world and is easily recognized by its colorful and ornamental flowers. The dried bulb scale is the medicinal part employed and the daodi area is in the mountains of northern Anwei and southern Hubei provinces.

This medicinal plant is also commonly used as a food. It can be found in a number of dishes in China, perhaps the most famous of which is a cold dish with sautéed celery, but it is also common in hot dishes and is frequently used in porridge recipes. In clinical Chinese medicine this herb is known for its ability to supplement lung qi, clear lung heat, and moisten the lung. It is commonly used during the dry autumn weather, boiled with pear, to help counteract the affect of the dry weather on the lungs. In medicine it is most commonly used to treat dry cough, although it is also an important medicinal used to clear the heart and calm the spirit, and nourish heart yin. Due to the latter set of functions, it is frequently used for anxiety disorders and sleeplessness.

There has been very little modern research on this herb, however some of its traditional uses have been supported with experiments suggesting anti-inflammatory activity in the lungs that may even potentially alleviate some of the negative effects of cigarette smoke when the herb is consumed prior to exposure to smoke.

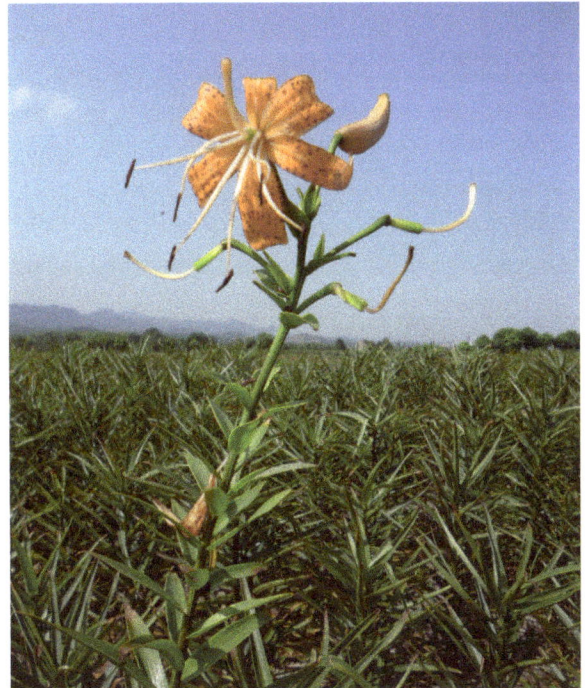

Contributing Authors

Duan Jin-ao, Qian Da-wei,
Yan Hui, Nie Hui

PRODUCTION SITE ECOLOGY

Elevation

Bǎihé is cultivated between 100–800 m elevation.

Temperature

Average temperatures within mountainous areas are 14.2–16.1°C.

Rainfall

Annual rainfall should be between 130–1800 mm.

Soil

Yellow-brown and brown soil with either sandy or clay soils are advantageous. Soils with high nutrient content, local hydrothermal conditions, and good water penetration are exceptional. Slightly acidic loam or sandy loam is ideal with pH 5.0–6.5, and soil organic matter content above 1.5% is best.

Topography

Bǎihé cultivation is best done in the basins and valleys within a mountain range.

PRODUCTION AREA ENVIRONMENTAL REQUIREMENTS

Site Selection

The site should have a deep layer of soil that is loose, drains well, and is slightly acidic. If the land was previously cropped, plants such as squash, beans, or paddy crops are acceptable. Avoid areas that may have previously grow Liliaceae family plants, and avoid continuous cropping.

Soil Preparation

Deeply plow, build beds 150–200 cm wide, with pathways that are 25–30 cm wide and 30–50 cm deep. Finally, use a cultivator to level and smooth the bed. Organic compost is applied at 15,000–18,000 kg per acre, cake fertilizer at 300–450 kg per acre, or general NPK fertilizer at 300–600 kg per acre. Compost or cake fertilizer should be tilled into the soil to incorporate it, while standard chemical fertilizer

should be added to ditches between the rows of planted seeds (8–10 cm deep). Do not allow the seed to come into immediate contact with fertilizer.

SOWING SEEDS & RAISING SEEDLINGS

Seed Quality Requirements

Seeds are collected in late August. A single plant has 3–5 flowering heads, bulbs should weigh 25–40 g, and should have no disease, visible insects, or rotting.

Sowing Seeds

Seeds are sown from mid-September through mid-November, do not plant them any later than mid-November. *Bǎihé* seeds are sown at a rate of 1200–1800 kg per acre. Seeds are often soaked in a general anti-fungal solution for 20–30 minutes, then dried in the shade before sowing. Trenches 25–30 cm apart are dug and seeds are sown, covering them with about 1–2 cm of soil. Bulbs are planted in the same manner, but should be buried with about 8 cm of soil and spaced 20–25 cm apart. Each acre should have 720,000-900,000 plants. After planting either seeds or bulbs, the field should be covered with straw at a rate of 2100–2400 kg per acre, to a depth of 3–4 cm. This will preserve moisture and temperature for the emerging plants.

FIELD MANAGEMENT

Cultivation and Weeding

Cultivation and weeding should begin when the seedlings reach 10 cm tall. During cultivation, great care must be taken around the plant, making sure that the soil is broken up well and all the weeds are removed without digging too deeply or damaging the seedling in any way. The seedling is very delicate, even small clods of dirt can hold down a young seedling and cause significant damage.

Irrigation and Top-Dressing

Bǎihé does not like to be waterlogged, and care must be taken to not allow water to accumulate in the field; therefore, site drainage must be carefully monitored, digging more drainage when necessary. When the seedlings have reached approximately 10 cm, a fermented manure solution or a diluted urea

(1%) spray at a rate of 6000 kg per acre with an added 25–30 kg of NPK compound fertilizer is applied. If compost is available apply it directly to the beds. After new bulb scales have developed, add 30 kg per acre of potash, buried in ditches along each row. In late May a 0.3% solution of potassium dihydrogen phosphate combined with a 0.3% solution of urea should be applied as a foliar feeding 2–3 times at intervals of 10 days.

Collection of Aerial Bulbs

Collect after *bǎihé* begins to bud, and the flowers have begun to change color but have not opened. The bulbs inflate quickly, so this is the time to pinch off flowers. About 10 days after the flowers are pinched off, the purple-brown bulbils begin to form at the leaf axils. When the aerial bulbs are fully mature they should knock easily from the stalk, this is the time to collect them.

PREVENTION AND TREATMENT OF DISEASE AND INSECT PESTS

Principles of Prevention and Treatment

When growing from either seed or transplanting, plants that appear weak or sick should be removed, and prescribed methods of application of fertilizer, field management, as well as proper encouragement or application of biological controls (including but not limited to diversity of species) should be adhered to. The most common diseases are sheath blight, grey mold, and anthracnose. The most common insect pests are grubs.

Anthracnose (*Colletotrichum lilii*)

Prevention and Treatment

Crop rotation with a grass family plant for three or more years. Keep the field clean of foreign matter. Timely drainage of excess water from rain or irrigation.

Sheath Blight (*Rhizoctonia solani*)

Prevention and Treatment

Crop rotation with a grass family plant for two or more years. Use soil and seedlings that are free of disease and apply an appropriate amount of fertilizers. Increasing compost and phosphorus can be helpful. Immediately cull out diseased plants and use lime in holes of diseased plants.

Gray Mold (*Botrytis cinerea*)

Prevention and Treatment

Using seeds and bulbils that are free of disease is essential. Make sure the field has good air-flow and plenty of sun. Do not crowd plants. Timely removal of diseased plants will reduce over-all disease problems.

Grubs & other Soil-Born Insect Pests

Prevention and Treatment

Deep plowing and fine harrowing along with well-composted compost help to prevent serious outbreaks. Use lights to trap and kill adult insects.

HARVESTING

Growing Period Before Harvest

Plants are harvested at the end of the first season

Harvest Season

The best time to harvest is on a sunny day during mid- to late August when the plants have withered.

Harvesting Method

Choose a sunny day. Using a digging fork, dig the entire bulb and root portion of the plant. Cut away the withered stalk and the fibrous anchor roots. After digging, place bulbs out of the sun in a well-ventilated area to dry.

ON-FARM PROCESSING

Peeling

The bulb scales are generally separated by hand, but one can use a knife to slice the base of the bulb to assist in the separation of the scales from the main bulb.

Sorting

Bulb scales are sorted according to their appearance, thickness, and there location at the outside, middle, or inside of the entire structure. These are all then washed clean and drip dried.

Soaking

Place *bǎihé* bulb scales in a pot with clean water and boil for at least 2 hours. In order to judge readiness, pick a big piece out and break it, then use a finger nail to pinch the inside; no sound should be heard. Drain and dry. Divide the bulb scale into categories of large and small for a second boiling process. Place 20–30 kg of bulb scales in the pot, with 100 L of water to just barely cover the herb. Use a stainless-steel rod to stir, making sure heat is evenly distributed. The bulb scales must be boiled again for 5 minutes (small bulb scales) to 10 min (large bulb scales). For this second boiling process, the bulb scales are added to already boiling water. When the edges of the bulb scales are soft and small cracks on the back side can be seen, remove them from the water, and rinse with cool water to wash away stickiness. Drain and dry. Each pot of water can be used 2–3 times for this process. When the water becomes unclear, it should be changed, then re-boil it to start a new round. Not

changing the water in this manner will negatively impact the color and quality of the herb.

Drying

Soaked pieces should not piled together; they should be spread out in the sun and dried immediately following the soaking process. Bulb scales can be flipped once when they are about 60% dry; choosing a clear day to dry completely is very important. If processing on a cloudy day, bulb scales should be put indoors in a room with good air-flow. Do not pile bulb scales as this will lead to the development of mold. Bulbs should be processed on the same day they are harvested, which should be on a clear, sunny day. External heating sources, such as a forced air drier can be employed if weather is inappropriate for sun drying. Many modern farms apply forced air-drying methods to process *bǎihé* to improve efficiency. When using this method, put drained bulb scales on trays, spread evenly without stacking, set in the drier, and use circulating hot air to dry. The temperature should be around 60–80°C. Bulbs are dried to 10% moisture. When physical examination yields a product that is hard but breaks easily with your hands, the drying process is done. Spread out in an appropriate location and allow to cool to room temperature.

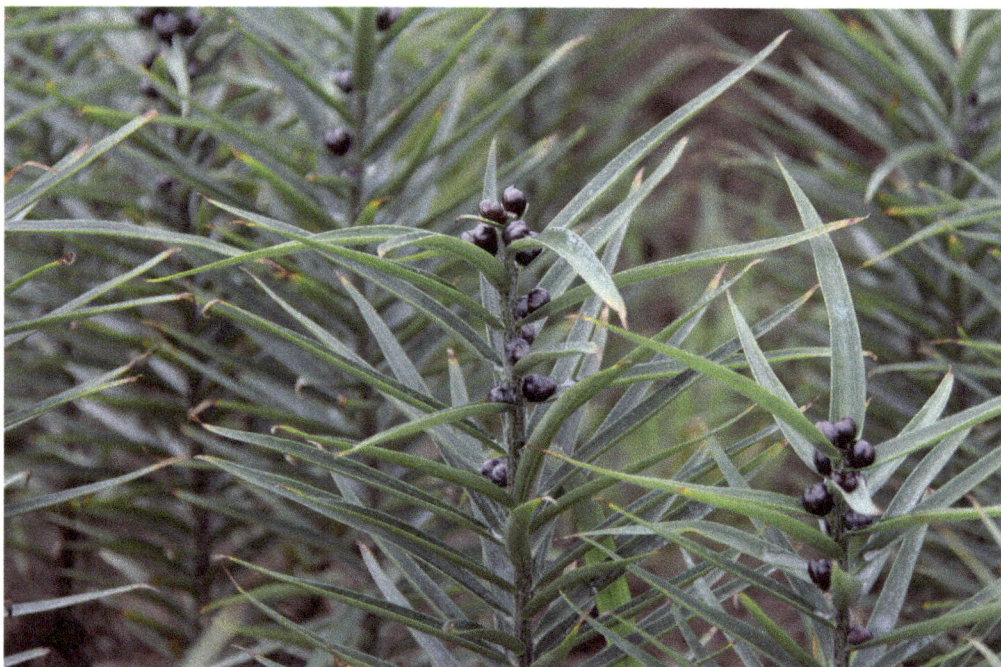

Aerial bulbs forming on *bǎihé* after the removal of flowers in Anwei province, China.

济银花
Honeysuckle Flower
Lonicera japonica

DISTINGUISHING FEATURES

This is the dried flower bud, or just opened flower, of the daodi herb *jì yínhuā* (*Lonicera japonica* Thunb.), known in China as *yínhuā* or *jīnyínhuā* (银花 \ 金银花), and is a member of the honeysuckle family (Caprifoliaceae). *Lonicera* is a genus with about 180 species in the northern temperate parts of the world. China has about 100 native species, this species grows throughout many areas of the country, as well as Korea and Japan, up to about 1500 m elevation. Material produced in Shandong Province in Linye, Jining, and surrounding area is considered the daodi medicinal for the cultivated *jìnyínhuā*. This plant is a known invasive species in both North America and Europe. This species should be properly managed to avoid escape and potential damage to the surrounding ecosystem.

This herb was first mentioned in materia medica literature during the Song dynasty (1220). Traditionally, *jìnyínhuā* has two primary actions: clear heat and resolve toxin, and clear heat and resolve the exterior. As such, it is used in many formulas for wind-heat invasion and other similar diseases. It is a very versatile herb and is often found in formulas to clear heat from the interior of the body when there are symptoms such as fever, boils, diarrhea, and other inflammatory type diseases. The herb is also applied externally for heat, swelling, and toxins.

Modern science has found a wide range of pharmacological activities in the plant. The ethanolic extract helped to reduce inflammation in fatty livers of experimental rats. The herb is known to have anti-inflammatory, antiviral, antibacterial, hepatoprotective, antioxidant, anti-tumor, hypoglycemic, and antithrombotic activities. These results suggest potential application for a number of "modern" diseases such as diabetes, metabolic syndrome, etc.

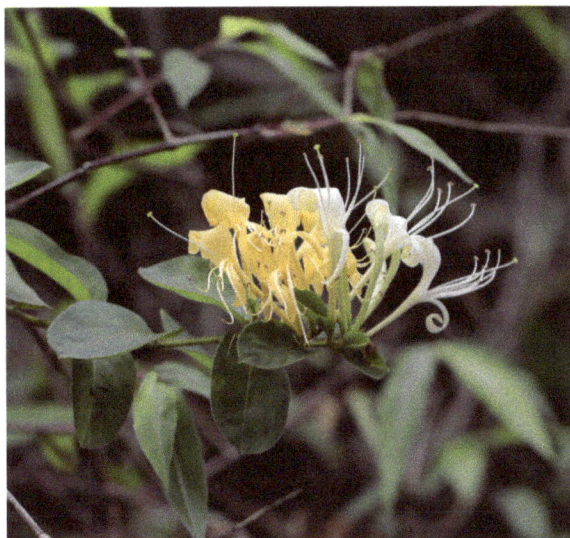

Contributing Authors

Huang Lu-qi, Guo Lan-ping,
Wang Xiao, Zhang Yan, Liu Wei,
Zhou Jie, Zhao Dong-yue, Hao Qing-xiu,
Sun Hai-feng, Zhang Xiao-bo

PRODUCTION SITE ECOLOGY

Elevation

Jīnyínhuā is cultivated between 50–1500 m elevation.

Temperature

The average annual temperature range is 13–16.7°C and the frost-free period is 150–230 days. During the flowering months, average sunshine is between 150–250 hours, with an average monthly temperature of 20–30°C.

Photo Period

Average annual sunshine ranges from 2290–2890 hours. Average daily sunshine is 58%.

Rainfall

Average annual rainfall is between 550–950 mm with an average monthly rainfall range during flowering at 40–220 mm.

Soil

Sandy-loam or loam soil with a deep layer of more than 60 cm. Soil pH should be neutral to slightly acid, a saline-alkaline soil can also be used for cultivation but is less desirable.

Topography

A southern, or at least half southerly gentle slope of less than 15 degrees is best; level areas can also be used.

PRODUCTION AREA ENVIRONMENTAL REQUIREMENTS

Site Selection

The soil layer should be deep with loose sandy-loam or loam soil. Water should drain easily.

Soil Preparation

Sometime between the end of February through the beginning of March the soil should be plowed deeply to more than 30 cm. This should be done in combination with the addition of 12,000–18,000 kg of well-composted manure or 1800–3000 kg of well-composted organic compost per acre. The addition of a NPK compound fertilizer is also recommended. Till in evenly and harrow smooth.

TAKING CUTTINGS FOR NEW PLANT STARTS

Quality Requirements

During the rainy season, cuttings are taken from the sections of the plant that are red (fresh growth) and have strong-thick wood development on the branch. A section of 20 cm should be cut (each section should have 2–3 nodes) with sharp, clean pruning shears and the leaves should be removed. Cuttings should only be taken from healthy mother plants that are free of disease.

Storage and Preservation of Cuttings

Cuttings may be stored at atmospheric temperature, in the shade, under moist conditions for up to one week, but it is best to plant them as soon as possible.

Nursery Area Selection and Preparation

The nursery has the same soil and drainage requirements as noted above, however 18,000 kg of well-composted manure or 3000 kg of organic fertilizer per acre are tilled into the soil before harrowing and building nursery beds.

Planting Cuttings

Cuttings are taken from August through October. Cuttings are planted at a rate of 48,000–60,000 per acre at a spacing of 20×10 cm. After planting, the cuttings should be watered; be sure the soil does not dry out. Once cuttings are in the ground, maintaining constant moisture levels is extremely important; weed as necessary.

Transplanting

Now rooted transplants are dug during early to mid-March and prepared for transplanting to a permanent location. After digging, any new shoots and buds are cut off and all leaves are removed (leaving 10 cm of the lower branch with the roots). After culling any low-quality cuttings, they are bundled in packs of 100 and stored in a shady area. It is best to wrap the roots with jut or other similar material and keep lightly moist during this storage period.

Transplanting into Field

Jīnyínhuā transplanting time is quite long, they may be transplanted any time between August and April, as long as the soil is not frozen. The best time is during the rainy season or early spring. Rooted cuttings are spaced from 1.2×1.5 m to 1.4×1.7 m apart in the field, at a depth of 30–50 cm, according the length of the roots. Dig each hole so that the sub-soil below and soil surrounding the hole is loosened before adding 5–7 kg of well-composted organic compost and mixing it into the soil. The top portion of the stem should be 15 cm below the top of the hole when planting, then covered with 5 cm of soil (this will leave a 10 cm indentation in the soil where it can easily be watered). Press the soil down firmly and water thoroughly; do not allow to dry out.

FIELD MANAGEMENT

Cultivation and Weeding

Cultivation and weeding should be done at the same time. Remove all weeds in a timely manner, especially around the holes where the plant is emerging; be careful of the tender shoots while working. Deeper cultivation can be used to ensure soil stays loose, always being careful of roots.

Irrigation and Top-Dressing

During its critical growth periods, e.g. after planting and during the spring and early summer, if there are dry spells *jīnyínhuā* should be thoroughly irrigated. Generally, each autumn in late October plants are fertilized with well-composted manure at a rate of 12,000 kg and 300 kg of NPK compound fertilizer per acre. When applying these amendments, the soil around the plants is loosened and the amendments are thoroughly combined into the soil. During the vigorous growth period, 120 kg of ammonium bicarbonate per acre is applied and immediately watered in. Also, potassium dihydrogen phosphate (diluted 500:1 in water) and a foliar trace mineral application (diluted 1000:1 in water, or according to the manufacturers specifications) can be sprayed on the plants at this time. Make sure that water drains properly after irrigation or heavy rains.

Pruning

Plants are pruned every year between late December and very early spring, prior to any bud-swell. Using a sharp pair of cutters, each branch should be cut by 1/3 to 1/2, leaving 3–4 sections on the branch where new growth can spring forth. Remove any small, rapid growing, spindly growth. Remove any diseased or insect infected growth including, dry, very thin, overlapping, entangled, or otherwise unhealthy branches. In the spring, remove any new sprouts coming from the main stem. Generally, a light trimming is also done after the harvest, but this is not always necessary.

PREVENTION AND TREATMENT OF DISEASE AND INSECT PESTS

Principles of Prevention and Treatment

The most common diseases affecting *jīnyínhuā* include, brown-spot disease, powdery mildew, leaflet disease, yellow leaf disease, fusarium wilt, etc., but these are not usually very serious and are relatively easily treated. Be sure to keep the area free from other diseased material and remove diseased plants in a timely manner. Make sure to keep weeds under control and soil around the plants properly aerated using the prescribed methods.

Aphids (Aphidoidea)

Prevention and Treatment

During the winter months it is important to clear and remove excessive weeds, dead branches, and other material that may be a vector for disease. Winter plowing is often performed to loosen soil and integrate well-composted manure. A lime-sulfur compound (used as recommended by the manufacturer) is sometimes applied once to the plant in the winter or very early spring before it has begun to bud.

Cotton Bullworm (*Helicoverpa armigera*)

Prevention and Treatment

All the same measures mentioned above for aphids can also be applied to bollworm. Additionally, corn or other crops that are likely to lure the bollworm to it can be grown in the vicinity to reduce damage to the *jīnyínhuā* crop. Interplanting of garlic or onions can also be helpful because the pungent odor of these plants tends to deter bollworms.

Biological Controls

Use 0.15% solution of *Bacillus thuringiensis* (Bt) in a spray in the afternoon (standard concentration is 8000 iu/mg).

HARVESTING

Harvest Season

Starting in the second year after transplanting cuttings, plants are usually harvested every year. *Jīnyínhuā* can be harvested during its four flowering periods during the year. 1) During early to mid-May, 2) during mid-June, 3) during mid- to late July, 4) during the month of August. Sometimes, the third period does not have significant flowering and yield may be low.

Harvest Method

Using one hand to hold the branch, use your other hand to pick the flower buds and put into an appropriate container. [Translator's Note: A basket

or other breathable container is best. Do not pile excessive amounts into the container when harvesting as this can damage the flower buds.

ON-FARM PROCESSING

Garbling

Prior to drying, remove any damaged flowers, leaves, or other debris.

Drying Method

Drying can be done either in the sun or in forced air driers. Forced air driers are preferred for high-quality finished product.

Sun Drying: Flowers should be spread out evenly on drying racks, avoiding stacking, and can be dried either in the sun or shade. Flowers should be disturbed frequently to ensure even drying. Avoid excessive heat, which will lower the quality of the herb. If drying outside, do not allow them to get wet from rain, dew, or to be otherwise affected by damp-cold weather conditions.

Drying Ovens: Place fresh flowers in a drying unit at 3–5 cm thickness, setting at a temperature between 40–50°C. The dried flower buds must have less than 12% moisture content.

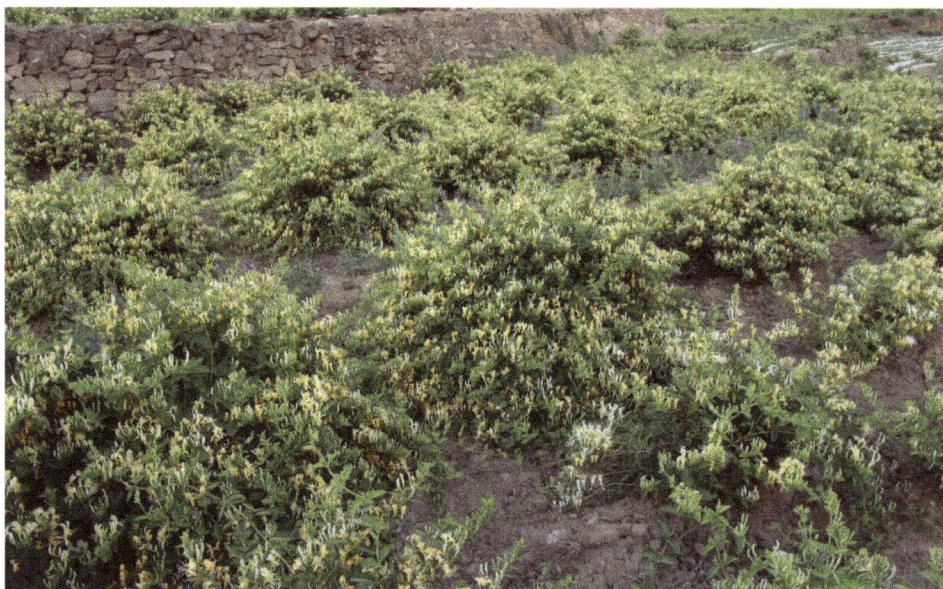

Commercial production of *jīnyínhuā* outside of Jining, Shandong province, China.

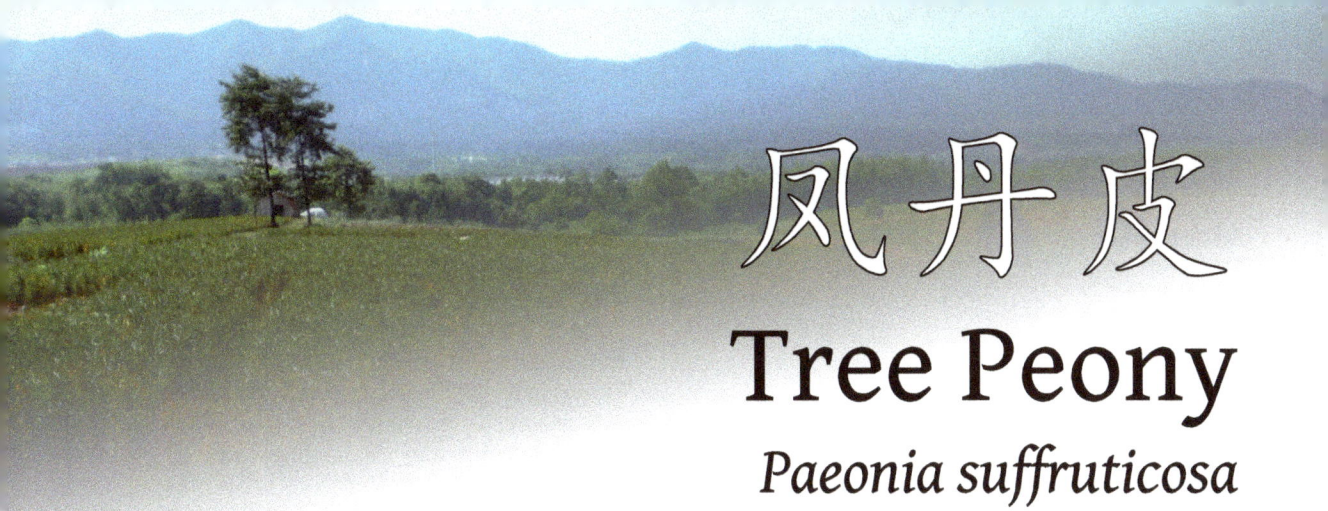

凤丹皮

Tree Peony

Paeonia suffruticosa

The dried root bark of the daodi herb *fēng dānpí* (*Paeonia suffruticosa* Andr.) is commonly known in China as *dānpí* (丹 皮) or occasionally *mǔdānpí* (牡 丹皮) or just *mǔdān* when emphasizing that this plant is a member of the peony family (Paeoniaceae) (*mǔdān* means peony). This plant family only has a single genus with about 30 species, half are native to China and one-third are endemic. This species takes a shrub form (as opposed to an herb form) and can still be found occasionally in the wild on cliffs; it is extensively cultivated around the world. It is native to central Anhui and western Henan provinces. In this text, *fēng dānpí* refers to the medicinal materials produced in Tongling and Nanling counties and the surrounding areas in Anhui province.

This herb has been used in medicine for over 2000 years and holds a prominent place in Chinese culture. The plant has been recorded in poetry and other literature throughout Chinese history and is a common subject of Chinese art. The herb is primarily used to clear heat and cool the blood when heat has entered the blood aspect with symptoms of bleeding due to frenetic movement of the blood. It also quickens the blood and can be found in many formulas for the treatment of menstrual disorders including painful menstruation and stopped menstruation due to heat.

Modern research has validated most of the traditional uses of *dānpí* but there is still a lot of work to be done. Laboratory confirmed activities include anti-oxidant actions, including applications for cigarette smoke-induced lung inflammation; anti-inflammatory effects, that can positively affect arthritis and liver inflammation; anti-tumor actions; and cardiovascular protective actions. It has also been shown to ameliorate acute myocardial infarction in rats and inhibit platelet aggregation and blood coagulation; it is potentially useful for diabetes, positively altering glucose uptake and preventing the development of nephropathy; and it has hepatoprotective and neuroprotective effects, mainly via anti-oxidant and anti-inflammatory activities.

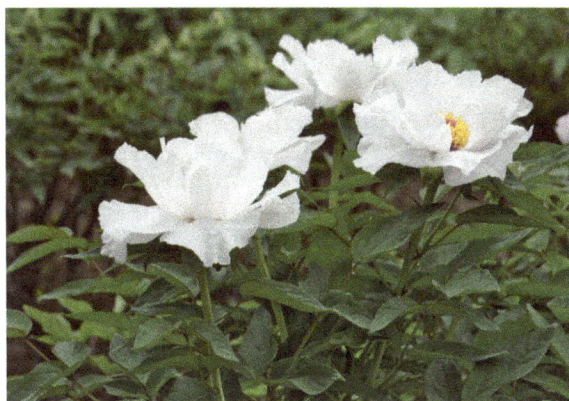

Contributing Authors

*Xie Dong-mei, Fang Cheng-wu,
Liu Shou-jin, Ji Kai-ming,
Jin Chuan-shan, Wu De-ling*

PRODUCTION SITE ECOLOGY

Elevation

Cultivation of *dānpí* works best in hilly or low mountainous areas with an elevation of 50–300 m.

Temperature

Growing *dānpí* is best in areas with an annual average temperature of 16–18°C. The area should have four distinct seasons and an annual average frost-free period of around 258 days.

Photo Period

Dānpí requires an average of 2000–2100 hours of annual sunshine, of which the most hours are accumulated in July and August, and the least in March.

Moisture

Dānpí requires an average rainfall of 1200 mm or more.

Soil

Cultivation of this plant is suitable in sandy loam soil (sandy soil), gneissic yellow laterite, thick, fine, yellow-red soil and middle gravel yellow-red soil; soil in sandy soil should be rich with organic matter, with a loose texture and slightly viscous. Soil must be acidic to slightly alkaline, and be able to retain water, not heavily compacted, low in sodium, and lo-cated on low lying land.

Topography

Sunlit areas on high terrain where water is easily drained and there is a slight slope to the south. The area should be easily irrigated with good drainage.

PRODUCTION AREA ENVIRONMENTAL REQUIREMENTS

Site Selection

Selected soil for field cultivation has a deep, loose texture that is slightly sticky, is able to retain water, and is a slightly acidic to slightly alkaline fertile sandy soil. Soil that is too sticky, too sandy, retains too much water, or has poor fertility should not be used. A site that has previously grown crops such as corn, peanuts, sorghum, sesame, etc. is considered best.

Soil Preparation

The land is plowed at least 30 cm deep in the autumn, winter or spring after 12,000 kg per acre of fully composted manure or 1800–3000 kg of other bio-organic fertilizer has been applied to the land. The ground is then harrowed level. Beds are built 40–80 cm wide and 25 cm high with 25 cm wide pathways between the beds.

SOWING SEEDS & RAISING SEEDLINGS

Seed Quality Requirements

Seeds are collected from late July to mid-August from plants that have grown for at least 3 years. Fruits are harvested when they turn yellow but before they split open, they must be full of seeds and be free of pests and diseases. The seeds are ripened in the husk until the husk breaks apart. Seeds begin a yellow-green color then turn to brown then black. Once they have all turned black, the seeds are removed from the husk. Seeds are placed in sand in single layers, then a layer of sand is added (about the thickness of the seeds), then more seeds, etc. The sand should have approximately 60% moisture (an easy test for this moisture content is to firmly grasp the sand, it should not have water dripping from it and should stay clumped after loosening one's grip). This process should be done in a cool dry area with good air circulation, where the seeds may be stored until they are planted.

Nursery Selection and Bed Preparation

The area should have irrigation available. Remove any grass or weeds, apply 12,000 kg per acre of composted manure, and plow deeply at least 30 cm, harrow and rake level.

Breeding

Before sowing seeds, it is necessary to stratify the seeds. The seeds are placed in a temperature range of 18–22°C for 30–40 days, then placed in a temperature range of 10–12°C for 30 days or 0–5°C for 20 days. After this process seeds are soaked in water, only seeds that swell and sink to the bottom are used, this should only take 1-2 hours. One-thousand seeds should weight 190–200 grams. Seeds that have not been sown in the current year may be placed in moist sand and stored in a cool place to be used the following year. Seeds should not be stored more than 2 years.

Sowing Seeds

Sow seeds in early September to early October. Seeds are sown at a rate of 360 kg per acre when row planting and 300 kg per acre when planting with a seed drill; broad cast sowing is done at a rate of 540 kg per acre. The soil should be moist when planting seed, therefore if it is dry it needs to be irrigated prior to sowing seed. Beds are built 80-100 cm wide with 10-15 cm deep pathways between rows. On each bed, rows should be 6-9 cm apart and seeds planted at a depth of 5 cm. Alternately, seeds can be planted on top of the bed and then covered with 3-5 cm of soil. Prior to sprouting and when the seedlings are young it is especially important to remember that moisture must be maintained in the soil, as plants will easily wither and die if the soil dries. If the temperature is expected to get very low or if the seeds were planted relatively late, agricultural film should be used to cover the bed. [Translator's Note: Agricultural film is most frequently used on the beds after sowing seeds. However, the use of this technique is not recommended due to the plastic waste and pollution it produces. Therefore, it is recommended to use straw or another appropriate mulch.]

Seedling Management

After sowing, roots should grow to 0.5 cm within 40–50 days and should achieve 7-10 cm within 90 days. By this time there may be threat of a freeze, so in order to protect the young plants the beds are covered with 3-5 cm thick humus soil or decomposed manure; plant-based mulch (such as straw) can also be used. After sowing, check the seedbed often for moisture content and germination. Depending on the amount of rain over the winter, you may need to maintain soil moisture with sprinkler irrigation. After the second year when the ground has thawed in the spring, promptly remove mulching and other coverings to facilitate the digging of seedlings for transplanting. Timely removal of weeds and maintenance of soil moisture is critical for seedling development. During the seedling cultivation period, a 0.02–0.05% compost solution is made and the equivalent of 1800–2400 kg of animal waste compost is applied per acre during the spring (late March and late April) and again in late summer (late June to early July), varying the amount based on the growth of the seedlings.

Seedling Development

Seedlings should be harvested in early September to late October (better in early October before it gets too cold); choose fully matured robust, pest-free roots and buds of at least 2-year-old seedlings, excluding sick seedlings and other substandard seedlings; separate the bigger seedlings from the smaller ones before tying them into bundles of 100 plants for transportation to the main field.

Transplanting to the Field

Transplanting is carried out in early September to late October. Large seedlings and small seedlings are planted in different field settings, but using the same technique. Rows are separated by 35×40 cm. Holes are dug lengthwise to a depth of about 10 cm and length of 20–25 cm, with two seedlings placed at opposite ends of each hole. *Dānpí* can be grown at a rate of 30,000 per acre, therefore seedlings need to be planted at a rate of 60,000 per acre. When planting a seedling, the root should be fully stretched out and tilted toward the slope. The buds should be at ground level and covered with soil, which should be gently compressed then covered with straw mulch.

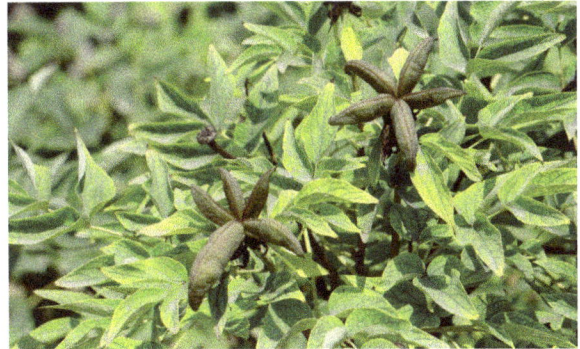

Swelling seed capsules on *dānpí*.

FIELD MANAGEMENT

Cultivation and Weeding

Cultivating the soil and weeding is generally done in the early rainy season to help loosen the soil and ensure the top of the soil is not compacted. During cultivation, make sure not to damage the roots. Before winter has settled in, it is necessary to hill-up soil around plants to prevent frost from damaging the roots.

Fertilizing and Irrigation

Fertilizers mainly include organic fertilizers, supplemented by trace element fertilizers; the use of nitrate fertilizer is prohibited. Organic fertilizers include mature animal manure compost, cake fertilizer, crop stalks, and so on. The traditional organic fertilizers were mainly decomposed cake fertilizer. The cake fertilizer is applied before budding (mid- to late February), compound fertilizer is applied after flowering (mid-June), and organic fertilizer around the time winter is setting in (October-November). The amount of phosphorus can be increased during the critical period of growth, since potassium fertilizer is conducive to improving the yield and quality of this medicinal plant. If using chemical fertilizers, they should be combined with organic fertilizer. Use 600 kg cake fertilizer, 15,000–18,000 kg manure, and 300–360 kg NPK fertilizer per acre. Fertilizers are applied around the plant about 10 cm from the root of the plant at a depth of 5–10 cm. Fertilizers can also be applied in a shallow ditch between the rows, which is then covered with soil and watered in. In case of drought in the growing season, ditch irrigation can be used in the morning or evening. After enough water has infiltrated, the remaining water can be promptly drained away. Irrigation is best done after the application of a thin layer of manure is applied, this will to enhance drought resistance.

Bud Removal

Flower buds are removed from plants for the first 1–2 years after transplanting to help reduce nutrient consumption. Choose a sunny day in early March, after the morning dew dries, using a sharp knife or pruners, carefully remove the flower buds.

Pruning

Before the end of autumn or beginning of winter, cut off thin or weak single stems at the base. This will encourage strong new growth in the following spring. Plants should have 3–5 stout branches. This process also promotes thick roots and increases production.

Exposing Roots to Sun

In April to May of the 3rd or 4th year, choose a clear sunny day to expose roots to the sun. Open the soil to allow sunlight to hit the roots, allow them to be exposed for 2–3 days to promote the growth of the root bark. Remove any roots that are diseased, have pests, or appear dead. Select 2–3 main roots that are thick, without a hollow center, and free of disease or pests to remain as the final medicinal. These roots will form buds that can be removed and transplanted for growing the next crop of *dānpí*.

PREVENTION AND TREATMENT OF DISEASE AND INSECT PESTS

Principles of Prevention and Treatment

Diseases of *dānpí* include rotting of the main root, spots on the leaves, gray mold disease, Sclerotium, purple line feather disease, and underground pests such as the python toad, and cutworm larvae. Most of these diseases are best managed with good water drainage and proper airflow in the field. Do not plant too closely together and pay close attention to areas that may pool water in heavy rainfall events; drain immediately if water stagnates.

Underground Pests (*Agrotis* sp., *Holotrichia* sp.)

Prevention and Treatment

Cultivate in winter and harrow finely to kill the source of insects and reduce the number of larvae. Also use fully matured organic compost. Before mature insects emerge, use light traps.

Peony Blotch (*Cladosporium paeoniae*)

Prevention and Treatment

Keep the area clean, avoiding dead or dying material on the ground around the plants. A grass family plant should be used as a crop rotation for at least three years before planting again. Use appropriate organic fertilizer, like phosphorus and potassium fertilizer. Spraying a 0.2–0.3% solution of potassium dihydrogen phosphate can be helpful.

Biological Controls

Pay attention to planting density, control of soil moisture, usage of compound and organic fertilizer, and appropriate amount of nitrogen fertilizer. Be mindful of observing disease and finding diseased plants. Dispose of diseased leaves immediately and carry out field and disease treatment as noted above.

Botrytis Fungus (*Botrytis* sp.)

Prevention and Treatment

Immediately remove known diseased leaves and diseased plants; once the disease begins to spread it is extraordinarily difficult to resolve with chemical remedies; therefore, diligence is required.

Southern Blight (*Sclerotium rolfsii*)

Prevention and Treatment

This disease occurs before and after blooming, during high temperatures and rainy season, and is considered a serious disease. It is a soilborne fungal disease that produces abundant white mycelium. Control methods include using rice or grass rotation. Diseased plants should be immediately removed, burn the soil, and treat sick areas with lime treatment.

Violet Root Rot Fungus (*Helicobasidium mompa*)

Prevention and Treatment

Crop rotation including corn, soybeans, and other crops is necessary. Strengthen field management, be vigilant about timely elimination of excessive field water, and thoroughly remove litter and burn it to reduce the source of disease. Diseased plants should be promptly removed, and 5% lime solution sprayed on the area for disinfection.

Root Rot (*Fusarium* sp.)

Prevention and Treatment

A crop rotation should be used for more than two years between harvest and planting of this herb. Use of a reasonable fertilizer formula, application of compost and cake fertilizer or an enzyme based compost is best; in extreme cases a compound fertilizer may be used. Use disease-free soil to cultivate seedlings and promptly remove seedlings if they become diseased. Use lime in the hole after removing the seedling to kill pathogens.

HARVESTING

Harvest Season

Transplant seedlings after 2 years, then cultivate the fields for 3–4 years before harvesting. Generally, in the spring and autumn, between autumn and the arrival of the first frost, which is generally from September to October every year, is considered the best time to harvest.

Harvest Method

On a sunny day, first rake away the yellow leaves on the ground, then dig around the root to expose the roots. The depth of digging is based on the length of the root, generally this is 30–50 cm. When digging, remove as much of the root as possible, then remove the soil from the roots. Do not dig and harvest roots during rainy periods or when the soil is wet.

ON-FARM PROCESSING

Grading and Sorting

After the fresh roots are dug out, remove non-medicinal parts such as the stems, soil, side-shoots, and other impurities. Cut away and discard any roots that are less than 0.5 cm in diameter.

Sweating

After sorting the roots, stack in a cool and ventilated place for 1–2 days for sweating, allowing the water to sweat from within the fresh roots. This process will help to separate the root bark from the woody center of the root and helps to ensure the root bark's appearance and medicinal quality.

Removing the Heart-Wood

After softening the root for removal of the heart-wood, grasp the root firmly and twist it to separate rootbark from the heart-wood. Once there is separation, one should be able to grasp a section of the heart-wood, if this is not possible, cut a small section of the bark away to expose a small section of the heart-wood. One hand twists the outer bark while another hand pinches the heart-wood. Continue this twisting motion until the heart-wood is completely separated from the rootbark, then pull the heart-wood free from the rootbark. After sorting the roots, stack in a cool and ventilated place for 1–2 days for sweating, allowing the water to sweat from within the fresh roots. This process will help to separate the root bark from the woody center of the root and helps to ensure the root bark's appearance and medicinal quality.

Drying Method

Choose a sunny day. After removing the heart-wood, place the root-bark in an open-air location exposed to the sun. During the drying process, protect the roots from exposure to rain and moisture, as such exposure will cause the roots to become red, which will negatively affect the quality of the final product. Final material should be below 12% moisture content.

Special Considerations

Dānpí has a strong aromatic smell, so it is best not to mix it with other herbs during transportation.

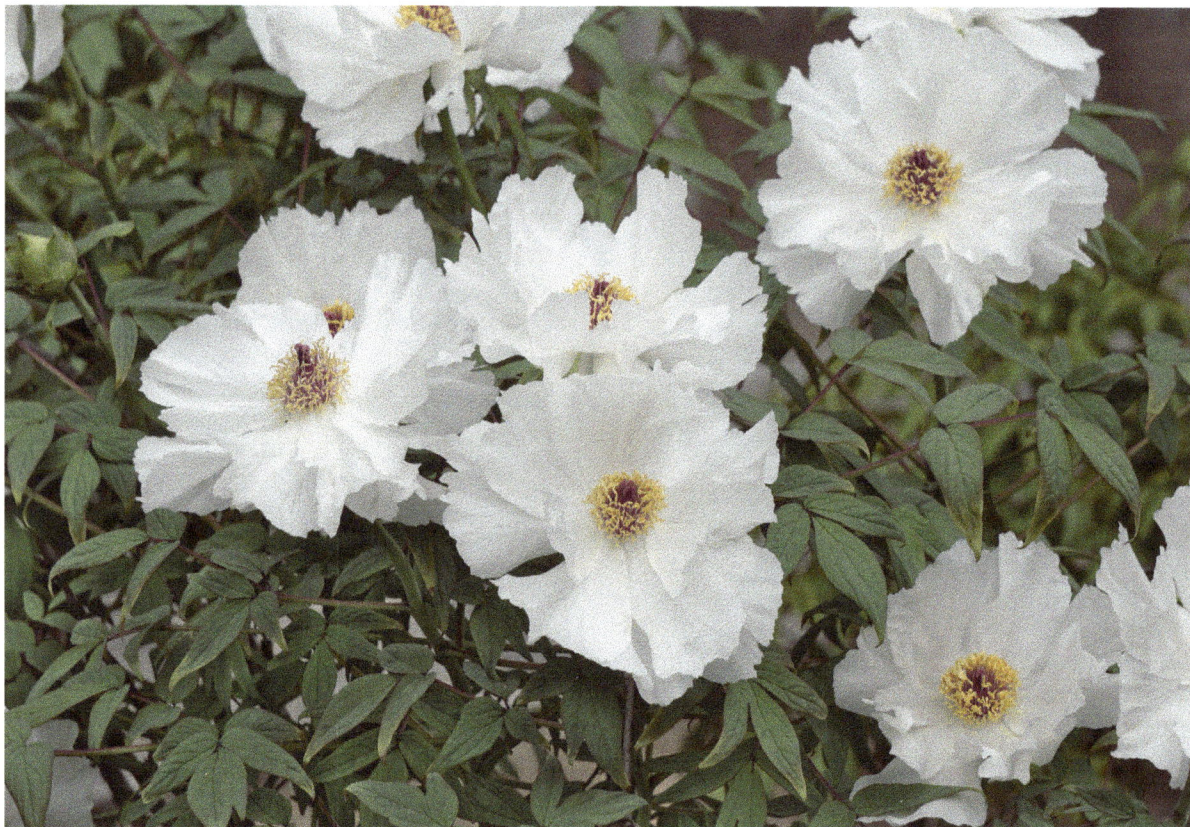

Flowering *dānpí* in Anwei province, China.

文山三七

Notoginseng

Panax notoginseng

DISTINGUISHING FEATURES

The dried root and rhizome of the daodi herb *wén-shān sānqī* (*Panax notoginseng* (Burk.) F.H.Chen), generally known as *sānqī* (三七) in China, is a member of the ginseng family (Araliaceae). This herb was native to southeast Yunnan and western Guangxi province, growing between 1200–1800 m, however there appear to be no remaining wild populations. The daodi location is in the southern part of Yunnan province in Wen-shan prefecture around Wenshan city, Yanshan county, Maguan county, and the surrounding area.

The history of *sānqī* is not very long, initially coming into use based on its traditional use in Guizhou for treating wounds due to swords and other weapons. It is the premier herb in Chinese medicine to stop bleeding and it also moves blood to treat pain. Therefore, it is most appropriate for bleeding conditions with blood stasis causing pain. Since *sānqī* is also warming, it is not appropriate for bleeding due to repletion heat patterns. Although *sānqī* is still the most important herb for stopping bleeding with concurrent stasis, its use has been expanded into gynecology, bi syndrome conditions, and it is especially popular for treating cardiovascular conditions in modern Chinese medicine.

Modern science has focused most research on *sānqī* and its activity on the cardiovascular system, yielding many positive outcomes. The herb and some of its constituents have shown promising results in protecting myocardial cells although the full mechanism of this action is still not completely understood. It

has shown potentially important protective effects for the endothelial cells lining the blood vessels. It exhibits an anti-atherosclerotic activity via at least three mechanisms. In addition to these, the traditional hemostatic and wound healing actions have been confirmed, along with anti-inflammatory, anti-oxidant, blood glucose lowering, neuroprotective, immune-stimulating, and certain renal- and hepato-protective activities that have been demonstrated either *in vivo* or *in vitro*.

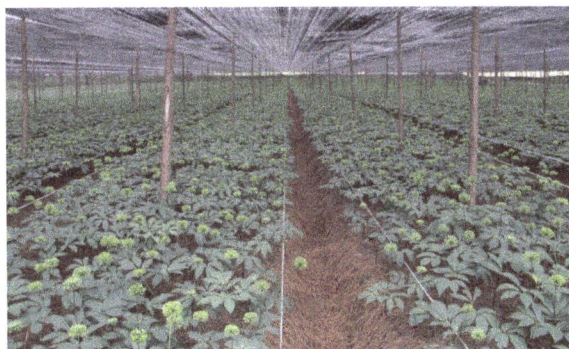

Contributing Authors

Zheng Yu-guang, Xie Xiao-liang, Guo Lan-ping, Huang Lu-qi, Hao Qing-xiu, Liu Ming, Song Jun-nuo, Wen Chun-xiu, Liu Ling-di, Gu Dong-sheng, Tian Wei

PRODUCTION SITE ECOLOGY

Elevation

Sānqī is cultivated between 1400–1800 m elevation.

Temperature

The area must have at least 300 frost free days. The temperature at the site can't go below -2°C and the high temperature should not go above 35°C. The average annual temperature at the daodi site is between 15–17°C. The average temperature during the coldest month is 8–10°C and the average temperature during the hottest months should be between 20–22°C.

Photo Period

Annual sunlight hours should be between 1516–2016 hours with average sunlight between 34–46%.

Moisture

Average annual rainfall of 900–1300 mm with average humidity between 75–85%.

Soil

Red, yellow-brown, etc. soils are acceptable. The soil structure should be loose, deep (at least 30 cm) with a pH of 5.5–6.5.

Topography

The site may have a slope of up to 15%. The slope may be facing anywhere in an arc draw from southeast to northwest. The site should allow for good air flow and drainage, and there must be access to irrigation.

Site Selection

The site should have appropriate slope, good drainage and air flow with sun exposure, an area close to headwaters is ideal. The soil layer should be deep with loose soil structure. The area cannot be allowed to become waterlogged. Virgin sites or those that were previously used to grow corn, wheat, dry-land rice, marigold, tobacco, or brassica family plants are all acceptable. Avoid areas where solonaceae or gourd family plants were previously grown. Avoid

continuous cropping, after harvest from a site it takes at least 10 years before the site can be used again to grow *sānqī*.

Soil Preparation

Before planting *sānqī* the land is plowed and harrowed three times. The first time is done in November of the year prior to planting, and then every 15 days after that to allow the soil to be exposed to the sun in an effort to reduce soil borne diseases and pests. Plowing should be at least 25 cm deep.

During the second or third tilling and harrowing in the month of October or November, 300–420 kg per acre of quick lime is added to kill any pathogens in the soil. [Translator's Note: This process effectively kills all or most of the soil biota, creating sterile soil. While this is a common practice in China, it is not recommended due to ecological concerns and a desire to use only sustainable practices. However, not practicing this method leaves open the possibility for soil-borne disease to overcome your crop. This issue has been the subject of significant research in China but has yet to be solved.]

BUILDING SHADE HOUSES

Timing

Shade houses should be built at least 20 days before planting *sānqī*, usually this is done some time from late November through late December.

Outlining the Beds

Lime is used to outline where the beds will be built according to the contour of the site (1.7–2.0 m wide), while marks are made to create an outline of the beds (2.0–2.2 m wide) where the poles will be placed to erect the shade house. The length of the bed is determined by the site and can be as long or short as needed.

Setting Posts

Posts must be at least 5 cm in diameter and 2.1–2.2 m long. Holes are dug 30–35 cm deep to set the posts, which should be 1.8 meters above the ground. Posts should be secured using wire or cable strong enough to stabilize them. The wire should be secured to the ground about a meter from the pole. The method of securing the wire to the ground is dependent on the site requirements; concrete, buried stones (~5 kg), or even buried logs can be used. Once the wire has been secured to the ground and poles, a turnbuckle should be used to tighten the wire/cable, adding stability to the structure. Be sure to tighten the turnbuckles evenly to ensure the poles are straight. The top of the shade house can be covered with plants such as tree fronds, corn stalks, or shade cloth. However, whatever is chosen must be somewhat adjustable since the sunlight requirements for *sānqī* change over the years. In the first year, plants should only receive 10–15% sunlight, this changes to 15–20% in the second year, then by the third year the requirement for light goes to 20–25%. If a shade cloth is used, generally two to three layers are used to achieve the desired shade, then in the years that follow a layer can be removed as the sunlight requirements shift to a higher percentage. The sides of the structure should also be covered with shade cloth or any other natural material.

The process is as follows. First, the posts should be secured and the material added to the outside of the structure, installing a door, which can be a simple hanging cloth or other material, in an appropriate area is necessary for access to the inside of the shade house. Install-ation of the sides is necessary to protect the plants from both sun and wind, especially when they are very young.

Building the Beds

After cleaning up from building the shade house, beds are built along the contour of the site 120–140 cm wide and 20–25 cm tall, according to the contour of the site. Paths 30–50 cm wide (at bed height) and 20 cm wide at the bottom are built between the beds. This creates a sloped edge on the bed which helps to drain water. Every 100 meters or so, there should be a drainage ditch from the inside to the outside to allow water to flow out of the shade house in the event of heavy rain. This ditch should be a little wider than the pathways inside the greenhouse to facilitate drainage.

Amending the Beds

The first time fertilizer is added to the edges of the beds at a rate of 210 kg per acre. Then, in August when the root is growing rapidly, a urea fertilizer is added at a rate of 120 kg per acre.

Bed Management

Modern *sānqī* cultivation basically uses various chemicals to sterilize the soil prior to transplanting. A number of different bactericides and fungicides are used to kill all the soil biota prior to planting. These chemicals have not been offered here because they are neither available outside of China nor are they approved for use on plants to be consumed by humans.

SOWING SEEDS & RAISING SEEDLINGS

Seed Collection Requirements

Sānqī seeds ripen during the month of November. Seeds are collected from plants that are at least three years old. Plants must be healthy and free from disease. When collecting seeds, plants that are tall with a strong stalk and present as a robust specimen should be chosen. Observing the scarlet red fruit, make sure that it is full and plump without signs of disease or damage. Clean and sanitized scissors should be used to cut the fruit cluster off the plant with approximately 10 cm of the stalk left attached to the fruit. Fruit clusters can be placed in baskets or other appropriate containers before transporting to the drying area. It is best not to pile the fruit clusters too deep in the basket because this may damage the fruits and could lead to disease.

Processing the Seed

Fruits are either mechanically or manually rubbed (between one's hands) to squeeze the seed from inside of the fruit. While doing this it is important to discard any immature, damaged, or otherwise imperfect seeds. The seeds are then rinsed with clean water before being placed in the sun until the water has dried from the seeds (do not allow the seeds to soak in the water). Seeds are then processed to reserve only the full and plump seeds. These seeds should be whitish in color and without any imperfections. Seeds are then soaked in a fungicide for 15 minutes then allowed to dry before storage. Seeds are stored for only about 45–60 days at a temperature of 20°C (slight variations are acceptable). After this initial storage period, fine river sand is moistened to 20–30% moisture. This sand is laid in baskets in layers (~1 cm thick) with the seed (a single layer), then repeated, one layer of sand, then one layer of seeds. The baskets should be checked every 15 days for mildew or rotting seeds. Any sign of disease must be treated immediately, discarding any seeds that may be compromised. Moisture level of the sand/seed mixture is also checked at this time. Water should be added to the mixture if necessary, to maintain the 20–30% requirement. The room where seeds are stored must have good air flow/ventilation to avoid stagnant air which can facilitate the growth of mold and mildew.

Seed Quality Requirements

One-thousand *sānqī* seeds should weigh at least 100 g. At least 90% of seeds should germinate and 80% of those that germinated should be able to thrive. Seeds should contain no more than 5% foreign matter.

Sowing Seed

Seeds are sown in mid- to late December through January. Before planting seeds, make 1 cm deep holes by pressing on the surface of the bed to create a de-pression to place the seed. The concave depressions are made in a 4–5×5 cm pattern. Seeds are sieved from the sand that was used to store them before sowing. After sieving, the seeds are mixed with a combination of fertilizer (calcium, magnesium, phosphorus — as above) and a fungicide (fungicide should be added at 0.5% of the total weight of the seeds) and mixed thoroughly. Seeds are then sown into the holes and covered with composted manure, just enough to completely cover the seeds. Beds are then covered with a layer of pine needles thick enough so that one cannot see the soil below. Finally, the beds should be watered.

Irrigation and Weeding

Beds should be watered once every 10–15 days in order to maintain a soil moisture content of 20% until the rainy season arrives. After seeds have germinated, weeding should be done on a regular basis to keep the beds free from competing weeds.

Common Disease Problems of Seedlings

Sānqī is prone to a number of diseases that have led to a general over-use of various fungicides, pesticides, and other chemicals. These diseases include seed rotting, "standing withered disease," sudden fall disease, black-spot disease, and "epidemic" mildew disease. Common pests include aphids, and cutworms. Careful monitoring and rapid treatment is highly recommended.

Fertilizer Application

Careful observation during the months of July and October is required to determine appropriate application of fertilizer. Generally, a standard NPK is used and is applied at a rate of 60–75 kg per acre. At this time careful observation of the plants should be employed and appropriate measures should be taken to treat any diseases discovered. Potassium dihydrogen phosphate is commonly used as a foliar feeding/fungicide.

Proper Drainage and Air-Flow

During the rainy season it is critical to check to make sure water is draining properly from the beds; any problems must be resolved immediately. Also, during the rainy season, it is important to reduce humidity in the shade houses by opening the sides to allow for good air-flow. This will reduce the likelihood of developing diseases and pests.

SPECIAL ATTENTION
During October through December adjust the shade houses so that sunlight penetration is around 20% and control the soil moisture at 15–20%. This will improve resistance to disease and pests as well as improve the quality of the seedlings.

TRANSPLANTING

Pricking Seedlings for Transplanting

Plants are transplanted during dormancy from the middle of December through the end of January. Using a narrow digging shovel, carefully loosen the soil from 2–3 sides, then gently lift the dormant root from the soil. Avoid damage to the root system and the bud. Each root should be carefully observed for any disease or damage; only transplant roots that show no signs of disease or damage. Any plants that are weak or diseased should be removed and discarded. A single root should weigh 1.25 g or more to qualify to be transplanted into the main growing area. Roots should be transplanted as soon as possible, or within 2–3 days. If the process takes longer than a few hours, measures must be taken to protect moisture levels in the roots. Do not leave them in the sun. *Sānqī* is planted in blocks ranging from 10-12×12.5-15 cm. This should allow for 150,000–192,000 plants per acre.

Preparation of Seedlings with Fungicide

A combination of oxadixyl-mancozeb is used at a concentration of 0.15–0.2% concentration in water and the roots of the seedlings are put in to soak for 15–20 minutes prior to transplanting.

Transplanting Seedlings

Planks 1.3–1.5 m long and 30 cm wide are fashioned with short dowels or other appropriate fixtures at intervals of 10×12.5–12×15 cm for quick and efficient digging of holes needed for transplanting. Dowels fixed in the planks for digging the holes are approximately 3 cm long and have a diameter of 0.5-1.0 cm. After seedlings have been treated with the fungicide, a single seedling is placed in each of the holes previously dug. Seedlings are placed in the holes according to the slope of the land. The first row is laid with the root pointing up-hill. Starting with the second row, the root is placed facing down the slope; but the bud should always be facing up the slope. At the sides of the bed, the roots should be facing toward the middle and the bud facing to the outside of the bed. This helps with air-flow and creates more optimal conditions for the plant to thrive. Transplants should be covered with a fine-grain soil, making sure that the dormant bud(s) is covered by 2–3 cm.

Mulching and Watering

The entire bed is covered with enough pine needles so that the soil cannot be seen through the needles, and the distribution of the pine needles should be even across the entire bed. Once all the seedlings have been transplanted and the bed is covered with pine needles, the bed should be watered enough that water penetrates and the transplanted roots are moist.

FIELD MANAGEMENT

Irrigation and Water Drainage

Watering should only be done to maintain the soil moisture at approximately 20%. During periods of rain, the site should be monitored closely and water should be properly drained with channels. During these periods of rain, the shade house should be

opened, allowing for good air-flow to reduce humidity and thus potential disease. Weeding should be done immediately after the leaves have completely matured; then as necessary.

Adjusting Shade Materials

In the early stage of *sānqī* growing, use Chinese fir fronds or other similar shading materials to maintain proper shade in the shade house. Thinning of the shade material needs to be done in the later stage of the third year. This process is done 3–4 times. The first time (mid-July) needs to be done at 3–4 pm on a clear day, using wood or bamboo stick to lightly slap the shading materials, causing leaves from the fronds to fall and exposing the area to increased light; the goal is to remove 1/3 of the material. The second removal of the shading materials should be done 20–30 days after the first time, giving the plants time to become accustomed to the new amount of light; this time another 1/3 of the total shading material is removed. The third time for removing the shading material is 20–30 days after the second time; this time the final 1/3 of the total shading material is removed. After removing the shading material, any remaining foreign materials that have fallen on the plant must be cleaned up. If shading net is used, 1–2 layers of shading net needs to be removed in the later stage for to adjust the shading.

Removing Buds

Flowering buds are removed from plants from mid- to late July to encourage root growth. These buds are used/sold as a flower tea. This time period is also the best time to pick flower buds that create the best quality tea. All pesticides, herbicides, and fungicides must be stopped at least 30 days prior to picking flower buds. Buds are removed by using a sharp, clean knife or scissors, cutting the bud 3–5 cm below the base of the bud. Buds are generally collected in baskets so the buds have good air-flow around them and do not begin to rot during the picking process.

Top-Dressing in the Second Year

Applications One & Two: The first top-dressing is done during early May when the plant leaves have fully matured, which is also the dry season. The crop should be watered 2–3 days prior to top-dressing. Fertilizer is applied in the late morning on a sunny day after all dew on the leaves has dried. The second application is in August when the flower buds are fully matured. This is during the rainy season and the fertilizer must be applied after 10 in the morning when all the dew on the leaves has dried. In both the first and second application of a top-dressing a NPK 10–10–15~20 is used at a rate of 75 kg per acre. After top-dressing an appropriate tool must be used to carefully brush away any fertilizer that may be on the leaves of *sānqī*. Alternately, a leaf blower can be used to accomplish this task.

Application Three: In late December or January after the plant withers, compost made with a combination of cow and goat manure along with grain stubble (6000 kg) that has been composted no less than three months is combined with fused calcium-magnesium phosphate (300 kg), potassium sulfate (60 kg), and carbendazim (6 kg). This combination and amount is applied to each acre. Finally, pine needles are used to mulch the beds. Once this is completed it is important to clean and tidy the area, being sure all the drainage ditches are clear and can easily drain water. All weeds and any remaining withered *sānqī* plants should be removed and disposed of properly.

Top-Dressing Year Three

Top-dressing in year three is done twice, once in late April or early May and the second time in mid- to late July. As above, the timing must be after 10 in the morning when all the dew has dried from the leaves. A 10–10–20 NPK compound fertilizer is applied at a rate of 120 kg per acre. As above, be sure to brush away any fertilizer that may have stayed on the leaves of the plants.

PREVENTION AND TREATMENT OF DISEASE AND INSECT PESTS

Principles of Prevention and Treatment

Because diseases can often spread through the crop very quickly, one must be mindful of any potential diseases and act quickly to avoid spreading of the disease using appropriate measures and quarantine if necessary. Watch the surrounding areas closely for any sign of pest or other potential threats and act swiftly. Setting up mouse or rat traps as a precaution is advised. Optimize the growing environment to stimulate *sānqī* growth and deter the growth of pathogens. When using quarantine as a measure, set up an area and move all plants affected by the disease to that area to avoid further infestation.

Prevention and Treatment

Crop rotation is essential. Always use seed and seedlings that are free from pests or disease. Manage and maintain the shade house meticulously, including shade and light penetration, humidity, and water drainage. Monitor the crop closely, at the first sign of disease or pests act swiftly to resolve the problem in an appropriate manner; keep the area clean and free of weeds. Be sure the compost is thoroughly composted, increase potassium and potash, magnesium, and boron. Make certain that drainage ditches are deep enough and remain free and clear. Use lime where disease arises.

Biological Controls

The use of biological controls is extremely important in the cultivation of *sānqī*. It is important to recognize disease, both insect and fungal, and provide appropriate controls to overwhelm the disease before the disease overwhelms the plants. These substances are antibiotics that are derived from natural non-plant sources for controlling diseases of *sānqī*, and include kasugamycin, avermectin, and polyoxin. However, none of these are approved for use in the US or EU. Measures for controlling pests include, Bt, *Beauveria* sp., *Metarhizium* sp., granulosis viruses, and nuclear polyhedrosis viruses. Compounds from botanical sources such as azadirachtin, pyrethrins, rotenone, nicotine, and marigold extracts are also commonly used.

Physical Means of Control

Use simple tools, light, heat, electricity, and control temperature and humidity to help control insect pests. Seeds should be soaked at 55°C for ten minutes to help disinfect them prior to planting. Deep plowing and heating the soil to sterilize it are often employed as a means of lessening the chances of disease. Yellow sticky boards for luring and trapping insects is a frequently used technique for controlling aphids and thrips. Black lights are used to lure and kill cutworms and scarab. Other tools such as mouse traps, etc. are also employed when necessary.

Root Rot (*Fusarium* sp.)

Prevention and Treatment

Ensure that the seed and transplants are free of disease. Sterilize all seeds and seedlings prior to transplanting. Watch the crop closely and immediately remove all diseased plants and use lime in and around the hole after digging out the diseased plant.

Black Spot Disease (*Alternaria alternata*)

Prevention and Treatment

Ensure that the seed and transplants are free of disease. Maintain the shade house to ensure the proper amount and evenness of light penetration, do not allow direct sun to penetrate the shade house. Proper management of air-flow is important, remove any plants or structures that may be impeding the air-flow in and around the production site. Thoroughly clean away any weeds or disease plants and dispose of them properly. Maintain proper water drainage, frequently check drainage during rainy season to avoid any stagnant water. Increase potash fertilizer but don't increase nitrogen.

Blight Disease (*Phytophthora cactorum*)

Prevention and Treatment

Starting in May and continuing through October, but especially during the months of May and June, careful attention must be paid to the management of blight; check the crop every day and act immediately if any disease is found. Any plants found infected with this disease must be immediately removed and destroyed. Make sure the shade houses are well maintained and neither too much nor too little sun is shining on the plants. Also, be sure proper air-flow is moving through the shade house.

Round Spot Disease (*Mycocentrospora acerina*)

Prevention and Treatment

Build the shade house on a northern slope. Maintain proper water drainage, frequently check drainage during rainy season to avoid any stagnant water. Open the doors and sides of the shade house to allow wind to flow freely through to help regulate humidity. Increase potash but not nitrogen fertilizer to strengthen the plants ability to resist disease.

Insect and Animal Pests

Underground Pests

If grubs (*Holotrichia* sp.) and cutworm (Noctuidae) numbers get high, the use of chemical controls may be necessary. An alternative is to shred vegetable leaves and put them out into the field in the evening at a rate of 300 kg per acre then collect them early in the morning and properly dispose of them.

Above-Ground Pests

Aphids (Aphidoidea) and scale insects (Coccoidea) may be treated with any appropriate chemical preparation. Mites (*Tetranychus urticae*), also known as red spider mites, are treated by chemical means but as above, none of these chemicals are approved in the US or EU. Daily observation and removal is critical. Vegetable scraps left around the surrounding area helps to lure slugs away from the *sānqī*. Lime can be spread in drainage ditches to deter them from entering the shade houses. Rats or Mice should be conroled by appropriate traps set as a matter of course to eliminate any potential damage by these animals. [Translator's Note: As noted elsewhere in the text, yellow sticky boards can be employed to control aphids. Neem oil is also effective for many of these pests, however there is no data regarding using it for *sānqī*. Introduction of natural predators indigenous to the area is also recommended.]

HARVESTING

Harvest Season

Sānqī is harvested after the third year; one year in the seedling beds and two years after transplanting. Spring *sānqī* should be harvested during the months of October and November. Winter *sānqī* should be harvested from December through February.

Harvest Method

Approximately 15 days prior to harvest, the entire covering of the shade house is removed to allow full sunlight. This is said to increase the weight of the root. Roots are dug on a sunny day with an appropriate digging tool. Be sure to keep the entire root system intact without damage to any portion thereof. Roots are laid in the sun for half a day before being turned once to allow even drying of the root. All soil is removed by shaking, and the stem is broken off from the root stolon; use baskets or other well-ventilated carrying device to transport the roots back to the processing area.

ON-FARM PROCESSING

Dividing for Further Processing

Roots must never be piled or stacked. The drying area must be clean and have good sunlight and airflow. Using shears or a sharp knife, separate the main root (1–6 cm long × 1–4 cm thick), tendon twig (large root) (2–6 cm × ~0.8 cm at the thickest point to 0.3 cm at the thinnest point), and hairy roots (fine roots).

Drying Method

After dividing the main and larger roots, they are placed in the sun for drying. The hairy roots are washed with clean water before placing in the sun for drying. Do not pile or stack the roots. Do not allow rain or dew on the roots. Roots should be turned 1–2 times per day, each time checking for mold or other diseases. Any roots found with any disease must be removed and disposed of immediately. Each evening before dusk, the roots are piled approximately 50 cm high and are covered with a plastic sheet and the

edges are sealed with sand. The plastic is removed in the morning and the roots are spread out to continue drying in the sun. This process allows the moisture from inside the root to move to the outside. This process is repeated until the roots are dry. When the roots have dried completely, they are placed in a sieve and shaken to allow for any dust or other foreign matter to be separated from the *sānqī* roots.

Polishing

This is an additional process that is not required. After the main root has been dried and sieved it can be polished with a tool, which is a cylinder that rolls the roots until the outside of the root is shiny and smooth. There are two methods of using material inside the cylinder to create the polished appearance. The first uses rice husks and pine needles, while the other uses buckwheat husks and pine needles.

Grading

The main root is graded according to size and density. Roots of roughly the same size are divided into piles and then divided as follows: the number of roots required to reach 500 grams is the number with which they are labelled: 20, 30, 40, 60, 80, 120, 160, 200, more than 200. This is normally done visually by an experienced person who gauges which roots should go into each category.

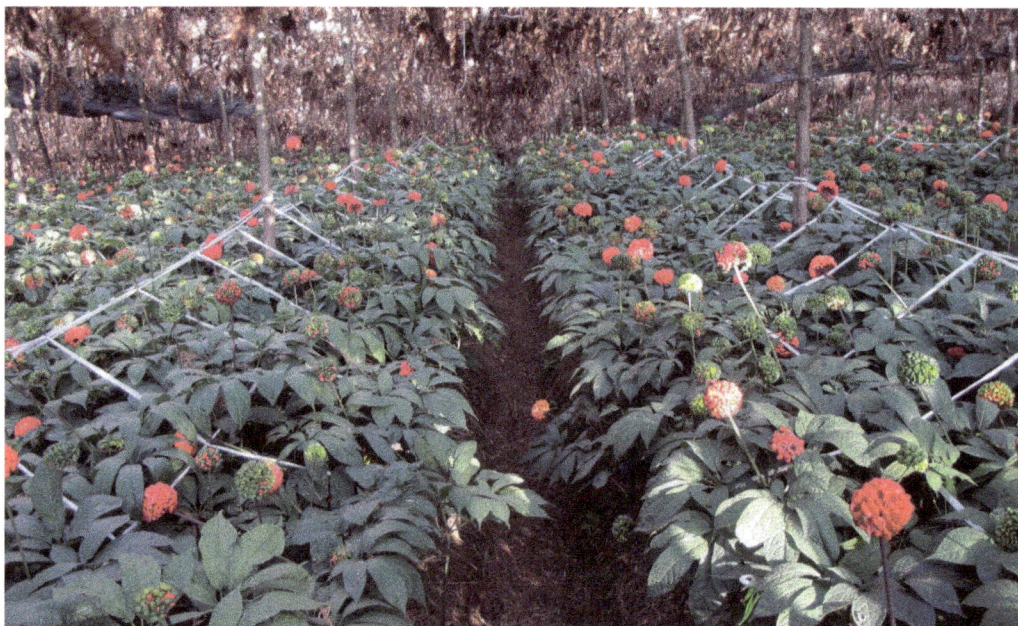

Three-year-old fruiting *sānqī* in Wenshan, Yunnan province, China.

太行山远志

Polygala Root
Polygala tenuifolia

The dried root of *tàihàngshān yuǎnzhì* (*Polygala tenuifolia* Willd. and *P. sibirica* L.) commonly known in China as *yuǎnzhì* (遠志 \ 远志), is a member of the milkwort (Polygalaceae) family, which includes around 500 species with 44 in China. There are two official species, the primary species, *P. tenuifolia*, is native to most of eastern and northern China as well as Mongolia, Korea, and Russia. *P. sibirica*, is also known as *xībóìyà yuánzhì* (西伯利亚远志). The daodi medicinal grows from 15–50 cm tall with purple flowers between 200–2300 m elevation. *P. sibirica* has a wider native range that includes most of *P. tenuifolia*'s range but is also found in the western part of the country and throughout much of Central Asia and into Europe. It has purple-blue flowers and grows from 1100–3300 m elevation. They both prefer grasslands and shrubby areas, although the latter is commonly found in forests. The daodi location is the Taihang Mountain area in Zanhuang, Lingshou, Shunping, and the surrounding area.

In Chinese medicine this herb is regarded as a special herb because is the only herb that calms the spirit while also improving memory. Although it is a warm herb, for this application it can be used for patients with either cold or heat conditions. Another function is to dispel phlegm and open the orifices. Although it can work on all the orifices, for this function, it is primarily used for the orifice of the lung for cough with abundant phlegm. However, in this situation, it is not particularly advisable to use it when there is pronounced heat in the lung. It is also commonly used externally for all types of abscesses, often mixed with honey.

Both species have shown wound-healing actions when the concentrated decoction is applied to infected wounds. The root also shows promising pharmacological activities for the treatment of Alzheimer's disease. Polysaccharides from *P. tenuifolia* have shown clear pharmacological activity in the treatment of ovarian cancer. The roots also show antidepressant, expectorant, and even antipsychotic activity.

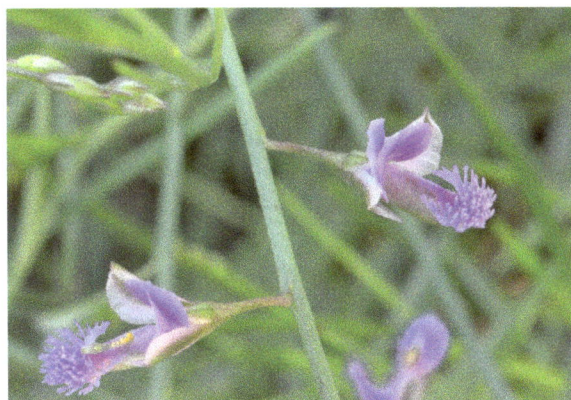

Contributing Authors

Tian Wei, Wen Chun-xiu, Xie Xiao-liang, Huang Lu-qi, Hao Qing-xiu, Guo Lan-ping, Liu Ming, Li Rong-xin, Liu Ling-di, Jia Dong-sheng

PRODUCTION SITE ECOLOGY

Elevation

Yuǎnzhì is cultivated between 50–500 m elevation.

Temperature

Cultivation of *yuǎnzhì* requires a minimum of 197 frost free days. Average temperatures in January are below 3°C and average temperatures in July range (low and high) between 18–27°C.

Photo Period

Average annual sunshine is between 2500–2757 hours. The sunshine percentage range is 35–70%.

Moisture

Average annual rainfall is 500–1000 mm with a relative humidity of 34–55%.

Soil

A deep (at least 30 cm), loose, and sandy soil with pH in the 5.5–6.5 range is ideal.

Topography

A mountain slope less than 15 degrees is ideal, but flat land can be used if there is adequate water drainage. If the field is sloped it should be facing either southeast or northwest to allow for proper drainage and wind-flow.

Site Selection and Soil Preparation

Select loose, sandy soil with good water drainage. Add 3000 kg per acre of organic fertilizer and 300 kg of compound NPK fertilizer, plow to at least 30 cm.

SOWING SEEDS & RAISING SEEDLINGS

Seed Quality Requirements

According to the *Pharmacopoeia of the People's Republic of China* (2015), seeds for *yuǎnzhì* (*P. tenuilolia*) or ovate leaf *yuǎnzhì* (*P. sibirica*) are the original source for these medicinal plants. Seeds should be black, full, and plump.

Pre-Treatment of Seeds

Prior to sowing seeds, soak in warm water (45°C) for 5–6 hours. After removing from the water, seeds are combined with a small amount of plant or wood ash, then they are sown.

Sowing Seeds

Seeds may be sown in the spring (April) or during the summer (June-July). After the bed is prepared, dig furrows 1 cm deep and 20–30 cm apart to create rows for planting. Seeds are placed evenly in the furrows, covered with soil and gently tamped down. Seeds are sown at a rate of 9–12 kg per acre.

After sowing seeds, beds should be covered with enough straw so that there is no soil showing. After seeds are sown, check every 5 days to ensure soil remains moist, if soil becomes dry, water enough to moisten soil. After true leaves have emerged from seedlings, gradually open up the mulch covering to allow the plants to receive full sun exposure. This should first be done on a cloudy day, or at the end of a sunny day to allow the plant ample time to adjust.

FIELD MANAGEMENT

Cultivation and Weeding

During the seedling stage, cultivation must be done shallowly, use a small hoe to lightly cultivate, keeping weeds at bay while loosening the soil. Cultivation can be done after watering or rains. It is important to keep the soil loose and free of weeds. [Translator's Note: This plant grows relatively slowly and weeds can easily overwhelm it, keeping the bed free of competing weeds is very important. Mulching can help this significantly, however adding mulch as a weed barrier is not a common practice in China.]

Irrigation and Water Drainage

During the seedling stage control the moisture level. Plants should be watered when they first begin to emerge and after top-dressing. Prior to harvest, only water when necessary. During the rainy season, or heavy rains, be sure that water is draining properly, do not allow water to accumulate and pool. [Translator's Note: Once established, this plant is relatively tolerant of dry conditions but does not like wet conditions, therefore it is suggested to err on the side of dryness.]

Top-Dressing

Starting in the spring of the second year (April and May) an application of a compound fertilizer should be added at a rate of 180-300 kg per acre.

PREVENTION AND TREATMENT OF DISEASE AND INSECT PESTS

Principles of Prevention and Treatment

Yuǎnzhì is a long-lived perennial and needs at least three years before harvest. For this reason, diseases such as root rot are very important to manage appropriately. This plant does not like to stay wet for extended periods of time, soil must drain well in order for it to grow and produce good medicinal material. Planting grass in the pathways may help manage some diseases and maintain soil health. Encouraging natural predators is recommended to control pests.

Root Rot (*Fusarium* sp.)

Prevention and Treatment

Using a crop rotation of a grass family plant [wheat, oats, etc.] every 3-5 years is recommended. Appropriate use of fertilizers, including combinations of elements of fertilization such as increases in phosphorus and potash to improve the plants ability to resist disease is strongly recommended. Timely removal of diseased plants, including using a 10% lime solution in the holes after removal of the plant and proper disposal of the diseased material, i.e. burning, is recommended.

Leaf Blight (*pathogen not identified*)

Prevention and Treatment

Doing crop rotation with grass family plants for two or more years is recommended.

Aphids (Aphidoidea)

Prevention and Treatment

Aphids are naturally attracted to the color yellow. Deploying "sticky yellow boards" or construction of areas with yellow painted boards will attract aphids where they can be killed. Boards are deployed at a rate of 180–240 per acre.

Biological Controls

Close monitoring of plants is important when using biological controls. At the first sign of aphid infestation lady bugs should be used to control the infestation. A 0.3% matrine solution is diluted in water to 0.075–0.1% or natural pyrethrins diluted to 0.01% in water; spray according to manufacturer's instructions. [Translator's Note: Lady bugs should be set out around dusk for best results.]

Bean Blister Beatle (*Epicauta gorhami*)

Prevention and Treatment

Plow deeply in the autumn to kill or disturb the larvae so that its ability to survive the winter is hindered.

HARVESTING

Harvest Season

Yuǎnzhì is harvested after 3 or more years of growth. *Yuǎnzhì* is havested in October when the above ground portions of the plant have withered.

Harvest Method

Choosing a sunny day, plants are dug with care to avoid damage to the root system. Allow to dry in the sun for about half a day then carefully remove any loose soil residues on the root before transporting for further processing. [Translator's Note: Using a digging fork rather than a shovel is recommended.]

ON-FARM PROCESSING

Drying and Removing Heart-Wood

Remove soil and any other material that may be within the root system, then place in the sun to dry. While the root is still soft, remove the remaining woody stem material from the crown area of the root and cut out the heart-wood from the root. When doing the latter, the roots are sometimes lightly beaten with a wooden stick or other appropriate tool to loosen the outer part of the root from the woody core. After the heart-wood is removed from the root, it is dried in the sun. Properly dried *yuǎnzhì* root should not exceed 12% moisture content.

Grading

Yuǎnzhì is usually divided into three classes according to size with the largest considered the highest quality (see table below). The largest roots with no heart-wood is the highest quality.

Specifications	Grade	Identifying characteristics	Differentiating characteristics	Diameter (cm)	Amount of heart-wood removed (%)
Yuǎnzhì tubes	very large	Dry material: Outer skin is a light-brown or gray-yellow color, the entire outside has relatively deep horizontal wrinkles, and has a brittle texture allowing for it to be easily broken. The cross-section is yellow-whitish in color, has a particular smell, and a bitter and slightly acrid flavor. The material should be free of foreign matter, damage by bugs, or mold.	Appears tubular without a core	>0.4	>95
	large			0.3–0.4	90–95
	medium			0.2–0.3	85–90
	small			<0.2	80–85
	ungraded			n/a	>80
Yuǎnzhì flesh	ungraded		Much of the material is broken with pieces of fleshy root mixed with whole root and irregular sizes	n/a	>80
Yuǎnzhì sticks	ungraded		Cylindrical with heart-wood present	n/a	n/a

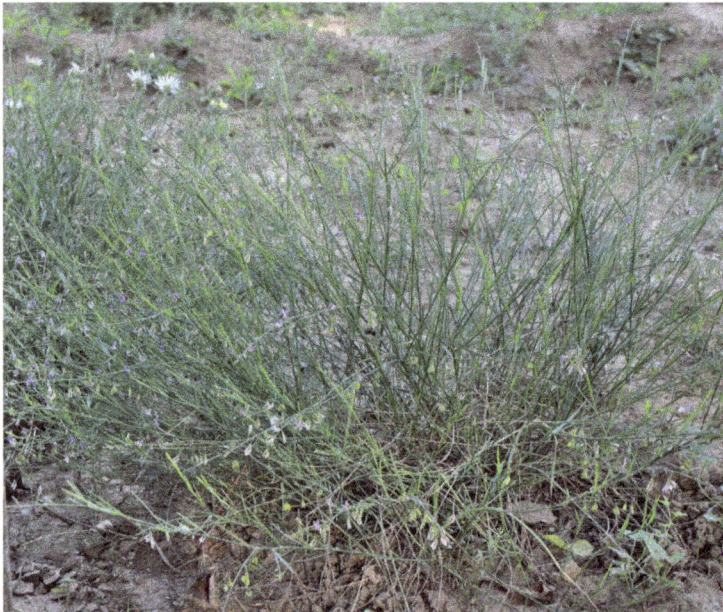

Yuǎnzhì flowering at the Institute of Medicinal Plant Development in Beijing, China.

施秉太子参
Prince's Ginseng
Pseudostellaria heterophylla

DISTINGUISHING FEATURES

The dried root of the daodi herb *shībǐng táizǐshēn* (*Pseudostellaria heterophylla* (Miq.) Pax ex Pax et Hoffm.), commonly known as *táizǐshēn* (太子参 \ 太子参) or *hái'érshēn* (孩兒参 \ 孩儿参) in China, is a member of the pink family (Caryophyllaceae). It is part of a genus comprised of 18 species, most of which are found in northern and eastern Asia. This species grows throughout most of central and eastern China from 800–2700 m elevation, it is also found in Korea and Japan. The daodi location for this medicinal is Shibing county in Guizhou Province as well as the 150 km surrounding area, which includes Huangping, Yuqing, and Zhenyuan.

A relatively recent addition to the Chinese materia medica, *táizǐshēn* was added during the Qing dynasty. The herb is sometimes thought of as a weak substitute for American ginseng because it supplements the qi and yin of the lung, spleen, and heart. However, it has no substantial supplementing action on the kidney. Both names (*táizǐ* -*shēn* and *hái'ér* -*shēn*) carry the meaning of children and were probably so named because this medicinal is commonly used in pediatrics as a supplementing herb. It is not a very strong herb and is very well suited to treating children. This is not to say it isn't used for adults, in fact it is very commonly used with adults and is particularly important when treating patients that have relatively minor vacuity as an underlying pattern.

There is a dearth of modern scientific literature regarding this medicinal plant. However, some research has shown the roots to have antitussive activity, be immune-stimulating, and show a number of promising benefits for the treatment of diabetes.

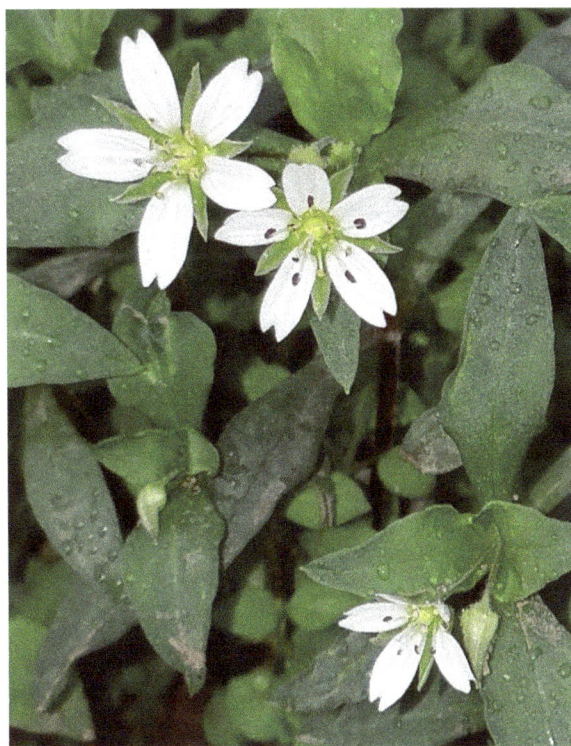

Contributing Authors

Xiao Cheng-hong, Zhou Tao,
Hong Wei-ke, Guo Lan-ping,
Huang Lu-qi, Yang Guang, Zhang Xiao-bo

151

PRODUCTION SITE ECOLOGY

Elevation

Táizǐshēn is cultivated between 650–1300 m elevation.

Temperature

January is the coldest month of the year but doesn't get below 2°C. The hottest month of the year is July but does not get above 28°C. Average annual temperature is 14–16°C. Annual frost-free days are between 255–294 days.

Photo Period

Annual sunshine range from 1060–1350 hours.

Moisture

Average annual rainfall is between 1000–1200 mm; 75% of the rainfall comes April through September.

Soil

Soils can be red, yellow, or brown at pH 6.0–7.2. A sandy or humus-rich soil that is fertile, deep, and loose with abundant organic matter is suitable for growing *táizǐshēn*. The upper soil level should be at least 30 cm deep.

Topography

Táizǐshēn prefers a relatively steep slope. In the wild it grows most frequently on slopes around 45 degrees. Because of this, the slope should be at least 10 degrees in a south-facing position or the top of a hill.

PRODUCTION AREA ENVIRONMENTAL REQUIREMENTS

Site Selection

To summarize, the site should mimic wild conditions as follows. The site should be in a hilly area with at least a 10-degree slope or the highest point on a rise. Virgin soil is best, or where a grass family plant has been grown for at least 3 years prior to establishing *táizǐshēn*. The soil layer should be thick and deep, fertile, loose, and drain very well. Clay soils or soils without significant organic matter are not suitable.

Soil Preparation

The soil is first tilled to 25–30 cm deep, then an application of Phoxim (40% concentration at 75 g per acre) is applied. After 20 days the soil is tilled to 20 cm deep. After this tilling 1500–2000 kg of aged manure or compost are added to the site and harrowed finely. Finally, a combination of NPK (20 kg), calcium 50 kg, and potassium sulfate 15 kg are spread on the top of the soil. Beds are then built 70–90 cm wide and usually not over 10 meters long with pathways dug to 25 cm deep. It is best to build beds according to the contour of the land, making sure that the pathways drain well.

Translator's Note: Phoxim is a non-persistent insecticide used to disinfect soils prior to planting. It is used due to the high susceptibility of *táizǐshēn* to soil-born insect pests. It is moderately toxic to earthworms and highly toxic to aquatic life with long-lasting effects. It is highly flammable and the fumes can cause dizziness, drowsiness, and other symptoms. Although it is registered and approved for use in the EU under limited use, it is not registered with the US EPA.

COLLECTING AND REPLANTING ROOT TUBERS

Collected and Saving Root Tubers

Root tubers are collected in the months of May and June from healthy disease-free plants. There are two methods of preserving the root tubers. The first method is the original local method where tubers are buried in the soil after harvest and left there until October or November when they are dug up and planted. In the second method the root tubers are dug during the months of July and August and combined with sand; sand to root tuber ratio is 3:1. Using this method the tubers are set on a layer of sand (2–3 cm thick), then another layer of sand is added, then tubers, then sand, etc., each layer of sand should be 2–3 cm thick. This can be done to create 4–5 layers before topping off with a good layer of sand. This process is done in a shady dry location. The system should be checked every two weeks to make sure there is no disease or pest intrusion. Any mold or other problems should be immediately addressed and eliminated. These can be planted in late October to early November at a rate of 240 kg per acre. Prior to planting, tubers can be dug up and inspected. Choose those with a plump healthy bud, a relatively well-proportioned body, absent of a forking root, without other damage including physical, insect, or other disease. Tubers are soaked in an all-purpose fungicide for 20–30 minutes, removed and allowed to drip-dry, then they are washed with clean water and allowed to dry until the surface of the tuber is dry.

Replanting Root Tubers

Rows are dug every 13 cm or so to a depth of about 10 cm. Tubers are planted every 5–7 cm with the bud facing upwards. Tubers are covered with fine soil 6–8 cm deep. This covering should form a dome that rises slightly above the level of the surrounding soil.

FIELD MANAGEMENT

Cultivation and Weeding

Cultivation should be done during early March, at which time any necessary weeding should be done. After all the sprouts have emerged (early May) cultivation should be halted but weeding should continue as needed.

Final Singling

During mid-April diseased or weak seedlings are removed and replaced with healthy plants.

Top-Dressing

Top-dressing should be coordinated with the first cultivation in March. A calcium magnesium phosphate fertilizer (25 kg) and a potash fertilizer (10 kg) are applied per acre. NPK fertilizer at a rate of 20 kg per acre is spread on the beds prior to cultivation, and this is best done on a day prior to forecasted rain. In mid-April a 0.5% solution of potassium dihydrogen phosphate is applied as a foliar application in the morning or evening at a rate of 30 kg per acre.

Irrigation and Water Drainage

Drainage is very important, regular inspection of drainage ditches should be done and any problem areas fixed. After heavy rains, it is prudent to inspect the site to ensure that all water has drained properly. Any problems should be resolved immediately. If there is any sign of leaves wilting early in develop-

ment the beds should be watered thoroughly, which should be done in the morning or evening.

SPECIAL NOTE

For fields where tubers will be harvested for future planting, a crop of corn or soybean can be planted.

SEEDS AND SEEDLINGS

Harvesting Seeds

During the months of April and May, select plants that are healthy and free of disease to harvest seeds. Seeds are collected from seed capsules that have partially fractured. Capsules are discarded. Seeds should be dried at 20–25°C, in the shade where there is good air flow.

Seed Requirements

Seeds should be full, plump, and all about the same size. 1000 seeds should weight more than 2.6 g, with 13% moisture, and no more than 15% foreign matter. Germination rate should be above 85%.

Seed Storage

Seeds are held under refrigeration around 0°C. Alternately, seeds can be combined with moist sand (3:1 ratio; sand to seed), then stored in a dry shady area under natural conditions.

Seed Stratification

Seeds can be planted in late September or early October to allow them to endure the cold of winter. Alternatively, seeds can be combined with moist sand (see above) and held at about 0°C for 45–50 days before sowing. Earlier sowing (before 45 days) or later sowing (after 50 days) will adversely affect germination rate.

Sowing Seeds

Autumn sowing is done in late September through early October. Spring sowing is done from late February to early March. When sowing seeds, the seeds are combined with wood ash (1:5, seed to ash) before being sown. The wood ash helps to both prevent fungal infections as well as assist in the even distribution of the seeds when sowing. Sow seeds evenly on beds approximately 30 cm wide. Seeds are sown at a rate of 600–1000 seeds per square meter, or 15–18 kg per acre, then covered with 0.5–1.0 cm of soil. After covering with soil, the beds are covered with straw (without seeds) about 2-3 cm thick before watering thoroughly.

Seedling Bed Management

After the seedlings have emerged and the first two true leaves are present, the straw is carefully removed. At this time a 1% foliar spray of mono-potassium phosphate (KH_2PO_4) is applied, then again 6–7 days later. Seedlings are thinned from March to May. During the initial thinning process, plants are thinned to about 5×5 cm with final distances creating rows 13–15 cm apart and spacing of 8×13 cm to 6×15 cm. [Translator's Note: Seedlings are very delicate; care must be taken during this step and it should be done before the seedlings get too tall and entangled with the straw.]

PREVENTION AND TREATMENT OF DISEASE AND INSECT PESTS

Principles of Prevention and Treatment

The most common problems when growing *táizǐshēn* are associated with retention of moisture in the soil and on the site. Remembering that this herb prefers steep slopes in the wild, it is paramount to choose appropriate sites and to assure that water does not stagnate at the site. Below-ground insect damage is problematic, which is why the pre-planting soil treatment has been developed. This is considered standard practice in China but is not ecologically friendly and farmers outside of China have an opportunity to test and develop other, more ecologically safe, methods.

Sheath Blight (*Rhizoctonia solani*) Purple Root Rot (*Helicobasidium mompa*)

Prevention and Treatment

Careful field management including being sure that rain water is draining properly, reducing humidity in the field by improving drainage and cultivating the soil, timely removal of any diseased plants, and using lime in and around any holes where diseased plants were removed.

Leaf spot (*Phyllosticta commonsii*)

Prevention and Treatment

Timely removal and proper disposal of any diseased plants. Continuous cropping not appropriate, a strict regime of crop rotation must be implemented.

Root rot (*Fusarium oxysporum & Verticillium alboatrum*)

Prevention and Treatment

Site selection and proper drainage are key factors to prevent this disease.

Virus diseases (*unidentified mosaic virus & wilt virus*)

Prevention and Treatment

Improve variety by careful selection of seeds from healthy plants. Increasing phosphorus helps to improve plants ability to fight viral diseases. Holding seeds below 0°C for 40 days before planting can help.

HARVESTING

Harvest Season

When growing from root tubers plants can be harvested the following year. The time from emergence of the plant in the spring to annual dieback is approximately 160 days. Root tubers are usually harvested during the beginning of July, 10 days after the plant has withered. Farmers should expect harvest 300–600 kg of dried root per acre.

Harvest Method

Clear away all withered plants, remove all weeds, then dispose of this material properly. Using a digging fork, locate where each plant was and dig 20–25 cm deep, carefully lift the soil with the root tubers, remove soil, then collect root tubers into a basket or other appropriate container (plastic bags and other non-breathable material are not recommended).

ON-FARM PROCESSING

Selection and Washing

After bringing in the harvest, carefully go through all the root tubers and remove any diseased or damaged material. Place root tubers in clean water and soak for 5–10 minutes. Then use running water to remove the rest of the soil from the root tubers before allowing to drip dry.

Drying Method

After washing, root tubers are laid on mats in the sun and dried to 70–80% dryness. At this point root tubers are rubbed between the hands to remove small fibrous roots before returning to the drying mat to complete drying. Final water content should not exceed 14%.

Final Cleaning and Processing

Once the root tubers have dried to under 14%, a fan is used to winnow away any dust, foreign plant matter, small roots, etc. After the material has been winnowed clean, the tail of the root tuber is cut away by hand with a sharp knife or scissors.

Grading

Grading is the final process before storage, although it is tedious, it is critical because it determines the final value of the root tubers. Grading is done by evaluating both the diameter of the upper-middle portion of the root tuber and the total number of root tubers needed to weigh 50 g. Top grade material has a diameter of at least 4.5 mm and 130 root tubers equaling 50 g (± 0.4 g). The middle grade material measures between 3.4–4.5 mm in diameter and 130–250 root tubers weighing 50 g (± 0.2–0.4 g). Lower grade material measures below 3.4 mm in diameter at the upper-middle portion of the root tuber and more than 250 are required to reach the 50 g mark (± 0.2 g).

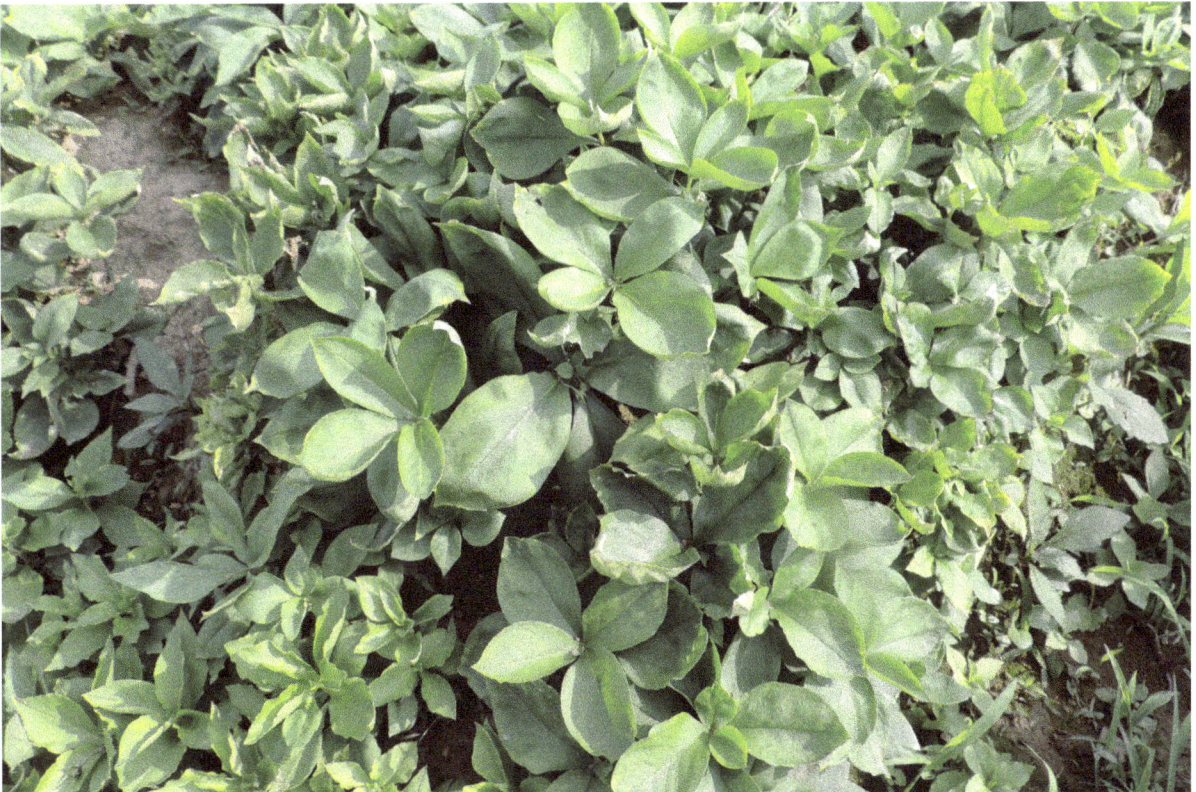

Second year *táizǐshēn* in Guizhou province, China.

怀地黄

Chinese Foxglove

Rehmannia glutinosa

The tuberous root of *huái dìhuáng* (*Rehmannia glutinosa* Libosch.), generally known as *dìhuáng* (地黄 ＼ 地黄) in China, is a member of the figwort family (Scrophulariacea) in a small genus of six species which are all endemic to China. This species is extremely common, often seen in waste places, roadsides, and on the edges of farms, and in the mountains up to about 1100 meters elevation. The plant is found in Gansu, Hebei, Henan, Hubei, Jiangsu, Liaoning, Inner Mongolia, Shaanxi, Shandong, and Shanxi provinces. Material produced in Wuzhi, Wenxiang, Qinyang, and Hemeng counties (and the surrounding region) in Henan Province is considered the daodi medicinal.

This plant is one of the most commonly used medicinals in Chinese medicine and is commonly processed in two distinct ways, giving it significantly different medicinal properties. The initial drying process (described below) produces what is known in China as *dìhuáng* (地黄) known in English as raw Rehmannia. The second requires further processing by soaking in wine and drying thus producing what is known as *shúdìhuáng* (熟 地黄), known in English as processed Rehmannia. While *dìhuáng* is primarily used to clear heat from the blood and construction levels of the body, it also nourishes yin and engenders fluids. However, *shúdìhuáng* enriches yin and supplements blood and essence giving the herb a prominent place in formulas for women and the elderly.

Modern science has found some fascinating pharmacological activities of both *dìhuáng* and *shúdìhuáng*, many of which seem to support traditional usage. It has been shown to improve the proliferation and differentiation of hematopoietic stem cells and bone marrow erythropoiesis progenitor cells. There are a significant number of studies that show the herb has multiple, positive actions on the immune system, the cardiovascular system, and the nervous system, with the potential to significantly reduce cognitive impairment. Most recent research has focused on its ability to promote the growth of bone and its positive effects for those suffering with diabetes.

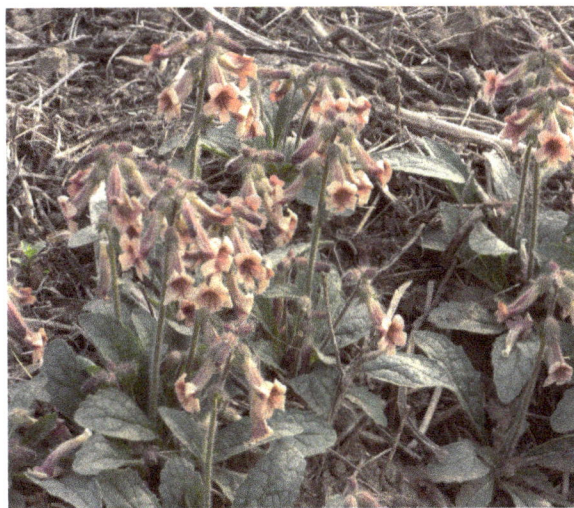

Contributing Authors

Gao Wen-yuan, Wang Ting-ting, Wang Hai-yang, Li Xia, Wang Juan

PRODUCTION SITE ECOLOGY

Elevation

Dìhuáng is cultivated between 150–300 m elevation.

Temperature

The average annual temperature is 14.1–14.9°C. There must be at least 210 frost-free days. The hottest month of the year is July and the coldest month is January.

Rainfall

The average annual rainfall is between 550–700 mm.

Soil

A thick, deep, and sandy soil layer that is loose with abundant humus is ideal. The land should be dry-arid with the excellent water drainage, but must have the ability to irrigate. Soil pH should be neutral to slightly acidic.

PRODUCTION AREA ENVIRONMENTAL REQUIREMENTS

Site Selection

The site should have a rich, mixed or sandy soil that is loose and deep. The site must have adequate drainage. Avoid sites that have grown *dìhuáng* within the last 10 years because of disease problems that arise with continuous cropping. Do not use sites that have recently grown cotton, sesame, or *guālóu* (see page 174). Previous crops that are suitable include soybean, vegetables, and corn.

Soil Preparation

During the autumn prior to planting, spread well-composted manure at a rate of 24,000 kg per acre, then plow deeply to 30 cm. Every year in late March organic fertilizer should be added as an amendment at a rate of 900 kg per acre. Prior to planting, the ground is watered, if necessary, so that it is moist, then it is shallowly tilled to 15 cm. Finally, it is harrowed and beds are constructed as follows: 120 cm wide, 15 cm tall, with 30 cm paths between them. It is common practice to build 60 cm raised pathways throughout the field in order to increase slow run-off and preserve water because *dìhuáng* requires a significant amount of water. However, these pathways must be built in a way that does not allow water to stagnate.

RAISING SEEDLINGS & TRANSPLANTING

Saving Tubers for Replanting

In selecting tubers for replanting it is important to observe the growth of the plants during the months of July and August. Mark plants that have vigorous growth and are free of pests and disease. These tubers are dug during the month of April for re-planting. Tubers may also be dug in the fall after one year of growth and stored as you would other tubers, such as potatoes, until the following April.

In the daodi region of *dìhuáng*, the upside-down planting method is adopted for seed-saving planting. The goal is to select the variety that seed in autumn and have high germination and low risk of pest disease. (In other words, those tubers from the ones planted upside down in July and August of the previous year can be dug out in April before planting). Also, keep the tubers in a cellar from the previous autumn. Before planting, choose 2 cm of good root as a starter, remove the head and end, use the middle part, and cut it into 3–6 cm pieces. Every piece should have more than 3 sprouts. Put them in an open place with no sun, and add plant ash to avoid rotting. The main variety from daodi regions are referred to (on the market in China) as 85-5, Beijing #3, Qinhuai #1.

Transplanting Tubers

Prior to planting, the stolons are broken into 3–4 cm lengths and soaked in a 50% solution of carbendazim for 15–20 minutes. At the end of this period they are placed in the sun to dry. Alternatively, the broken ends of these lengths can be covered with lime. The primary function of this process is to stop potential infections by fungi, bacteria, etc. In the daodi area planting commences in late April.

FIELD MANAGEMENT

Seedling Management

After *dìhuáng* tubers are planted, water thoroughly. Immediately following irrigation, a film mulch is used to cover the plantings. During the first 20–30 days (when the seedlings are 3–4 cm tall and have 2–3 true leaves), the film is only removed to irrigate as necessary, or to replant areas where plants failed to emerge. Any sprouting plants that are weak are removed, only one seedling per hole should remain. If there are holes where plants failed to sprout, these should be immediately re-placed with new tubers; preferably this is done on a cloudy, or even rainy day. If it is not raining, then make sure to water-in the new plantings.

Cultivation, Weeding, and Hilling

Shallow cultivation and weeding is generally done soon after tubers are planted, this loosens the soil and prevents weeds from getting established in the beds. The second time is after the plants have emerged and are approximately 6–9 cm tall. At this time, cultivation can be done more deeply, being careful not to get too close to the plants. Once the plants are well established and are growing vigorously, there is no need for cultivation.

Bud Removal

In order to concentrate the plant's energy on producing a large and healthy tuber, flowering stems are pinched off as soon as they emerge from the rosette of leaves. Also, during the month of August, yellowing leaves from the rosette are removed.

IRRIGATION AND FERTILIZATION

Foliar Feeding

Foliar feeding with a urea solution (0.35%) is done after the plants have at least 5 true leaves. This is done for 3-4 days, then repeated once after 7-10 days. [Translator's Note: Urea is a common agricultural pollutant. Compost tea sprays are advised, however there is no data to support its use on this plant.]

Top-Dressing

Top dressing is generally done three times. Each application should contain nitrogen 240 kg per acre, calcium phosphate 120 kg per acre, and potassium sulfate 240 kg per acre. [Translator's Note: While this is common practice in China, the use of composted manure is recommended as an alternate to these fertilizer applications.]

Irrigation and Water Drainage

Prior to planting *dìhuáng* the field should be watered 1–2 times to ensure the soil is very moist, but free of stagnate water. However, do not water at the time the plant is emerging from the soil as this can easily cause disease. It is best not to water after the hottest days of summer have begun. If watering must be done during this time, it is important to use the following protocol. When to irrigate: 1) Always water after top-dressing, 2) if the fields are dry for three days without rain, irrigate, 3) after torrential rains in the heat of summer, irrigate. When *not* to irrigate: 1) if the soil surface is not dry, do not irrigate, 2) if there is rain in the forecast within 3 days, do not irrigate, 3) Do not irrigate during the hottest part of the day, the best time to water is early morning before 9:00 or in the evening after 17:00. This protocol is extremely important during the hottest period of the summer (mid-July through mid-August). Not following this protocol will lead to leaf wilting.

PREVENTION AND TREATMENT OF DISEASE AND INSECT PESTS

Cultivation of *dìhuáng* has a number of significant disease and pest problems. Heavy rainfall and high humidity are major contributing factors to most of these problems. Good drainage is essential as a preventative measure. Also, proper spacing helps to minimize the problems and, if they arise, the spread of disease or pests. Leaf borne diseases and pests are most common.

Spot Blight (*Septoria lycopersici*)

Treatment and Prevention

Cover cropping with a grass family plant after 2 years. Identify and eliminate any plants showing early signs of disease. Destroy any diseased plants found during harvest.

Fusarium Wilt (*Fusarium* sp.)

Treatment and Prevention

Use of a grass family plant to cover crop every 3-5 years helps to resolve this problem. More and deeper cultivation, appropriate use of top-dressing and watering are also important. Be sure that water is draining properly after rain. Promptly remove any diseased plants and destroy them.

Red Spider Mite (*Tetranychus cinnbarinus*)

Prevention and Treatment

The original text only offers chemical treatments for this pest although it also suggests the use of pyrethrins at a 0.05% concentration sprayed on plants. [Translator's Note: In our experience at our farm planting too close together can lead to problems with this pest. Also, the timely removal of yellowing leaves helps to control it. Finally, the use of neem oil can be very useful to control this pest, especially in its early stages.]

Cutworm (*Agrotis ypsilon*)

Treatment and Prevention

The use of black light traps is employed to attract and kill the adult moth before it lays its eggs.

Mole Cricket (*Gryllotalpa* sp.)

Treatment and Prevention

The use of black light traps is employed to attract and kill the adult moth before it lays its eggs.

HARVESTING

Growing Period Before Harvest

Plants should be harvested within one year from the time the tubers are planted. The optimal time is between 140–160 days.

Harvest Season

The optimum time for harvesting *dìhuáng* is during the last 10 days of November. At this time the leaves should have withered and yellowed, growth has stopped, and the root has stored its maximum potential. If, during the months of September and October, the fruiting seed capsule has split open and its seeds have fallen, the herb can be dug.

Harvesting Method

Digging by Hand: Shovels or digging forks may be used to dig the tubers. Harvesters should be careful to dig beyond the depth of the tuber (approximately 35–40 cm) to avoid damage to the tuber during digging.

Digging by Machine: Larger excavators are used in large fields. Attachments used for digging roots should be used to ensure proper depth and reduced risk of injury to tubers.

ON-FARM PROCESSING

Traditional Oven Baking

In the corner of an appropriate room, a rectangular drying oven is built with brick and adobe; 116 cm high, 117 cm wide, and 226 cm long. After completion, the wall is fortified with adobe, and baked. In the middle of the outer wall there are two openings, 30 cm high and 30 cm wide; these are built and connected internally. Within these areas (under where the *dìhuáng* will be dried) a fire is started and six or seven sticks of sorghum stalks are laid horizontally to reach a height of 90 cm from the ground of the baking wall.

Add 200–300 kg of freshly picked *dìhuáng* to the built oven. The basic baking principle is to lay the tubers so that they are no more than 30 cm thick (as they lie on top of each other) and they are basically of uniform thickness. The temperature should not be too high nor too low, too high and they will be baked dry, too low will cause juice to ooze from the tubers. Both conditions will reduce the medicinal value of *dìhuáng*. The temperature should be about 50°C for the initial phase of roasting. This temperature is maintained for 2 days and then increased to 70–75°C until roots reach that temperature, then the temperature is decreased to 40–45°C, which is achieved by smothering the fire and allowing the oven to cool.

After the *dìhuáng* is put in the oven, it should only be turned once in the first two days until it reaches the maximum temperature (70-75°C). Once the oven has reached this temperature, the tubers are turned 2 times a day. During this process, if the tuber is found to be dry on the exterior, gently press with your hand to see if the entire tuber is soft all the way to the center, when it has achieved this softness it is done. Generally, 4–5 days are needed to bake the tubers.

After the *dìhuáng* is baked to dryness on the exterior, but the interior is soft, the roots are piled and allowed to "sweat,"* usually 3–4 days, allowing the moisture from the interior to move to the exterior so that the entire tuber is equally moist. Then the roots are baked in the oven for another 3–4 hours at a temperature of 50°C; after this the process is complete.

Once the roots have cooled, the final step is to knead the root tubers into round balls by hand. Finally, transfer them to the oven at a temperature of 45°C for 3–4 hours, but not so long that the balls lose their shape. Once removed, the drying process is complete.

*Sweating is a process to allow the moisture in a plant part, usually a root or tuber, to become evenly distributed. The reason this is important is because causing the exterior to become overly dry while the interior remains moist can cause damage to the medicinal quality of the herb. Note that sweating does not entail causing moisture to ooze from the plant material as humans do when they perspire.

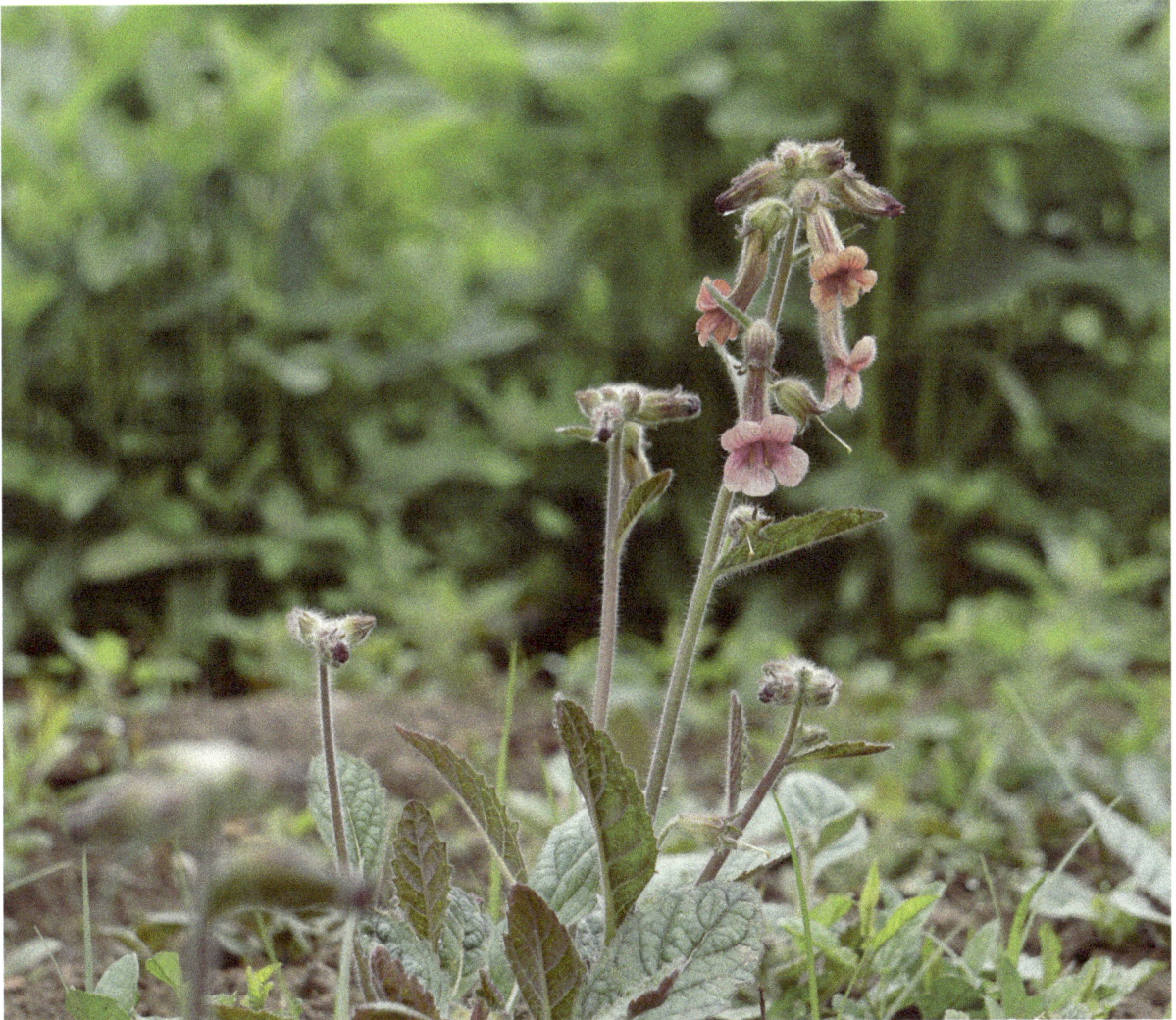

Wild *dìhuáng* in Henan province, China.

山东丹参

Red Sage Root
Salvia miltiorrhiza

The root of *shāndōng dānshēn* (*Salvia miltiorrhiza* Bunge), commonly known as *dānshēn* (丹参 ＼ 丹參) in China, is a member of the mint family (Lameaceae). The genus (*Salvia*, commonly known as sage) is the largest genus in the mint family with close to 1000 species throughout the world. This species is common throughout much of eastern China and is found growing along streams, on hillsides, and in forests from 100–1300 m elevation. Many different types of sages are used in cooking, medicine, perfumery, and ornamental gardening and are often aromatic, although this species has little to no aroma. The daodi location for this medicinal is in Linyi, Jinan, Tai'an, and surrounding areas of Shandong Province in northeastern China.

This extremely important medicinal was first recorded nearly 2000 years ago and has likely been used for much longer. Chinese medicine uses this herb to quicken and cool the blood, expel blood stasis, and stop pain. It is used for blood stasis and treats nearly any type of pain including chest pain, menstrual pain, and pain from physical trauma. *Dānshēn* is commonly used in gynecology to regulate menstruation and relieve menstrual pain. Because this root is cooling, it is a preferred choice when there is heat combined with pain syndromes.

This is an extensively studied medicinal plant and some of its compounds have been developed into standard drugs. The root of this herb has been found to have pharmacological activities including antioxidant, anti-inflammatory, antibacteria, anti-

tumor, anxiolytic, and cardioprotection. The herb can be used to treat a wide range of illnesses including coronary heart disease, angina pectoris, cerebrovascular diseases, ischemic stroke, hepatitis, hyperlipidemia, Alzheimer's disease, Parkinson's disease, diabetes, and insomnia.

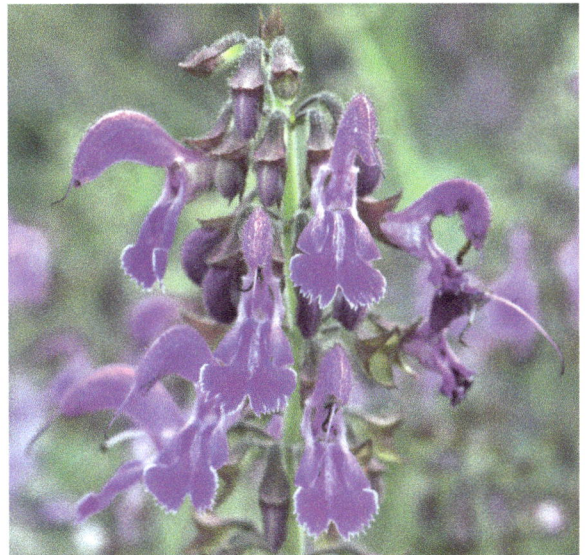

Contributing Authors

Huang Lu-qi, Guo Lan-ping, Zhang Yan, Zhao Dong-yue, Hao Qing-xiu, Sun Hai-feng, Yang Guang, Wang Xiao, Zhou Jie, Liu Wei

PRODUCTION SITE ECOLOGY

Elevation

Dānshēn is grown between 60–1000 m elevation.

Temperature

Cultivation of this medicinal requires 170–220 frost-free days with an average annual temperature range between 11–16°C. January is the coldest month, averaging between -4–0.2°C and July is the hottest month averaging between 21.5–27.5°C.

Photo Period

Annual sunshine range should be 2290–2890 hours.

Rainfall

Average annual rainfall range should be between 550–950 mm.

Soil

A sandy loose soil with a pH close to neutral is best. It can be either slightly acidic or slightly alkaline.

Topography

Dānshēn must have good water drainage and can be grown on mountain slopes, gentle hilly slopes, or flatlands.

PRODUCTION AREA ENVIRONMENTAL REQUIREMENTS

Site Selection

The top layer of the soil should be loose and tilled to a depth of at least 40 cm. A fertile, sandy soil with good water drainage is important. Clay or saline-alkaline soils are not appropriate for cultivation of *dānshēn*. Continuous cropping must be avoided. A crop rotation of millet, corn, onion, garlic, coix, castor, etc. all can be used. It can also be used for inter-cropping in fruit orchards, but it is not suitable for growing with legumes or other root crop herbs. [Translator's Note: Inter-cropping with *Calendula officinalis* has also been successful and could help prevent root-knot nematodes.]

Soil Preparation

Soil should be prepared in late February or March by deep plowing (more than 30 cm) after applying ample nutrition at a rate of 12,000–18,000 kg of compost (or 1800–3000 kg organic fertilizer), or NPK fertilizer 300–600 kg per acre. After this plowing, the field is harrowed, beds are formed, and then raked smooth until there are no hilly areas. Beds should be 40–80 cm wide and 25 cm tall, with 25 cm pathways between the beds.

SOWING SEEDS & RAISING SEEDLINGS

Seed Quality Requirement

Select the current year's seed with no more than 5% foreign matter. Seeds should have a 75% or higher germination rate.

Seed Saving Requirements

Seeds are saved from healthy mature plants that are free from disease. If seeds are sealed in a bag and kept at room temperature for one to two years, expect a reduction in germination rate of between 5–7%. Liquid nitrogen canasters have been utilized to keep the seeds at approximately -196°C as a method of preserving seeds for extended periods of time.

Seed Storage

Seeds should be stored in a dry room with good air circulation and normal atmospheric temperatures. Seeds stored for extended periods of time will have reduced germination rates; even short storage periods, such as storing until the next season, can result in a drop in germination rates of 5–7%.

Nursery Soil and Bed Preparation

Beds should be deeply plowed to at least 30 cm. Well-composted manure should be added at a rate of 18,000 kg per acre (organic fertilizer 3000 kg), combined well, and raked smooth.

Sowing Seeds

Seeds are sown from mid-July through the end of August at a rate of 21–30 kg per acre. Seeds are surface sown and raked in, being sure they are evenly distributed on the bed. The bed is covered in a light organic mulch (straw is often used) and watered appropriately to maintain soil moisture.

Management of Seedling Beds

After sowing, beds should be inspected once a day to assess soil moisture and degree of germination. If the weather is dry during this period, be sure to water beds appropriately, do not allow the soil to dry out. Any weeds should be removed immediately after they emerge. Once seeds have germinated, the thin layer of straw mulch should be removed from the bed.

Emergence of Seedlings

Seedlings generally emerge within the first 20 days of March and continue afterwards. Once they have emerged, they are dug and tied in small bundles of 100 plants to be taken to the field for transplanting. Any particularly small, malformed, or otherwise sub-standard plants should be discarded.

Transplanting to Field

Transplanting can occur in the spring or autumn. Spring transplanting happens during mid-March, autumn transplanting happens during late October or early November, before the first heavy frost. Plants are transplanted in rows 25 cm apart with 30 cm between each row. A hole or trench is dug for transplanting and must be deep enough for the entire root to stretch to the bottom; do not allow the root to be bent inside the hole. Fill in and mound the soil around the above ground portions of the plant. Water after transplanting is complete. Each acre should have 48,000–60,000 plants.

FIELD MANAGEMENT

Cultivation and Weeding

Generally, this is done 2–3 times during the months of May and June. After this time there is generally little need for weeding because the plants shade out weeds.

Irrigation and Top-Dressing

While *dānshēn* is growing it should have ample irrigation and not be allowed to dry out. During vigorous growth, fertilize with 120 kg urea per acre and give it ample water. During the month of August, when root growth becomes expansive, apply 120–180 kg per acre of diammonium phosphate complex. If rain is extended or very heavy be sure there is proper drainage so that water is not allowed to stagnate.

Removing Flowers

Only the flowering stalks of plants that are being reserved for seed harvest should remain, all others are removed during the months of May and June to encourage growth of the leaves and roots.

PREVENTION AND TREATMENT OF DISEASE AND INSECT PESTS

Principles of Prevention and Treatment

Dānshēn tends to be relatively free of diseases or pests, and serious or contagious problems are rare. In most cases proper management and attending to any problems with proper physical or biological treatments can readily resolve problems. When growing from either seed or transplanting, plants that appear weak or sick should be removed, and prescribed methods of application of fertilizer, field management, proper encouragement or application of biological controls (including but not limited to diversity of species) should be followed.

Root Rot Disease (*Fusarium* sp.)

Prevention and Treatment

After two years of harvesting, a crop rotation with a grass family plant should be done. Be sure not to use seedling beds that have known diseases present. Use appropriate fertilization, and appropriate organic fertilizer with phosphorus and potash. Remove any diseased plants in a timely manner and use lime in the holes to kill pathogens.

Leaf Spot (pathogen not confirmed)

Prevention and Treatment

Pathogen may be *Cercospora salviola* and/or *Alternaria zinnia*. After three years of harvesting, a crop rotation of a grass family plant should be done.

Keep fields free from disease-causing residue such as infected plants, etc. Appropriate use of organic fertilizer, including phosphorus and potash, is helpful. A 0.2–0.3% solution of monopotassium phosphate can also be sprayed on plants.

Root-knot Nematode (*Meloidogyne* sp.)

Biological Controls

The use of *Paecilomyces lilacinus* (200 million spores\g) is employed with two applications over a week. For agricultural controls see root rot above.

Below Ground Insect Pests

Prevention and Treatment

Use simple methods such as meticulous plowing and fine harrowing, deep plowing and tilling, and be sure to use thoroughly decomposed compost. These are generally sufficient to control these pests. Light traps can be used during the insects' adult stage.

HARVESTING

Growing Period Before Harvest

Dānshēn can be harvested after a single season.

Harvest Season

Generally, the plant is harvested in the months of October and November, but they can be harvested in the spring just as they begin to emerge.

Harvesting Method

Digging by Hand: Hand tools or small machines can be used for small quantities, or in areas machines cannot easily reach. It is important to do one's best to keep the entire root system intact. [Translator's Note: *Dānshēn* can have very deep roots, digging can be very arduous, for this reason building slightly taller beds can be helpful during digging process when it is time to harvesting.]

Machine Harvesting: In large fields a root excavator can be used for harvesting *dānshēn*.

ON-FARM PROCESSING

Initial Processing and Drying

After digging, roots are separated from any foreign matter, soil, non-medicinal parts, etc. and sun-dried. Care must be taken to turn root regularly to avoid collection of moisture and for even drying. Do not allow them to get wet from rain or morning dew. After the roots reach 50% dryness, the roots are loosely piled in 70 cm high and 50 cm wide rows. The roots remain this way for about 10 days before being turned and piled. This is repeated 2–3 times. This helps to draw the moisture from the inside of the roots out and hastens the drying process. During this process it is important to be careful not to break the small roots. Final moisture content must be below 12%.

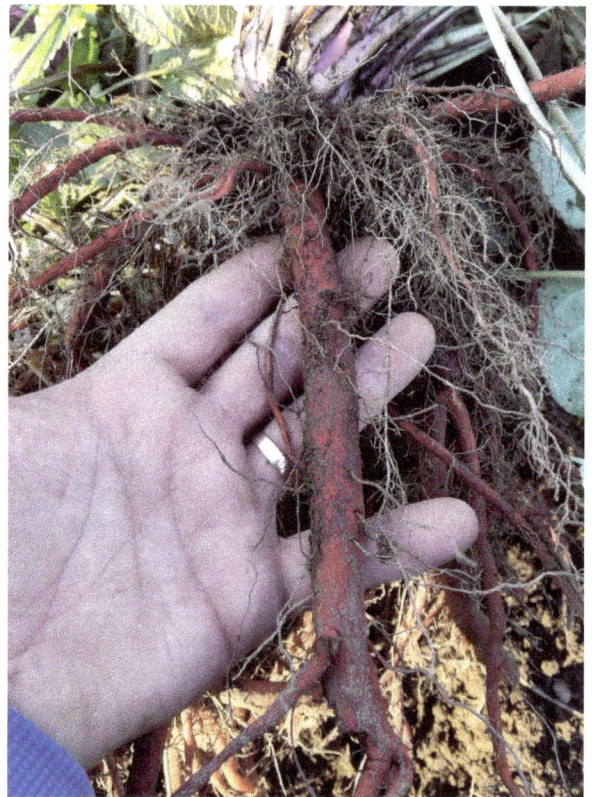

Fresh *dānshēn* root from our farm in Beijing, China.

祁荆芥
Japanese Catnip
Nepeta tenuifolia

The dried herb or dried flowering stalks of *qí jīngjiè* (*Schizonepeta tenuifolia* Briq.*), commonly known as *jīngjiè* (荆芥 / 荊芥) in China, is a member of the mint family (Lamiceae). This plant is native throughout much of China excluding eastern and southeastern provinces, although it is cultivated in much of that area. The plant grows 30–100 cm tall with a terminal spike of small violet flowers. In its native habitat it grows along sloping forest margins and in valleys from 500–2700 m elevation. Daodi *jīngjiè* refers to the area of Anguo in Hebei Province.

*Translator's Note: Although *Schizonepeta tenuifolia* is the name listed in the original text and in the *Pharmacopoeia of the People's Republic of China* (2015), the name has been changed to *Nepeta tenuifolia* Benth.

This herb is traditionally used to dispel wind and resolve the exterior for both wind-heat and wind-cold exterior invasions such as the common cold and influenza. Although it is warm in nature, this quality is not strong and it is frequently used for both wind-heat or wind-cold without regard for its warm nature. The herb is also frequently used to dispel wind and resolve the exterior for skin conditions with itching. It is especially frequently used as an herb of choice for allergic skin conditions with itching and raised bumps on the skin. Although the entire herb is used, the flower spike, *jīngjièsuì* (荆芥穗), is generally considered the best part.

The water extract of *jīngjiè* has shown both in vitro and *in vivo* (mouse) inhibition and significantly im-

proved outcomes for hand, foot, and mouth disease. The herb has shown immunomodulating activities specific to allergic dermatitis significantly lowering a number of inflammatory markers; in the experiment, markers of inflammation and allergic reaction, IFN-γ, TNF-α, IL-4, and IL-6, were suppressed. The herb and its essential oil have also shown anti-inflammatory, antioxidant, and antibacterial activities.

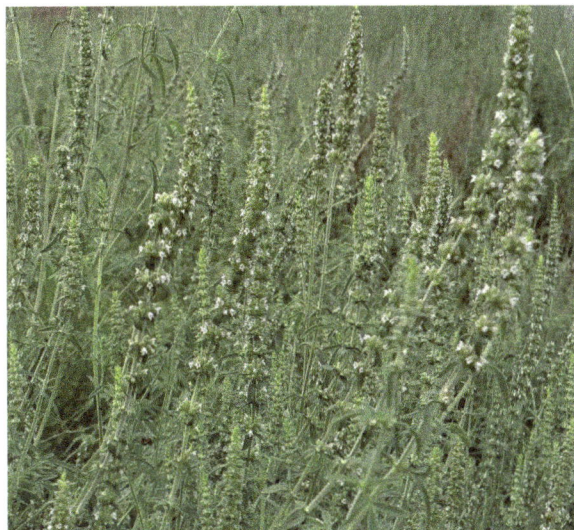

Contributing Authors

Zheng Yu-guang, Xie Xiao-liang, Guo Lan-ping, Huang Lu-qi, Hao Qing-xiu, Liu Ming, Song Jun-nuo, Wen Chun-xiu, Liu Ling-di, Gu Dong-sheng, Tian Wei

PRODUCTION SITE ECOLOGY

Elevation

Jīngjiè is cultivated between 50–500 m elevation.

Temperature

At least 197 frost free days. January is the coldest month with average temperatures below 3°C. July is the warmest month with average temperatures ranging between 18–27°C.

Photo Period

Average annual sunshine is between 2500–2757 hours. Sunshine percentage range 35–70%.

Moisture

Average annual rainfall 606–1000 mm with relative humidity of 34–55%.

Soil

A loose sandy soil with a depth of at least 30 cm is ideal, and pH should be in the 5.5–6.5 range.

Topography

The field can be either level or have a slope up to 15 degrees. A sloped field should be facing either southeast or northwest to allow for proper wind-flow.

PRODUCTION AREA ENVIRONMENTAL REQUIREMENTS

Soil Preparation

Soil is prepared by adding 12,000–18,000 kg of composted manure per acre, or 1800 kg of organic fertilizer, superphosphate 50 kg, and urea 20 kg per acre, then plowing 20–30 cm deep before harrowing.

SOWING SEEDS & RAISING SEEDLINGS

Seed Quality Requirements

According to the *Pharmacopoeia of the People's Republic of China* (2015), the source of seeds for the mint family plant *jīngjiè* is *S. tenuifolia*; they should be thoroughly dried and mature. The seeds have three ridges and an ovoid shape. It should be 1.4–1.7 mm long and 0.5–0.8 mm wide. Seeds are brown to brownish-black color and should be somewhat glossy in appearance. Dense pockmarks are visible under a microscope.

Sowing Seeds

In the spring seeds are sown in mid-April. When growing for *jīngjièsuì*. Seeds are sown in late June or early July if is not desired. Some farms sow seeds in September and October for harvest in the following year. Rows are spaced 20–25 cm apart. *Jīngjiè* seed is sown in rows 0.5 cm deep and 5–7 cm wide. Seeds are sown at a rate of 3 kg per acre.

FIELD MANAGEMENT

Cultivation and Weeding

Timely cultivation, keeping the soil loose and free of weeds, is important. [Translator's Note: Because *jīngjiè* grows very quickly from seed, sowing seeds in excess of the prescribed rate can be used to overcome weeds. However, this will require thinning once the plants have reached 2–4 cm tall.]

Top-Dressing

When the plants reach a height of approximately 15 cm, top-dress with urea at a rate of 120 kg per acre. [Translator's Note: Alternatively, composted manure can be used to top-dress (horse, cow, and goat are all appropriate, chicken and pig mature are not).]

Irrigation and Water Drainage

While *jīngjiè* does not require a lot of water, be sure to water if there are extended periods without rain. Irrigate after top-dressing. Be sure that there is proper drainage during heavy rain periods.

PREVENTION AND TREATMENT OF DISEASE AND INSECT PESTS

Principles of Prevention and Treatment

Generally, *jīngjiè* has very few disease problems. The primary diseases are caused by over-crowding and continuous cropping. Pests are usually most problematic during the early growing season, however mole crickets could affect mature plants as well.

Silver Lined Noctuid (*Argyrogramma agnate*)

Biological Controls

During seedling and young plant growth, watch closely for the larvae stage and manually eliminate them. During larvae and early life stages use 100 million spores per gram of *Bacillius* (Bt) at a 0.5% dilution in water and apply accordingly. Natural pyrethrums (5%) in a 0.05–0.1% dilution in water can also be used. These treatments should be applied once a week for 2–3 weeks to kill the insects.

Mole Cricket (Gryllotalpidae)

Use black light to trap and kill adult insects.

Stem Blight (*pathogen not identified*)

Prevention and Treatment

Crop rotation after 2 years is an effective method for prevention and treatment of this problem.

Damping-off Disease (*Rhizoctonia solani*)

Prevention and Treatment

Utilizing crop rotation with a grass family plant, aggressive cultivation, and making sure there is proper drainage during heavy rains are important methods for avoiding this problem.

Powdery Mildew (*pathogen not identified*)

Prevention and Treatment

Appropriate spacing of plants is important, along with increased application of phosphorus and potash to improve the plant's ability to fight the disease. Be sure that water does not accumulate and stagnate.

HARVESTING

Harvest Season

Jīngjiè is an annual, plants are harvested in the same year they are sown; time from sowing seeds to harvest is 120–150 days. However, seeds sown in the autumn may overwinter and plants are harvested the following year.

Jīngjiè is harvested in the autumn of the same year it is planted (October) when the flowering stalks are half in bloom and half past bloom (it will have seeds). At this stage the plant's essential oil is at its peak, averaging 0.97%. Plants that have completed flowering should not be used as medicine. According to the *Pharmacopoeia of the People Republic of China* (2015), the minimum amount of essential oil required in the dried herb is 0.60%. The half-blooming/half-past-bloom inflorescence (*jīngjièsuì*) and leaves harvested at that time have the highest quantity of essential oil and are generally considered the best medicine. It should be noted that stems only have about 0.14% essential oil at this time, so excessive stems mixed in with inflorescence (*jīngjièsuì*) and leaves is considered poor quality product. Seeds sown in April are harvested in September. Seeds sown in the summer are harvested in October, and seeds sown in autumn are harvested in late May to early June of the following year.

Harvest Method

Choose a bright sunny day for harvesting. The plant can be either cut off at the base or pulled from the ground.

ON-FARM PROCESSING

Drying Method

The entire plant is hung to dry. If growing for *jīngjièsuì* (flowering spike), these parts are removed and the remaining parts are reserved for *jīngjiègěng* (stem with some leaves, this material is low quality and rarely used in modern practice). If growing for *jīngjiè*, the entire herb is dried and only the thickest, woody stems are discarded after drying. If a dryer must be used because of atmospheric conditions, low temperatures should be used (preferably <40°C).

Further Considerations

After harvest, avoid exposure to sunlight, place in a cool shady location with good air circulation. A dryer can be used; however, this changes the chemical composition of the dried material significantly. In particular, there are two monoterpenes (cotonone and menthone) whose ratio changes significantly. This has a negative effect on the herbs anti-inflammatory activity. Therefore, traditional drying in a cool shady location is preferred. Dried material should not exceed 12% moisture content.

Packaging and Storage

Both *jīngjiè* and *jīngjièsuì* are bundled with twine to avoid breakage of the material, this also discourages mold and loss of essential oils during storage.

Jīngjiè should be stored at temperatures not exceeding 20°C and ambient humidity of 65%.

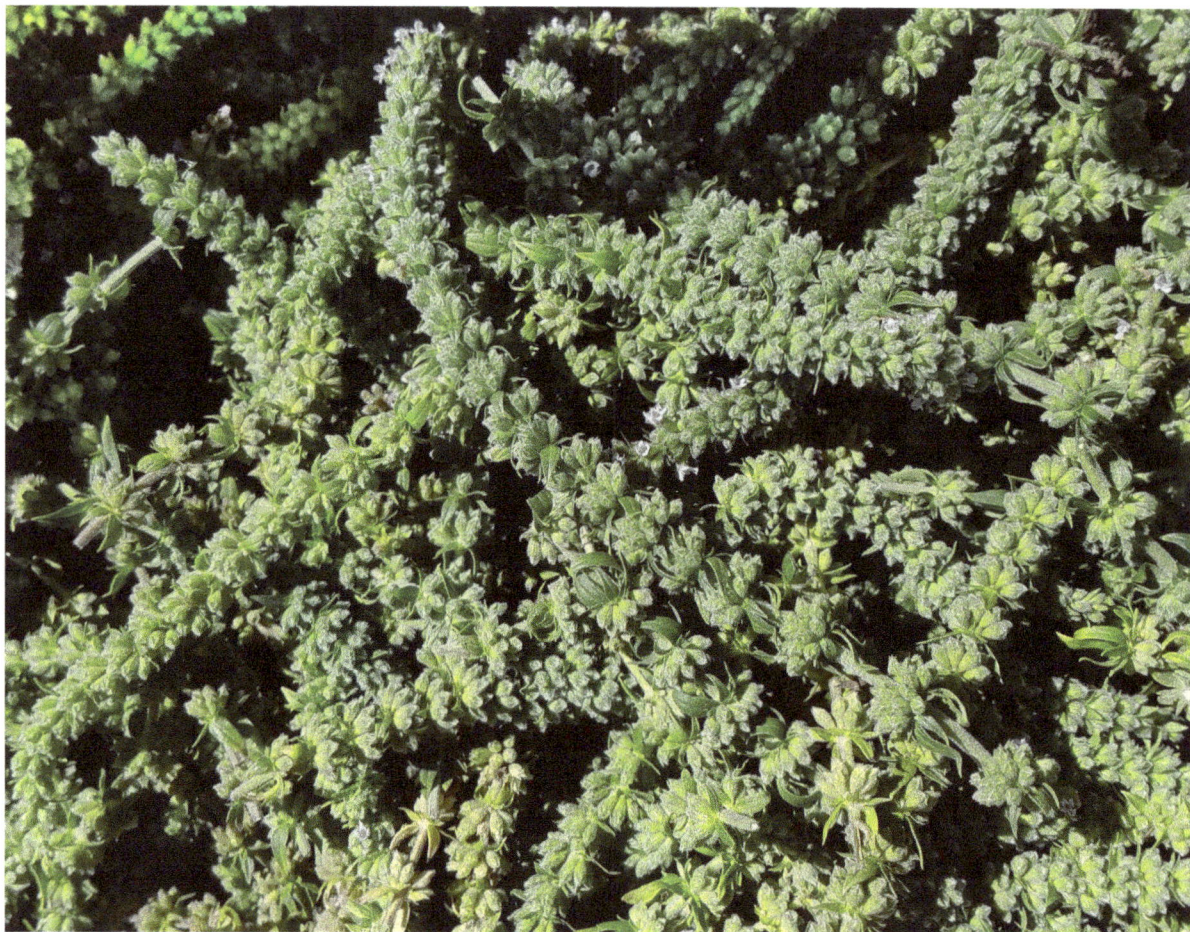

Fresh *jīngjièsuì* from our farm in Beijing, China.

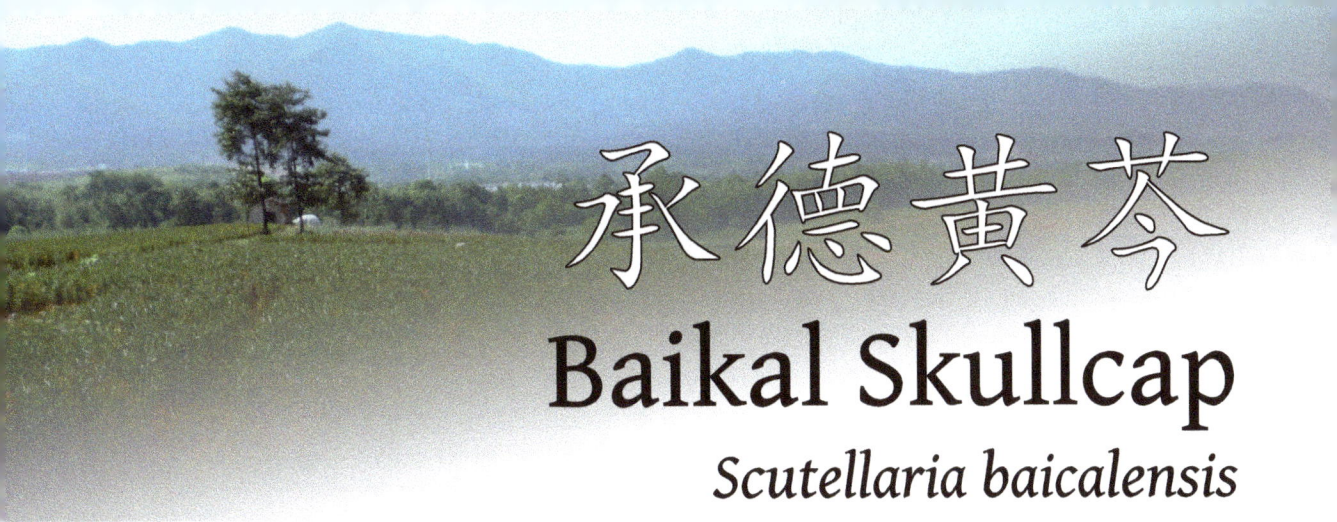

承德黄芩
Baikal Skullcap
Scutellaria baicalensis

DISTINGUISHING FEATURES

The dried root of the daodi medicinal *chéngdé huángqín* (*Scutellaria baicalensis* Georgi), known as *huángqín* (黃芩 \ 黄芩) in China, is a member of the mint family (Lamiacea). Scutellaria is a large genus of about 350 species, almost one-third of which are found in China. It grows mostly on grassy slopes from 100–2000 m elevation throughout much of central, eastern, and northern China and can also be found in Mongolia, Russia, Korea, and Japan. Material produced in the Chengde district in Hebei Province (north of Beijing) is considered the daodi medicinal.

This herb has a long history in Chinese medicine and is among the most commonly used herbs today. Traditionally, it is used to clear heat and dry dampness and can be used in almost any pattern where there are heat and dampness pathogens. Although some say that it is most useful for upper burner patterns such as lung infections, it is also extremely beneficial for conditions of the liver and gastrointestinal diseases. It is commonly used to clear heat and drain fire, and specifically to clear heat and drain fire from the qi aspect. It is also used to calm the fetus when a pregnant mother has a febrile condition, as it has the functions of both clearing fire and calming the fetus. The alcohol processed root is best for treating upper burner conditions.

Modern science has done extensive research on this plant. The whole root and several of its flavonoids have shown significant anti-inflammatory, antibacterial, antioxidant, hepatoprotective, antitumor, and anti-HIV pharmacological activities. Extracts of the roots have been shown to have a synergistic action when combined with some antibiotics, which could lead to combination drugs in the future.

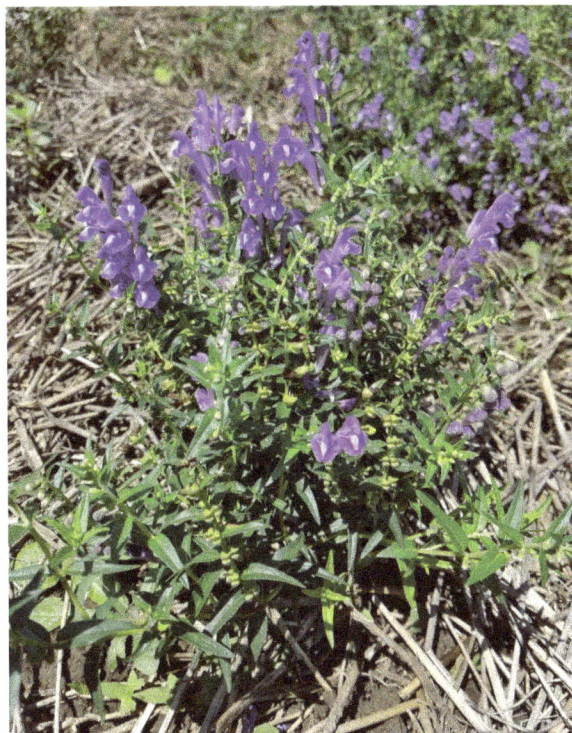

Contributing Authors

Zhao Run-hui, Zhang Xue-wen, Wang Ji-yong, Zeng Yan

PRODUCTION SITE ECOLOGY

Elevation

Huángqín is cultivated between 300–1000 m elevation.

Temperature

The average annual temperature is 8.9°C with a frost-free period of 160 days.

Photo Period

Annual sunshine hours should range from 2600–3100 hours.

Moisture

Suitable average annual rainfall is 402.3–882.6 mm.

Soil

Loam and sandy loam are preferred, with pH neutral to slightly alkaline (7.0–8.5).

Topography

Southeast, south, southwest slopes are all appropriate, with direct south facing areas being ideal. Although slope is not required for growing *huángqín*, it naturally grows on slopes and does not like stagnant water or overly wet soils, so it a slope up to 20° is recommended.

PRODUCTION AREA ENVIRONMENTAL REQUIREMENTS

Site Selection

A slope facing the sun (SE, S, SW) with good soil structure that is deep with good drainage. Problems with continuous cropping do not appear to be significant, based on the experience of growers, but it is recommended that growers rotate crops with a suitable cover-crop or fodder, recommended crops are soy, corn, potato, etc.

Soil Preparation

Soil preparation can begin either in the fall after harvest, or as soon as the ground has thawed in the spring. Thoroughly composted manure is applied at a rate of 21,000–24,000 kg per acre, or diamine phosphate is applied at a rate of 120–180 kg per acre. Plow to a depth of at least 30 cm to integrate compost or fertilizer, harrow, and rake smooth.

SOWING SEEDS & RAISING SEEDLINGS

Seed Quality Requirements

Seeds should be selected from plants that are at least 2 years old. High quality seeds have at least a 75% germination rate and produce plants with at least 85% vitality. Seeds should not have more than 5% foreign matter.

Sowing Seeds

Seeds are sown in the early spring or late autumn. Sow between March and the beginning of May if in the spring being sure that the temperature of the soil at 5 cm deep has reached 15°C or higher. Seeds sown in autumn should be during mid- to late October before the ground freezes. A seedling bed (for later transplanting) can also be used for growing during the months of June and July when there is ample rain. Field sowing is done by creating furrows 1.5–2.5 cm deep, mixing seed at a ratio of 1:1–1.5 with millet or fine sand, then hand sowing into the furrows. Seeds are covered with 0.5–1.5 cm of soil. Seeds are sown at a rate of 6–9 kg per acre.

FIELD MANAGEMENT

Thinning and Final Singling of Seedlings

Furrows are thinned 1–2 times; gaps in planting can be filled during this time. The first thinning should commence when seedlings are between 3–5 cm tall. The second thinning is when they reach 8–19 cm tall. Generally, thinning means eliminating every other seedling, more or less, leaving the tallest and strongest plants. Final spacing should be 10–15 cm. Any areas within the rows with poor germination or excessive numbers of poorly growing plants should be replaced by this time with plants from the thinning process. Plants are not generally transplanted after this stage is complete.

Dunmiao

This is a traditional process to encourage root growth during the early growing stage of the plant. A clear sunny afternoon should be selected. Gently press the soil around the seedling. This is done 2–3 times at 8–10-day intervals. On larger, modern farms this is done at the same time weeding is done.

Top-Dressing

During the bud and flowering period (mid-June to mid-August), and after irrigation, applications of a compound fertilizer (10–10–10) may be added as top-dressing at a rate of 60–120 kg per acre. This can be done 3–5 times every 10 days.

Removing Flowers

If there is no intention of collecting seed, flower buds are removed between July through mid-August to encourage root growth. Traditionally, on small-scale farms this was done by hand with scissors, 3–5 times with 10–15 days between cuttings. However, on larger farms this is generally done once or twice with a sickle or other appropriate tool to cut the majority of the flowers off the plant.

Cultivation, Weeding, and Hilling

Cultivation and weeding should be done 3–4 times each year. The first time should be in early spring when weeds first begin to get established. The second time should be done when beds are built. The third time should be done before weed seeds can ripen. Cultivation, weeding, and hilling should be done at the same time. After 3 years, cultivation and weeding should only be needed 1 or 2 times per year. [Translator's Note: Hilling is the process of pushing soil around growing plants, "hilling-up" the soil around the plant to stabilize it and encourage lateral root grown from the lower stem. This helps to give the plant an up-right growth and develops lateral roots that will be harvested later.]

Irrigation and Water Drainage

During the period after sowing seeds, the soil must remain moist, if the soil moisture seems to be insufficient after the seeds have sprouted, watering may be done once. After this, especially once the roots have established to a depth of 10 cm or more, they should basically not be watered. Watering is reserved for times when there are significant dry spells and after top-dressing. Watering can also be done after 2 years of growth in order to encourage root growth. If sowing seeds during the rainy season watering is probably unnecessary. If there is water accumulation in the field during the rainy season, the water should be drained off. Because *huángqín* does not like water accumulation, planting in beds is generally considered the method of choice since you avoid potential water accumulation altogether.

Harvesting Seeds

Seeds ripen in succession between July and September, therefore harvesting in batches is required. Sometimes farmers simply wait until the first 20–30% of seeds are ripe to harvest the first time, then wait until 60–70% are ripe to harvest the second time. This ensures that there is minimal loss in the field, but also yields immature seeds that need to winnowed out later. Seeds are dried in the sun, then threshed and saved in bags. Harvesting of seeds may be done by cutting off the flowering branch after the flowers have fallen and the seeds begin to ripen, or one may wait until the majority of the seeds have ripened and harvest the seeds by hand into a container. At this time the seed capsules should be dry and easily come off the branches. If there are capsules that have not broken open, lightly rolling over them with a roller on a flat surface will break them without damaging the seeds. Then use a fan to thresh the seeds. Generally, seeds are warehoused at temperatures between 10–25°C with little adverse effect on germination rate during short-term storage (<1 year). However, storing between 0–10°C allows for long-term storage. Temperatures over 25°C quickly have an adverse effect on germination rates.

PREVENTION AND TREATMENT OF DISEASE AND INSECT PESTS

Principles of Prevention and Treatment

The most common diseases affecting *huángqín* are root rot and powdery mildew. The most common insect problems are the turnip sawfly (*Athalia rosae*) and grubs. Water drainage is critically important to avoid root rot and to improve root development. Planting on a slope can help with water drainage, but a loose soil is strongly recommended. Overcrowding plants should be avoided.

Root Rot (*Fusarium* sp.)

Prevention and Treatment

First consider whether there is a lack of soil aeration, and, if necessary, you can help the soil to ventilate by digging away sections near the plants. This is the primary reason why growing this plant on a slight slope is recommended. Reasonable crop rotation is also a consideration. Appropriate fertilizer application is important, but overuse of fertilizer may encourage root rot. Any plants showing signs of withering should be checked for root rot; any plants found with root rot should immediately be removed and the entire crop should be monitored, perhaps taking preventive measures noted above to prevent any further damage.

Powdery Mildew (*Oidium* sp.)

Prevention and Treatment

Be sure the plants are not planted too close together. Be sure to drain any excess water accumulation. Remove any infected leaves in a timely manner. Any diseased leaves discovered during harvest should be disposed of properly.

Grub (*Holotrichia* sp.)

Prevention and Treatment

Before winter and subsequent to transplanting, plow deep (perhaps several times) to destroy the insects. During the time of pest incursion, use black lights, or a combination of black and green lights to lure the grubs to traps.

Biological Controls

Use *Bacillus popilliae* and *Beauveria bassiana* as non-toxic spray controls.

HARVESTING

Harvest Season

Autumn harvest commences when the plant has withered. If harvested in the spring, plants should be dug before they reach 10 cm tall. Plants are generally harvested at the end of the third year but can also be harvested in the fourth or fifth year. [Translator's Note: Many farmers harvest *huángqín* after the second year, however this yields an inferior product and is not recommended. The main root harvested in the fourth and fifth year is likely to begin to become hollow and have some minor rot. Roots harvested at this time are called *kūhuángqín* (枯黄芩) (ku means "dry and withered") and were traditionally used to drain lung fire and clear heat from the muscle and exterior layers. However, any *kūhuángqín* on the market today is most likely wild since the extra time and risk of crop damage is not generally considered worth it for farmers.]

Harvest Method

Choose a sunny day, dig the roots, and rid the plant of all dirt and the buds present (what would have been the following year's growth) on the crown of the root.

ON-FARM PROCESSING

Drying Method

The whole roots are generally dried in the sun before slicing; if there is an appropriate location they can also be dried in the shade.

Electric Drum Roller Processing

Once the root has reached 20–30% dryness on the outer cork-like root bark, roots are loaded into a drum and spun to remove the outer cork-like bark. Roots are removed and allowed to continue to dry in the sun. When the roots have reached 50–60% dryness they are loaded into the drum and spun again to further remove the cork-like bark. When this is done correctly the root will turn a red-yellow color. After this process roots must be sun-dried in a clean location. When the roots have reached 70-80% dryness they are spun for a 3rd time. This time, the roots should come out looking yellowish. Roots are removed and placed on drying racks to dry in the sun until they reach 90% dryness. During this process it is important to protect the root's integrity; be careful not to damage the outer parts of the root. When sun-drying, be sure to turn the piles regularly, and carefully, to avoid uneven drying, mold, etc. Do not allow roots to get wet from rain or morning dew.

山东瓜蒌

Trichosanthes Fruit

Trichosanthes kirilowii

DISTINGUISHING FEATURES

The dried, mature fruit of the daodi medicinal *shāndōng guālóu* (*Trichosanthes kirilowii* Maxim.), commonly known as *guālóu* (瓜蒌 \ 瓜蔞) in China, is a member of the cucumber family (Cucurbitaceae). The *Trichosanthes* genus has about 100 species in Asia and Australia with 33 species in China (14 are endemic). This species is dioecious, meaning that it has both male and female plants, is native to eastern and central China, and grows in open forests, areas with scrub, and grasslands that are between 200–1800 m in elevation. Material produced in Shandong province in the Changqing, Feicheng, and the surrounding regions is considered the daodi medicinal.

Guālóu has been used for a very long time, however at different points in history different parts of the fruit (i.e. rind or seed) were considered to be the most potent, medicinal part. Today, the fruit is a separate medicinal, while the rind and the seed are considered to be medicinals in their own right with different therapeutic actions. However, the whole dried fruit is not frequently used; instead the rind or seeds, used separately, are the most commonly used parts of this medicinal plant. The whole fruit is primarily used to clear heat and transform phlegm and is frequently used with phlegm-heat and cough. The seeds are used when an intestine moistening action is needed, as can be quite common in lung heat conditions. The rind is more frequently used in general; its action is to disinhibit qi and relax the chest, and is frequently used for chest impediment and other similar ailments.

Modern science has focused on researching the cardiovascular activities of this herb. While it is primarily known as an herb to clear heat and resolve phlegm, the additional actions of the rind to disinhibit qi and relax the chest has led researchers to investigate cardiovascular effects. A great deal of research has shown very interesting results, with demonstrated pharmacological activities including; protecting ischemic myocardium and endothelial cells, calcium antagonistic effects, and promoting coronary blood flow. Expectorant, anti-inflammatory, and antioxidant activity has also been shown.

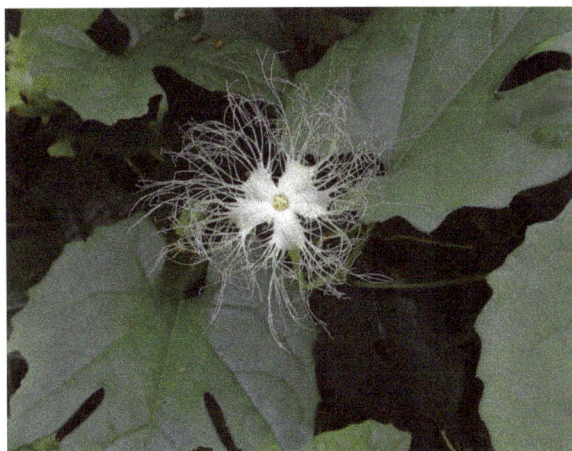

Contributing Authors

*Chao Zhi-mao, Sun Wen,
Wu Xiao-yi, Yu Li, Guo Lan-ping*

PRODUCTION SITE ECOLOGY

Elevation

Guālóu is cultivated from sea level to 200 m elevation.

Temperature

An average annual temperature range of 11–15°C is suitable with a frost-free period of 190–220 days.

Photo Period

Annual sunshine hours range from 2300–2800 hours.

Moisture

Average annual rainfall is between 520–680 mm.

Soil

A loose soil high in organic matter including brown soil, sandy soil, gray-brown soil, yellow soil, etc. can all be used for the cultivation of *guālóu*. Soil pH can vary greatly from strongly acidic to strongly alkaline.

Topography

Flat or up to 25 degrees of slope is suitable. If sloped, the slope should be south-facing. Avoid the north slope or places where sunshine is limited by other factors. Avoid areas where water can stagnate such as near bodies of water or low-laying areas.

PRODUCTION AREA ENVIRONMENTAL REQUIREMENTS

Site Selection

The site should not have been previously cultivated or, if it has, it should have had several seasons of rest. The soil layer should be deep, with a rich loose soil and plenty of humus. The site should have good drainage. Brown soil and a rich sandy soil are highly desired with a neutral or slightly acid or slightly alkaline pH. The site should have excellent sun exposure.

Soil Preparation

Soil should be plowed at least 25 cm and then 15,000–18,000 kg per acre of well-composted manure should be tilled in. Beds are made 25 cm tall and 1.5 m wide with 30–40 cm pathways for working and drainage.

PROPAGATION FROM RHIZOMES

Propagation

The tuber of the plant is dug as soon as the soil is no longer frozen. Select rhizomes that are 2–6 cm in diameter and cut off 3–6 cm sections. These are then immersed in an all-purpose fungicide for 30–60 minutes. The rhizomes are then dried in the sun, and, once dry, they can be prepared for planting. Rhizomes can be planted as soon as they are ready, generally this is in April or May.

Planting Method

Rhizomes are planted in holes dug 15 cm deep. Rows should be 1.2 m apart and in-row spacing should be 0.8–1.0 m. After placing the rhizome in the hole, it should be covered with soil and the soil should be firmly pressed. [As noted above, *guālóu* is a dioecious plant, both male and female plants are needed in the field in order to achieve a fruit set.] Generally, male plants are only 2–5% of the total plants in the field (fruits are borne on the female plants).

Trellis Construction

Any kind of trellis can be used. Wooden trellises are most commonly used. Another commonly used method is employing 2-meter concrete posts (sunk to 0.5 m) along either side of the beds, placed every 4 meters. These posts are wired with 0.3–0.4 mm wire every 20 cm (starting about 20 cm above the ground), which is then used to affix bamboo, wood, or other appropriate material for the *guālóu* to climb on. The slats of wood, or other material, should be placed every 15–20 cm apart. This allows the plant to easily climb and makes harvesting of the fruit convenient.

FIELD MANAGEMENT

Trellising Vines

Once the plant begins to emerge, watch for unhealthy vines and gently remove them. From each transplanted rhizome, only the strongest, healthiest vine should be maintained. Once that vine has grown more than 0.5 m, it can be easily trained onto the trellis.

Cultivation and Weeding

Cultivation between the plants should be done periodically during the growing period to avoid excessive weeds.

Irrigation and Top-Dressing

Top-dressing should be done during the period of vigorous growth to ensure plentiful flowers. This is generally done with a compound fertilizer at a rate of 120 kg per acre. Top-dressing with a P-K compound fertilizer at the same rate during fruiting season is also common practice. Foliar spray of a P-K compound will help to minimize flower drop and premature dropping of ripening fruits. Be sure to water after top-dressing. *Guālóu* does not like to be water-logged, therefore fields must be well-drained and water must not be allowed to stagnate.

Winter Survival Management

Around October 1st, after the fruit is all harvested, all the withered vines and leaves are removed from the growing area. Before the ground freezes, each hole where the shoots emerge should be covered with 10 cm of soil. Any diseased roots, or plants that showed weakness, poor fruit production, etc. should be removed and discarded, making sure to mark the hole clearly so that the during the following spring a new rhizome can be planted in that location.

PREVENTION AND TREATMENT OF DISEASE AND INSECT PESTS

Principles of Prevention and Treatment

After transplanting, plants that appear weak or sick should be removed, prescribed methods of field management, and proper encouragement or application of biological controls should be used. Most common diseases seen in *guālóu* include clearwing moth, anthracnose, root rot, and root-knot nematode.

Clearwing moth (*Melittia bombyliformis*)

Prevention and Treatment

Removing the larvae by hand is the most effective measure to managing this pest.

Anthracnose (*Colletotrichum lilii*)

Prevention and Treatment

Crop rotation using a grass family crop every 3–5 years is recommended. Appropriate use of organic fertilizers, including phosphorus and potash fertilization, is important. Maintaining clean fields, free of diseased plants, and making sure that water is draining properly after heavy rains will contribute substantially to a reduced incidence of disease. A copper sulfite, quick lime, and water mixture (1:2-3:200-240 ratio) can be sprayed on the plants as a protective measure. A lime-sulfur compound (used as recommended by the manufacturer) can also be applied to treat this disease.

Root Rot Disease (*Fusarium* sp.)

Prevention and Treatment

Cover cropping with grass family plants, avoiding transplanting of diseased rhizomes, appropriate combinations of fertilizers, appropriate increases in organic fertilizer, including phosphorus and potash, and early removal of diseased plants all help to contain this problem.

Root-knot Nematode (*Meloidogyne* sp.)

For prevention and treatment, see root rot above.

Biological Controls

Use *Paecilomyces lilacinus* (2 million spores per gram) and pour at the base of the plant. Two applications one week apart.

HARVESTING

Timing of Harvest

Guālóu is a perennial vine. Fruits are harvested each year from late September to early October; fruits can be picked as late as mid-November as long as there has not been a significant frost. While there is no standard for size, the fruits can't be young and tender; the skin must be firm.

Harvesting Method

When harvesting fruits at least 30 cm of the vine should be left attached, but all the leaves and leaf petioles should be removed from the vine. Do not allow the fruits to drop to the ground or otherwise be damaged as this may have significant impact on the quality of the final product.

ON-FARM PROCESSING

Braiding

Any fruits with damaged skins or bruising should be discarded. Once fruits have been picked, they are returned to the working area to be braided. Fruits are stacked and covered with a tarp and can remain that way for up to 3 days while awaiting braiding. The vines are braided with the fruits every 120°, creating a circle with every three fruits, being sure that fruits are not touching each other.

Shade Drying

The braided fruits are then hung in a shaded area, being sure not to knock them into each other or hang them in such a way that they are pushed together. The area should be shaded and cool with good air flow. If this is an outside area, care must be taken to protect the fruits from extreme cold or snow (humidity). In general, fruits hung in October are dry and ready for further processing in April of the following year. Translator's Note: The daodi region has a very dry winter season with humidity generally around 25–40%.

Cutting the Fruit

When the following criteria are met the fruit is ready for use as a medicine: the fruit skin has turned yellow, wrinkled, and crispy; the inside pulp is caramel colored with a caramel smell; the seeds have turned a light gray to gray color; and the fruit is completely dried. Leaving 1 cm of the vine for a handle, cut the fruits from the braid. Discard any fruits with mold or mildew, or damaged skin. Fruits can then be pressed and sliced for use as medicine.

Storage Note

Because *guālóu* is a fruit it tends to have problems with insect pests. For this reason, long-term storage is not recommended. Storage temperature should never be above 20°C and the ambient humidity should never go over 65%.

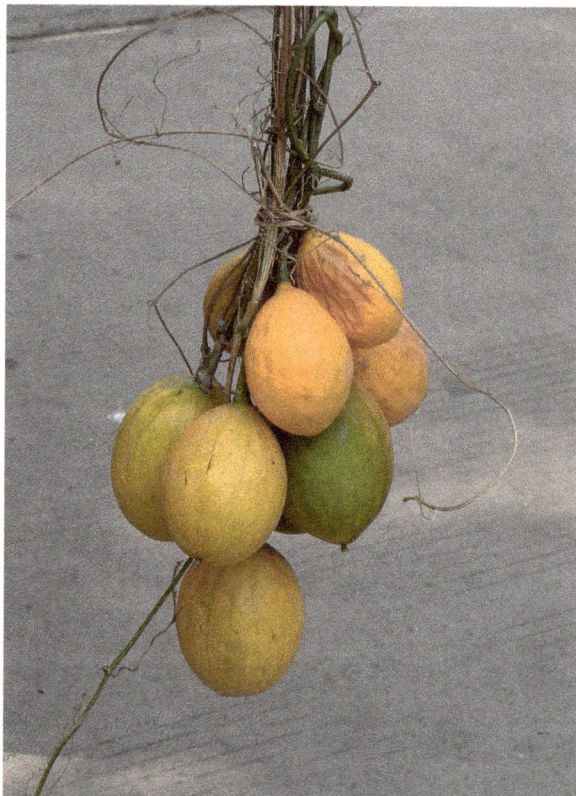

Ripe *guālóu* fruits braided and set to dry.

承德金莲花

Trollius Flower

Trollius chinensis

The dried flower bud of the daodi medicinal *chéngdé jīnliánhuā* (*Trollius chinensis* Bge.) is commonly known as *jīnliánhuā* (金莲花 \ 金蓮花) and is a member of the crowfoot family (Ranunculaceae). The *Trollius* genus has 30 species in the northern hemisphere with 16 species in China and eight endemic species. The species, which can grow to 80 cm at fruiting time, is native to the northeastern part of China and is found growing on grassy slopes between 1000–2200 m elevation. Material produced in the Chengde district in Hebei Province (north of Beijing) is considered the daodi medicinal.

This is a relatively new addition to the Chinese materia medica, having been first mentioned in the literature in the early Qing dynasty. It is an effective herb for clearing heat, resolving toxin, and dispersing swelling. It is used for common cold with fever, sore and swollen throat, mouth sores, swollen and painful teeth and gums, red and swollen eyes, and toxic swelling with redness and pain. It is also sometime used for lung heat and toxin. It can also be used externally. The flowers have become somewhat popular in parts of China as a daily tea to brighten the eyes.

The plant has recently gained a significant amount of attention due to its high content of flavonoids. The whole flower extract and many of its chemical compounds have shown excellent antioxidant and anti-inflammatory activities. Experiments have shown good antibacterial activity. In another study, ultrasonic assisted ethanol extraction was significantly better than any other extract for this antibacterial activity. This activity is thought to be from several of the flavonoids present in the flower. One of the flavonoids, orientin, which is also found in other medicinal plants such as holy basil (*Ocinium sanctum*) and *Passiflora* sp., has been studied extensively for its pharmacological activities. To date, it has shown significant potential as an antioxidant, anti-aging agent, cardioprotectant, vasodilator, antiviral and antibacterial agent, and neuroprotective agent.

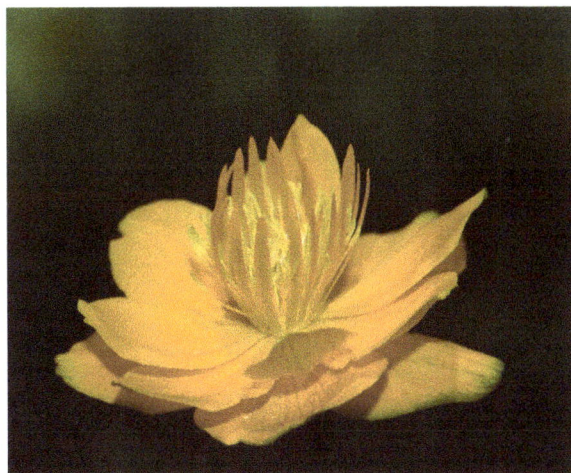

Contributing Authors

Xie Xiao-liang, Liu Ming, Guo Lan-ping, Huang Lu-qi, Hao Qing-xiu, Wen Chun-xiu, Liu Ling-di, Jia Dong-sheng, Tian Wei

PRODUCTION SITE ECOLOGY

Elevation

Jīnliánhuā is cultivated between 1200–2000 m elevation.

Temperature

Growing *jīnliánhuā* requires at least 135 frost free days. January is the coldest month with average temperatures below 3°C. July is the hottest month with average temperatures in the range of 18–27°C.

Photo Period

Annual sunshine hours range from 2600–2700 hours. Sunshine percentage range 56–70%.

Moisture

Average annual rainfall is 402.3–882.6 mm. Average humidity is 15–35%.

Soil

Sandy soils with a large quantity of organic matter and a pH of 5–6 are suitable.

Topography

Mountain-side grassy slope, open forest, or moist grass pasture land are all appropriate locations for growing *jīnliánhuā*.

PRODUCTION AREA ENVIRONMENTAL REQUIREMENTS

Site Selection and Soil Preparation

Select a site with sandy soil and add 12,000–18,000 kg per acre of well-composted manure, then harrow smooth.

SOWING SEEDS & RAISING SEEDLINGS

Seed Storage and Pre-Treatment

After harvest, seeds may be stored at room temperature for 4.5 months to more than 6 months. After this period, the seed should be stored in sand at 50–60% moisture and held at 0–4°C for 30–50 days prior to sowing. Seeds may also be immediately stored in moist sand, as above, and will be ready for sowing in about 75 days. [Translator's Note: This latter method is used for early sowing in greenhouses, allowing young plants to be trans-planted into the field in the spring.]

Sowing Seeds

Seeds are sown during mid-March after the ground has thawed. Beds are built 1.3–1.5 m wide. Seeds are mixed with 10 times their volume of fine sand and sown using the broadcast method. After they are sown, they are covered with 3–5 mm of soil, then another 2–3 cm of straw, then watered (agricultural plastic is also used as an alternative to straw). Seeds are sown at a rate of 9–15 kg per acre.

Transplanting

After plants have grown for one year, prior to emerging in the early spring they may be dug and then transplanted in a permanent location. They should be planted in rows 30 cm apart with plant spacing of 20 cm.

FIELD MANAGEMENT

Cultivation and Weeding

Before plants are developed, it is important to keep the beds free from weeds and loosen the soil by cultivation with a hoe.

Irrigation and Water Drainage

Careful observation during early watering will help to find possible areas that need to be managed so that water does not accumulate, this will be important during the rainy season to prevent plants from becoming waterlogged.

Top-Dressing

Top-dressing with appropriate amounts of compost, as needed for your farm, is performed after flowering has completed. [Translator's Note: Because this is a relatively newly cultivated plant, there is no traditional information or research data suggesting amounts of compost needed. If your soil is fertile, minimum amounts of compost should be sufficient.]

PREVENTION AND TREATMENT OF DISEASE AND INSECT PESTS

Principles of Prevention and Treatment

Jīnliánhuā is a relatively new crop, previously coming solely from wild sources, and has not shown any signs of succumbing to soil-borne or above-ground diseases, thus it is potentially a good intercropping plant that might attract beneficial insects for other crops. However, some pests do seem to be problematic, particularly below-ground pests such as grubs and mole crickets. Aphids can also be a problem, but early detection and treatment should be sufficient to allay any significant crop losses.

Grubs (*Holotrichia* sp.)

Prevention and Treatment

Before the winter freeze, deep plowing and harrowing is performed to reduce numbers in the soil and minimize their ability to over-winter. Adult insects are attracted to black light, so one platform with a black light trap can be put out every 8 acres.

Mole Cricket (Gryllotalpidae)

Prevention and Treatment

Use black light to trap and kill adult insects (as above). Before the winter freeze, deep plowing then harrowing is performed to reduce the numbers and minimize their ability to over-winter.

Silver Looper Moth (*Argyrogramma agnata*)

Manual Catching and Killing

While the plants are seedlings, look for the larva and remove it from the plant.

Biological Controls

When the eggs are hatching the use of Bt (100 million spores) is combined to form a 0.5% solution with water and sprayed on the plants. Spray every 10 days, 2 to 3 times per day.

Aphids (Aphidoidea)

Prevention and Treatment

Aphids are naturally attracted to the color yellow. Deploying "sticky yellow board" or construction of areas with yellow painted boards (60×40 cm) will attract aphids where they can be killed. The oil can be applied to the surface of these boards so the aphids get stuck there. Check to see when the board is coated with aphids, and when it is the board can be scraped and more oil can be added. Boards are deployed at a rate of 180–240 per acre.

Biological Controls

Introduction of lady bugs early can be a very effective control for aphids. A 0.3% solution of matrine diluted to a 0.075–0.1% concentration in water. Natural pyrethrin may also be used at a 0.01% concentration. Azadirachtin (0.3%) is diluted to a 0.2% solution is also effective. [Translator's Note: Azadirachtin is the active compound in neem oil, one might also find that neem would be effective here.]

HARVESTING

Years of Growth Before Harvest

When growing from seed, a small harvest can be brought in during the second year. Starting in the third year, and continuing each year, a full harvest should be expected. If plants are grown from root divisions, a full harvest can be expected in the first year.

Harvest Season

Jīnliánhuā flowers during the months of July and August. Flowers should be harvested every 3–5 days during the flowering period to optimize yield and flavonoid content.

Harvest Method

Flowers should be cut with a clean knife or scissors, do not snip with your fingers. Be careful to keep flowers intact and do not pile excessive numbers of flowers in a basket or other means of carrying them as this could lead to spoilage and low-quality herbal product.

ON-FARM PROCESSING

Drying Method

Flowers should be dried in an area that is cool, shaded, and has excellent air circulation. Avoid piling them up together, which can lead to mold and mildew damage. Be sure to flip them over so that their position is changed regularly. Research has shown that drying at 50°C in a dryer produces a better product than traditional air-drying techniques. Dried *jīnliánhuā* should not exceed 12% moisture content.

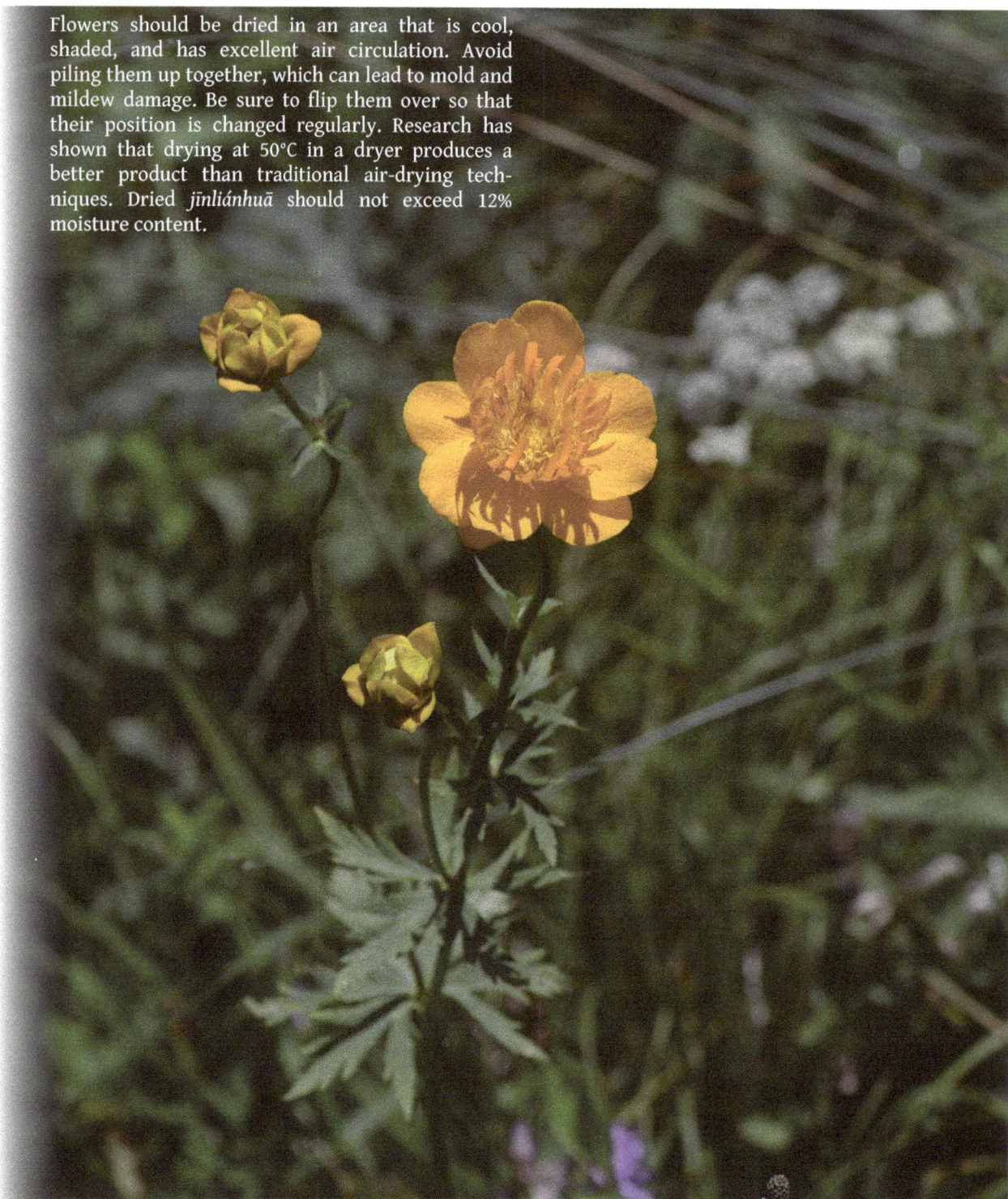

蔚县款冬花

Coltsfoot

Tussilago farfara

The flower bud and stem of the daodi herb *wèixiàn kuǎndōnghuā* (*Tussilago farfara* L.), commonly known as *kuǎndōnghuā* (款冬花) in China, is a member of the aster family (Asteraceae) and is native in areas from Asia to Europe. The plant has also naturalized in north-eastern North America. It is considered an invasive species in North America because of its aggressive stolon growth in native moist habitats. Although there were once a number of other species classified as part of this genus, *Tussilago* is now considered a monotypic genus. The daodi location for this herb in China is in Wei county in Hebei province south of Beijing.

This herb is primarily used for cough in Chinese medicine. Because its action indicated for treating phlegm are not particularly pronounced, it should always be combined with herbs that transform phlegm if the cough is accompanied by phlegm. This herb is also sometimes used for other types of panting and wheezing patterns when coughing is one of the symptoms. The honey mix-fried and licorice mix-fried versions of this medicinal are frequently prescribed. The leaves, however, are the part traditionally used in Western herbal medicine.

Modern science has identified many pharmacological activities, including neuroprotective, antioxidant, antimicrobial, and anti-inflammatory. Unfortunately, modern chemistry has also identified toxic compounds known as pyrrolizidine alkaloids in this plant, and these are also in the flower buds. These alkaloids are known to cause damage to the liver and therefore extended use of this herb is not recommended. However, some Chinese research has shown that when using the traditional licorice mix-fried processing technique, total alkaloids are reduced significantly. This suggests that using this method would be safer, however further research is needed.

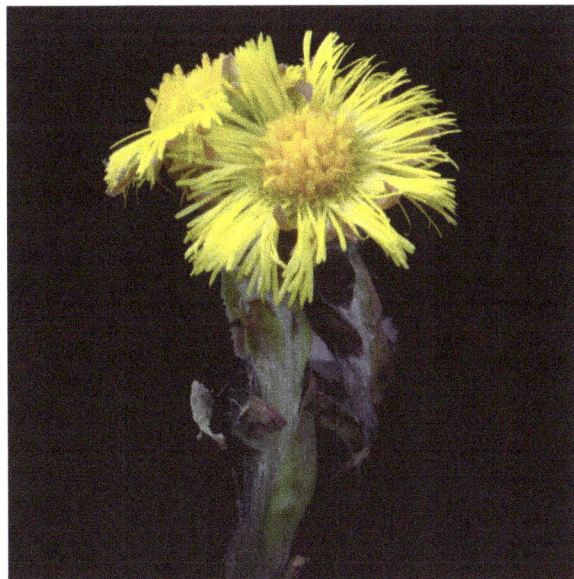

Contributing Authors

Xie Xiao-liang, Liu Ming, Guo Lan-ping, Huang Lu-qi, Hao Qing-xiu, Wen Chun-xiu, Liu Ling-di, Tong Zai-li, Gu Dong-sheng, Tian Wei

PRODUCTION SITE ECOLOGY

Elevation

Kuǎndōnghuā is grown between 600–2800 m elevation.

Temperature

A frost free period of 128 or more days is required to cultivate this herb.

Photo Period

Required annual sunshine hours range from 2800–2950 hours and a sunshine percentage range of 60–75%.

Moisture

The average annual rainfall should be 300–500 mm with a relative humidity of 75–85%.

Soil

A sandy, slightly acidic soil is ideal with pH in the 5.5–6.5 range.

Topography

Kuǎndōnghuā can be grown on flat agricultural land, in the mountains, or in forested land. The land should have good air circulation and adequate water drainage.

PRODUCTION AREA ENVIRONMENTAL REQUIREMENTS

Site Selection and Soil Preparation

Kuǎndōnghuā cultivation is most appropriate between 1000–2000 m elevation. Select an environment that has about 50% shade, with loose, moist, fertile top-soil, and good air movement through the land, i.e. an open forest.

PROPAGATION

Seedling Preparation

The *Pharmacopoeia of the People's Republic of China* (2015) stipulates that the fresh stolon of the aster family plant *kuǎndōnghuā* (*T. farfara*) is to be used for propagation of this medicinal.

Stolons are used for reproduction. Stolons are dug in late October and early November. Strong plants that bore many flowers are chosen. Stolons should be mostly white and free of disease or insect pests. After they are dug up, stolons are cut into 6–9 cm sections, with each section having 2–3 joints.

Planting

The period for planting the stolons is quite long, ranging from December through April (as long as the ground is not frozen). The best time is during the winter or early spring.

Generally, the planting time and the time the plant starts to emerge from the ground is the same, so one can freely dig and plant during this time. Space rows 24–30 cm apart and dig a trench 6 cm deep. Place the prepared stolons in the trench at 6–9 cm intervals, cover, then firmly press the soil. In non-irrigated land, the soil should be watered thoroughly after planting, being sure that water completely permeates the soil. After this the soil should be raked to loosen the top soil if there is crusting so that new growth can easily grow through it.

FIELD MANAGEMENT

Cultivation and Weeding

In early April, after the leaves of *kuǎndōnghuā* have emerged, any gaps in the rows should be filled by new plants. This is also the time to cultivate and eliminate weeds for the first time. During this period roots grow slowly and loosening the soil can help them develop faster, but it is important to be careful not to damage the young roots. The second time should be during the month of June or July as needed. The leaves are fully developed at this time and roots are growing more rapidly; deeper cultivation is appropriate. The third time should be done in early September. At this time, leaf growth is gradually slowing, flower buds are falling apart, and the field should be maintained free of weeds. The exact timing for cultivation to eliminate weeds should be based on the development of *kuǎndōnghuā*, the rate of growth of weeds, and other factors including pests and disease.

Top-dressing and Hilling

Top-dressing is not employed during the early stages of development, however during early September top-dressing with well-composted manure is applied at a rate of 6000 kg per acre. In late September or early October, urea is applied at a rate of 90 kg per acre and diammonium phosphate at a rate of 45 kg per acre. Regardless of whether compost or chemical fertilizers are used, controlling weeds and loosening the soil with cultivation are important management techniques, as well as integrating fertilizer into the soil when performing hilling around the plants to improve their growth.

Irrigation and Water Drainage

During the dry spring months, irrigate 2–3 times to ensure the proper growth and development of the young plants. Prior to the summer rainy season be sure to properly prepare fields for good drainage so that plants do not become flooded and waterlogged.

Cutting Leaves to Improve Air Circulation

During the months of June and July when temperatures get high, *kuǎndōnghuā* develops leaves very quickly, especially when grown with Chinese sorghum or corn,* creating dense foliage, which does not allow proper air flow, leading to insufficient sunlight. This situation can be improved by cutting leaves at the base of the petiole, and removing any yellow or withered leaves, as well as any leaves that show any sign of disease. The rule of thumb is to avoid having leaves that are overlapping. Do not attempt to break off leaves by hand, and use clean (sterilized) tools.

*[Translator's Note: *Kuǎndōnghuā* is often grown in fields with Chinese sorghum or corn. This is a method of intercropping that has become popular as a way to combine food production with medicinal plant production.]

PREVENTION AND TREATMENT OF DISEASE AND INSECT PESTS

Principles of Prevention and Treatment

Kuǎndōnghuā has minimal disease problems, but when disease occurs it can be serious. Good water drainage is critical to avoid fungal diseases, which can dominate this herb. Removing leaves during its primary growth is also important to allow for good air-flow. Although *kǎndōnghuā* prefers wet conditions, standing water can easily lead to disease, therefore slope and soils that easily drain are preferred, clay soils, especially on flat land, are not good for growing this herb.

Brown Spot Disease (*Stagonospora tussilaginis*)

Prevention and Treatment

During the initial stages, affected leaves are removed, and this can also be done during the winter months. If this progresses to the point that leaves are dropping, the field should be completely burned or buried deeply with soil. Improve field management, make sure to drain excess water after heavy rains, remove all weeds growing around the plants, make sure to allow for proper air flow and sunlight, and increase the application of compost to help strengthen the plants ability to resist diseases. These are all important preventative measures.

Leaf Withering Disease (*pathogen not identified*)

Prevention and Treatment

Appropriate autumn cleanup of fields, removing dead leaves and branches that may harbor disease and burning them is a common practice.

Aphids (Aphidoidea)

Prevention and Treatment

Timely weeding and eliminating withered branches and leaves. Hanging 5 cm wide strips of silvery-gray plastic is a method used during the early stages when aphids still have wings to discourage them from colonizing the plants. Aphids are naturally attracted to the color yellow. Deploying "sticky yellow boards" or areas with yellow painted boards (60×40 cm) will attract aphids to places where they can be killed. Oil applied to the surface traps the aphids. When the board is coated with aphids it can be scraped and more oil added. Boards are set up about 30 cm from the ground and deployed at a rate of 180–240 per acre.

Biological Controls

Early introduction of lady bugs can be a very effective control for aphids. A 0.3% solution of matrine diluted to 0.10–0.16% concentration in an emulsion, natural pyrethrins diluted to a 0.05% concentration, or osthol diluted 0.2% concentration can all be sprayed according to manufacturer's instructions.

Grubs (*Holotrichia* sp.)

Prevention and Treatment

Before the winter freeze, deep plowing and harrowing is performed to reduce the numbers and minimize their ability to over-winter.

Biological Controls

Adult insects are attracted to black light, so a platform with a black light trap can be used at a rate of one per 10 acres. *Bacillus popilliae* can be applied at a rate of 9 kg of spores per acre. *Beauveria brongniartii* can also be employed at the rate prescribed by the manufacturer.

HARVESTING

Harvest Season

In Wei County, *kuǎndōnghuā* is harvested during early April. Plants may be harvested in the same year they are transplanted. Plants transplanted in the spring can be harvested in late October and early November of the same year. Flower buds should be harvested before they have opened, when they are purplish-red colored.

Harvest Method

The entire plant is dug and the flowering stalk (2–3 cm) with the bud is removed. Do not pile too many in a single basket or other container, and do not wash, as this will help to prevent the buds from turning black, which decreases their value and quality.

ON-FARM PROCESSING

Drying Method

The flower buds should be laid out only one layer thick in a shaded area with good air circulation. After 3–4 days when they have dried a significant amount, they are sifted to eliminate dirt and clean the flowering stalk, and then put back into the drying area until completely dry. Or, if a drier is available, they can be dried at 40–50°C until dry, approximately 3 hours, stacking no more than 5–7 cm thick, until about 90% dry, then removed and put in a natural setting to complete drying. During the drying process avoid moving the bud as much as possible because this can damage them and affect their medicinal quality. The moisture content of dried *kuǎndōnghuā* should not exceed 12%.

内丘王不留行

Vaccaria Seed

Vaccaria segetalis

DISTINGUISHING FEATURES

The seed of the daodi herb *nèiqiū wángbùliúxíng* (*Vaccaria segetalis* (Neck.) Garcke), known as *wángbùliúxíng* (王不留行) in China, is a member of the pink family (Caryophyllaceae). The plant is native throughout Eurasia and has naturalized in eastern North America. The daodi location for this medicinal plant is in Neiqui county and the surrounding area in Hebei province.

[Translator's Note: Although the *Pharmacopeia of the People's Republic of China* (2015) still lists *V. segetalis* as the scientific name for this plant, it is currently accepted in the monotypic genus *Vaccaria* as *V. hispanica* (Mill.) Rauschert.]

In Chinese medicine this medicinal is said to "free the three," which means it frees the menses, breast milk, and strangury. *Wángbùliúxíng* quickens the blood and frees the menses for stopped menstruation or painful menstruation. It can also be used to facilitate birth in difficult labor. It helps with the initial milk "let down" after birth, disperses abscesses in swollen breasts, and is helpful for insufficient milk after giving birth. Finally, *wángbùliúxíng* disinhibits urine and frees strangury. This seed is also commonly used for the "ear seeds" attached to the ear points for auricular acupuncture therapy.

Modern science has studied this plant extensively both for its medicinal activity and its impact on agriculture as a weed and potential alternative crop. Pharmacological activities found in the seed include galactopoietic, antitumor, reduce blood viscosity, and antioxidant activities, and it has also been shown to have an ameliorative effect on osteopenia. Animal experiments show that *wángbùliúxíng* can increase milk production in healthy cows and rats, suggesting this seed could be used in the dairy industry. The seeds have also been shown to be efficacious for treating sudden deafness in humans because they increase the microcirculation in the inner ear.

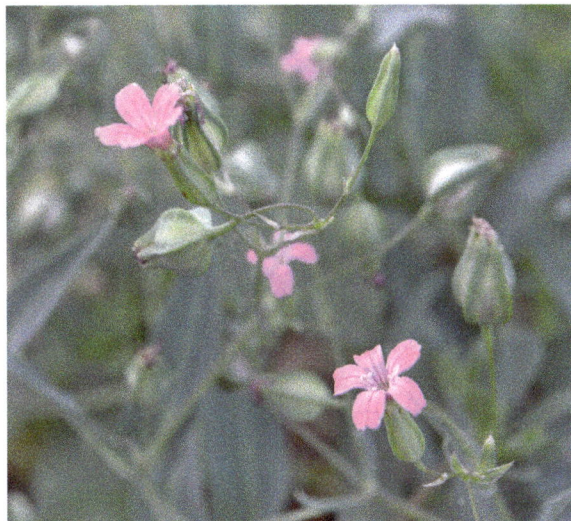

Contributing Authors

Xie Xiao-liang, Yang Tai-xin, Huang Lu-qi, Guo Lan-ping, Hao Qing-xiu, Wen Chun-xiu, Liu Ling-di, Liu Ming, Tian Wei, Gu Dong-sheng

PRODUCTION SITE ECOLOGY

Elevation

Wángbùliúxíng is cultivated between 20–500 m elevation.

Temperature

The site should have at least 178 frost free days. The average annual temperature should be 12–14°C with average lows in January of -2°C but potentially as low as -20°C. Average temperatures in July are 27°C but may get as high as 41°C.

Photo Period

Annual sunshine is between 1998–2956 hours. Daily average sunshine average of 49%.

Moisture

Average annual rainfall 500–800 mm with relative humidity of 35–55%.

Soil

A loose structured soil with pH in the 5.5–6.5 range.

Topography

Field can be either level or a slope below 15 degrees. The planting area must have irrigation, proper drainage, and good wind-flow.

Site Selection & Soil Preparation

A sandy loose soil with good fertility and water drainage is best. Apply 15,000 kg per acre of either well composted manure or compost, then harrow finely.

SOWING SEEDS & RAISING SEEDLINGS

Seed Quality Requirements

Seeds for *wángbùliúxíng* should be dry and ripe with a germination rate greater than 80%.

Sowing Seeds

Seeds are sown in the latter two-thirds of September or the first 10 days of October in rows 25–30 cm apart. Shallow trenches of 3 cm are dug with a hoe and seeds are sown in the trench at a rate of 9 kg per acre. The trench is then filled with 1.5–2 cm of soil and the field is watered.

FIELD MANAGEMENT

Cultivation and Weeding

When plants have reached a height of 7–10 cm the first round of shallow cultivation is executed; any larger weeds are generally removed by hand. At the same time weak seedlings can be thinned out and gaps filled with the strongest seedlings; spacing of 15 cm between plants is desirable. The second round of cultivation is done the following year during the months of March and April; during this time final thinning (singling) is performed. After this, cultivation or weeding is only done as necessary to keep soils loose and fields free from weeds.

Irrigation and Water Drainage

Irrigation is appropriate in early spring and early winter. Be sure that water is well drained during rainy season.

Top-Dressing

Generally top-dressing is done 2–3 times. The first time is when seedlings are 7–10 cm tall. Cultivation is first performed to rid the fields of weeds, then a dilute manure tea (9000 kg) or urea (30 kg) per acre is applied. The second time is in the spring of year-two. As before, cultivation is performed, then either a dilute manure tea (12,000 kg) or superphosphate (120 kg) per acre is applied. Alternately a one-time application of monopotassium phosphate is applied via foliar feeding in a 0.2% solution.

PREVENTION AND TREATMENT OF DISEASE AND INSECT PESTS

Principles of Prevention and Treatment

Wángbùliúxíng is generally easy to grow and there are few disease problems. Pests can be a problem so careful monitoring is advised so that appropriate measures can be taken early. An ecologically diverse agriculture ecology is less likely to sustain major impacts from these pests.

Black Spot (*pathogen not identified*)

Prevention and Treatment

Eliminate diseased branches and leaves; pay attention to timely drainage of stagnant water; increase organic fertilization to enhance the plant's ability to resist disease.

Aphids (Aphidoidea)

Prevention and Treatment

Aphids are naturally attracted to the color yellow. Deploying "sticky yellow boards" or construction of areas with yellow painted boards (60×40 cm) will attract aphids to places where they can be killed. Oil can be applied to the surface of these boards so the aphids get stuck there, check to see when the board is coated with aphids, at which time the board can be scraped and more oil can be added. Boards are deployed at a rate of 180–240 per acre. Another method is to place 5 cm wide "flags" of silvery-gray plastic dispersed within the field, at a rate of about every 30–40 plants, during the early winged stage to deter aphids from the plants.

Biological Controls

Introduction of lady bugs early can be a very effective control for aphids. A 0.3% concentration of matrine diluted in a solution to 0.1–0.17%; or natural pyrethrins diluted to a solution 0.05–0.01%; spray according to manufacturer's instructions.

Caterpillars (*Anomis flava* and related moths)

Prevention and Treatment

During adult mature stages use black light traps to lure moths during the evening; they will die in the trap during the heat of the day.

Biological Controls

During the egg hatching period, use 10 billion live spores/g *Bacillus thuringiensis* (Bt) diluted to a solution of 0.15%, or with fluoxifen (5% anti-CPIC) or 25% urea suspension diluted to 0.035%, or 25% of the insecticidal urea suspension diluted to 0.01%, or in the young larvae with 0.36% matrine diluted in water at a concentration of 0.17%, or natural pyrethrins (5% pyrethrins) diluted to 0.05–0.1% concentration. Spray once per week, 2–3 applications should control aphids.

HARVESTING

Harvest Season

Seeds planted from mid-September into the beginning of October are harvested the following year. Seeds are harvested near the end of May when the calyx turns yellow; as soon as the seed turns black it may be harvested.

Harvest Method

Seeds are harvested on a bright sunny day; the entire field is harvested at one time and seeds are transported to an area where they can be dried in the sun; a combine harvester can be employed for large fields.

ON-FARM PROCESSING

Drying Method

Calyces are laid in the sun until they are dried, at which point any seeds that have not fallen can easily be winnowed by hand or with a thresher. Seeds should be shriveled and shrunken to no more than 12% moisture.

Experts and Contributors

The original text was a collaborative work written by 19 recognized experts, assisted by 105 special contributors. All of the original contributors to this text, their home institutions, and the herbs they contributed to are listed below.

Expert	Affiliated Institution	Herb(s)
Huang Lu-qi	China Academy of Chinese Medical Sciences	jinyinhua, danshen, cangzhu, honghua, sanqi, qumai, kuandonghua, baizhi, shegan, wangbuliuxing, beishashen, chaihu, lianhua, lianqiao, huainiuxi, yuanzhi, ziwan, juhua, jingjie
Guo Lan-ping	China Academy of Chinese Medical Sciences: Institute of Materia Medica Resources	jinyinhua, gualou, honghua, canzhu, danshen, huanglian, sanqi, tianma, longdancao, muxiang, qumai, kuandonghua, baizhi, shegan, wangbuliuxing, beishashen, chaihu, lianhua, lianqiao, huainiuxi, yuanzhi, ziwan, juhua, jingjie
Xie Xiao-liang	Hebei Academy of Sciences: Research Institute of Agriculture and Forestry	qumai, kuandonghua, baizhi, shegan, wangbuliuxing, beishashen, chaihu, jinlianhua, lianqiao, huainiuxi, yuanzhi, ziwan, juhua, jingjie
Qian Da-wei	Nanjing University of Chinese Medicine	danggui, baihe
Wang Wen-quan	Beijing University of Chinese Medicine	*gancao, zhimu*
Gao Wen-yuan	Tianjin University	*shānyao, dihuang*
Zeng Yan	China National Traditional Chinese Medicine Corporation	*huangqin*
Zhang Yan	China Academy of Chinese Medical Sciences: Institute of Materia Medica Resources	*honghua, danshen, cangzhu*
Chao Zhi-mao	China Academy of Chinese Medical Sciences: Institute of Materia Medica Resources	*gualou*

Fang Cheng-wu	Anwei University of Chinese Medicine	*mudanpi*
Zhou Ning	Guizhou Tong Ji Tang	*yinyanghuo*
Zheng Yu-guang	Hebei Medical University	*baizhu, qumai, baizhi, chaihu, ziwan, juhua, jingjie*
Song Liang-ke	School of Life Science and Engineering, Southwest Jiaotong University	*huanglian*
Yang Feng-qing	Chongqing University	*yujin*
Liu Da-hui	Yunnan College of Agriculture: Institute of Medicinal Plants	*sanqi, tianma, longdancao*
Li Min-hui	Inner Mongolia Medical College at BaoTou	*huangqi*
Sun Hai-feng	Shanxi Medical University	dangshen
Li Min-hui	Inner Mongolia Medical College at BaoTou	*roucongrong*
Li Lin-yu	Yunnan College of Agriculture: Institute of Medicinal Plants	*muxiang*

Special Contibutors	**Affiliated Institution**	**Herb(s)**
Duan Jin-ao	Nanjing University of Chinese Medicine	*danggui, baihe*
Yan Hui	Nanjing University of Chinese Medicine	*danggui, baihe*
Nie Hui	Nanjing University of Chinese Medicine	*baihe*
Wei Sheng-li	Beijing University of Chinese Medicinee	*gancao*
Hou Jun-ling	Beijing University of Chinese Medicine	*baihe, zhimu*
Huang Ming-jin	Beijing University of Chinese Medicine	*baihe*
Yu Fu-lai	Beijing University of Chinese Medicinee	*baihe*
Liu Ying	Beijing University of Chinese Medicine	*baihe*
Chen Qian-liang	Beijing University of Chinese Medicine	*zhimu*
Zhong Ke	Beijing University of Chinese Medicine	*zhimu*
Xie Jing	Beijing University of Chinese Medicine	*zhimu*
Wang Ting-ting	Tianjin University	*shānyao, dihuang*
Xie Jing	Tianjin University	*shānyao, dihuang*

Li Xia	Tianjin University	*shanyao, dihuang*
Wang Juan	Tianjin University	*shanyao, dihuang*
Zhao Run-huai	China National Traditional Chinese Medicine Corporation	*huangqin*
Wang Ji-yong	China National Traditional Chinese Medicine Corporation	*huangqin*
Zhang Xue-wen	China Medicinal Plant Group, Chengde LLC	*huangqin*
Zhao Dong-yue	China Academy of Chinese Medical Sciences: Institute of Materia Medica Resources	*cangzhu, danshen, jinyinhua, honghua*
Hao Qing-xiu	China Academy of Chinese Medical Sciences: Institute of Materia Medica Resources	*cangzhu, danshen, jinyinhua, qumai, kuandonghua, baizhi, shegan, chaihu, wangbuliuxing, beishashen, lianhua, lianqiao, huainiuxi, yuanzhi, ziwan, juhua, jingjie*
Sun Hai-feng	China Academy of Chinese Medical Sciences: Institute of Materia Medica Resources	*cangzhu, danshen, jinyinhua, honghua*
Zhang Xiao-bo	China Academy of Chinese Medical Sciences: Institute of Materia Medica Resources	*cangzhu, jinyinhua*
Kang Li-ping	China Academy of Chinese Medical Sciences: Institute of Materia Medica Resources	*cangzhu, honghua*
Zhu Shou-dong	China Academy of Chinese Medical Sciences: Institute of Materia Medica Resources	*cangzhu*
He Ya-li	China Academy of Chinese Medical Sciences: Institute of Materia Medica Resources	*cangzhu, honghua*
Wang Ling	China Academy of Chinese Medical Sciences: Institute of Materia Medica Resources	*cangzhu*
Ge Xiao-guang	China Academy of Chinese Medical Sciences: Institute of Materia Medica Resources	*cangzhu*
Wang Xiao	Shandong Academy of Sciences: Testing & Analysis Center	*danshen, jinyinhua*
Liu Wei	Shandong Academy of Sciences: Testing & Analysis Center	*danshen, jinyinhua*
Yang Guang	China Academy of Chinese Medical Sciences: Institute of Materia Medica Resources	*danshen, honghua*
Zhou Jie	Shandong Academy of Sciences: Testing & Analysis Center	*danshen, jinyinhua*

Zhu Shou-dong	China Academy of Chinese Medical Sciences: Institute of Materia Medica Resources	*honghua*
Wang Ling	China Academy of Chinese Medical Sciences: Institute of Materia Medica Resources	*honghua*
Wu Hui-xiao	China Academy of Chinese Medical Sciences: Institute of Materia Medica Resources	*honghua*
Sun Wen	China Academy of Chinese Medical Sciences: Institute of Materia Medica Resources	*gualou*
Wu Xiao-yi	China Academy of Chinese Medical Sciences: Institute of Materia Medica Resources	*gualou*
Yu Li	China Academy of Chinese Medical Sciences: Institute of Materia Medica Resources	*gualou*
Xie Dong-mei	Anwei University of Chinese Medicine	*danpi*
Liu Shou-jin	Anwei University of Chinese Medicine	*danpi*
Ji Kai-ming	Anwei University of Chinese Medicine	*danpi*
Jin Chuan-shan	Anwei University of Chinese Medicine	*danpi*
Wang Qian	Anwei University of Chinese Medicine	*danpi*
Wang Qian	Hebei Medical University	*baizhu*
Hou Fang-jie	Hebei Medical University	*baizhu*
Li Jing	Hebei Medical University	*baizhu*
Liu Zhen-yi	Hebei Medical University	*baizhu*
Zhao Man-qian	School of Life Science and Engineering, Southwest Jiaotong University	*huanglian*
Tan Rui	School of Life Science and Engineering, Southwest Jiaotong University	*huanglian*
Wang Yan	School of Life Science and Engineering, Southwest Jiaotong University	*huanglian*
Zuo Hua-li	Chongqing University	*yujin*
Li Feng	Chongqing University	*yujin*
Cui Xiu-ming	Kunming University of Science and Technology	*sanqi, tianma, longdancao*
Yang Ye	Kunming University of Science and Technology	*sanqi, tianma, longdancao*

Fang Yan	Yunnan College of Agriculture: Institute of Medicinal Plants	*sanqi*
Wang Jia-jin	Yunnan College of Agriculture: Institute of Medicinal Plants	*sanqi, tianma, longdancao*
Zhang Zhi-hui	Yunnan College of Agriculture: Institute of Medicinal Plants	*sanqi, tianma, longdancao*
Wang Li	Yunnan College of Agriculture: Institute of Medicinal Plants	*sanqi, tianma, longdancao*
Li Peng-zhang	Yunnan College of Agriculture: Institute of Medicinal Plants	*sanqi*
Xu Nuo	Yunnan College of Agriculture: Institute of Medicinal Plants	*sanqi*
Zheng Dong-mei	Yunnan College of Agriculture: Institute of Medicinal Plants	*sanqi*
Shi Ya-nuo	Yunnan College of Agriculture: Institute of Medicinal Plants	*sanqi*
Zuo Zhi-tian	Yunnan College of Agriculture: Institute of Medicinal Plants	*sanqi, tianma, longdancao, muxiang*
Zhang Chun-hong	BaoTou Medical College	*huangqi, roucongrong*
Zhang Ai-hua	BaoTou Medical College	*huangqi*
Cui Zhan-hu	BaoTou Medical College	*huangqi*
Li Zhen-hua	BaoTou Medical College	*huangqi*
Gao Jian-ping	Shanxi Medical University	*dangshen*
Cao-ling-ya	Shanxi Medical University	*dangshen*
Zhao Guo-feng	Shanxi Medical University	*dangshen*
Wang Li	Yunnan College of Agriculture: Institute of Medicinal Plants	*tianma*
Fang Wei	Yunnan College of Agriculture: Institute of Medicinal Plants	*tianma*
Li Peng-zhang	Yunnan College of Agriculture: Institute of Medicinal Plants	*tianma*
Xu Nuo	Yunnan College of Agriculture: Institute of Medicinal Plants	*tianma*

Shi Ya-nuo	Yunnan College of Agriculture: Institute of Medicinal Plants	*tianma, longdancao*
A Si Ba Te Er	Inner Mongolia Medical College at BaoTou	*roucongrong*
Wu Li-ji	Inner Mongolia Medical College at BaoTou	*roucongrong*
Zou De-zhi	Inner Mongolia Medical College at BaoTou	*roucongrong*
Liu Bo	Inner Mongolia Medical College at BaoTou	*roucongrong*
Bai Bing	Inner Mongolia Medical College at BaoTou	*roucongrong*
Zhao Zhen-ling	Yunnan College of Agriculture: Institute of Medicinal Plants	*longdancao*
Yang Mei-quan	Yunnan College of Agriculture: Institute of Medicinal Plants	*longdancao*
Ji Peng-zhang	Yunnan College of Agriculture: Institute of Medicinal Plants	*longdancao*
Fang Yan	Yunnan College of Agriculture: Institute of Medicinal Plants	*longdancao*
Li Shao-ping	Yunnan College of Agriculture: Institute of Medicinal Plants	*muxiang*
Yang Li-ying	Yunnan College of Agriculture: Institute of Medicinal Plants	*muxiang*
Yang Bin	Yunnan College of Agriculture: Institute of Medicinal Plants	*muxiang*
Wang Xin	Yunnan College of Agriculture: Institute of Medicinal Plants	*muxiang*
Dong Zhi-yuan	Yunnan College of Agriculture: Institute of Medicinal Plants	*muxiang*
Ma Wei-si	Yunnan College of Agriculture: Institute of Medicinal Plants	*muxiang*
Yan Shi-wu	Yunnan College of Agriculture: Institute of Medicinal Plants	*muxiang*
Li Jia	Yunnan College of Agriculture: Institute of Medicinal Plants	*muxiang*
Tong Zai-li	Hebei Academy of Sciences: Research Institute of Agriculture and Forestry	*kuandonghua*

Liu Ling-di	Hebei Academy of Sciences: Research Institute of Agriculture and Forestry	*qumai, kuandonghua, baizhi, shegan, wangbuliuxing, beishashen, chaihu, lianhua, huainiuxi, yuanzhi, ziwan, juhua, jingjie*
Liu Ming	Hebei Academy of Sciences: Research Institute of Agriculture and Forestry	*qumai, kuandonghua, baizhi, shegan, wangbuliuxing, beishashen, chaihu, lianhua, huainiuxi, yuanzhi, ziwan, juhua, jingjie*
Wen Chun-xiu	Hebei Academy of Sciences: Research Institute of Agriculture and Forestry	*qumai, kuandonghua, baizhi, shegan, wangbuliuxing, beishashen, chaihu, lianhua, huainiuxi, yuanzhi, ziwan, juhua, jingjie, lianqiao*
Tian Wei	Hebei Academy of Sciences: Research Institute of Agriculture and Forestry	*qumai, kuandonghua, baizhi, shegan, wangbuliuxing, beishashen, chaihu, lianhua, huainiuxi, yuanzhi, ziwan, juhua, jingjie, lianqiao*
Gu Dong-sheng	Hebei Academy of Sciences: Research Institute of Agriculture and Forestry	*qumai, kuandonghua, baizhi, shegan, wangbuliuxing, beishashen, chaihu, lianhua, huainiuxi, yuanzhi, ziwan, juhua, jingjie, lianqiao*
Song Jun-nuo	Hebei Academy of Sciences: Research Institute of Agriculture and Forestry	*baizhi*
Liu Zhi-miao	Hebei Academy of Sciences: Research Institute of Agriculture and Forestry	*shegan*
Bo Jian-ying	Hebei Academy of Sciences: Research Institute of Agriculture and Forestry	*beishashen*
Hou Fang-jie	Hebei Academy of Sciences: Research Institute of Agriculture and Forestry	*chaihu*
Gao Xiu-qiang	Hebei Academy of Sciences: Research Institute of Agriculture and Forestry	*lianqiao*
Li Rong-xin	Hebei Academy of Sciences: Research Institute of Agriculture and Forestry	*yuanzhi*
Zheng Kai-yan	Hebei Academy of Sciences: Research Institute of Agriculture and Forestry	*jingjie*
Yang Tai-xin	Hebei Agriculture University	*wangbuliuxing, juhua*

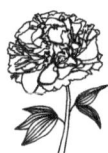

Appendix II
Ecological Conditions
Organized by Botanical Latin Binomial

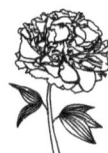

Botanical Latin Binomial	Chinese Name	Elevation (m)	Frost-Free Period (days)	Photo Period (lx)	Annual Rainfall (mm)
Achyranthes bidentata	niúxī	50–500	>197	2500–2757	500–1000
Anemarrhena asphodeloides	zhīmŭ	100–1000	8–12°C*	n/a	150–300
Angelica dahurica	báizhĭ	50–500	>190	2500–2757	500–1000
Angelica sinensis	dāngguī	2000–2500	4.5–5.7°C*	n/a	570–650
Aster tataricus	zĭwăn	50–500	>197	2500–2757	500–1000
Astragalus membracaceus var. mongholicus	huángqí	1000–1500	>95	2500–3100	250–350
Atractylodes lancea	cāngzhú	100–1000	~220	~2000	~1000
Atractylodes macrocephela	báizhú	500–800	200–260	~2000	1200–1500
Aucklandia lappa	mùxiāng	2700–3300	150–180	n/a	800–1000
Belamcanda chinensis	shègān	100–1000	~200	1516–2016	300–1200
Bupleurum chinensis & B. scorzonerifolium	cháihú	260–1500	181–204	1998–2957	331–1032
Carthamus tinctorius	hónghuā	100–1000	8–12°C*	n/a	150–300
Chrysanthemum morifolium	júhuā	50–500	>197	2500–2757	500–1000
Cistanche deserticola	ròucōngróng	800–1400	120–180	3000–3700	80–220
Codonopsis pilosula	dǎngshēn	1000–3200	157–182	1800–1900	500–1000
Coptis chinensis	huánglián	1100–1800	170–220	1100–1400	1300–1600
Curcuma phaeocaulis	yùjīn	450–550	>290	1100–1200	950–1000
Dianthus superbus & D. chinensis	qúmài	50–500	~197	2500–2757	500–1000
Dioscorea opposita	shānyao	150–300	~210	n/a	550–700
Epimedium wushanense	yínyánghuò	300–1700	>270	200–1500	~1000
Forsythia suspensa	liánqiáo	300–2200	>196	1916–3216	300–800
Gastrodia elata	tiānmá	1400–2300	7.9–12.5°C*	n/a	972–1125
Gentiana rigescens	lóngdǎn	1700–2500	7–21°C*	n/a	800–1400
Glehnia littoralis	shāshēn	50–500	>197	2500–2757	500–800
Glycyrrhiza uralensis	gāncǎo	1000–1500	6–8°C*	n/a	150–300
Lilium lancifolium	bǎihé	100–800	14.2–16.1°C*	n/a	1300–1800
Lonicera japonica	yínhuā	50–1500	150–230	2290–2890	550–950
Paeonia suffruticosa	dānpí	50–300	~258	n/a	>1200
Panax notoginseng	sānqī	1400–1800	>300	1516–2016	900–1300
Polygala tenuifolia	yuǎnzhì	50–500	>197	2500–2757	500–1000
Pseudostellaria heterophylla	táizǐshēn	650–1300	255–294	1060–1350	1000–1200
Rehmannia glutinosa	dìhuáng	150–300	>210	n/a	550–700
Salvia miltiorrhiza	dānshēn	60–1000	170–220	2290–2890	550–950
Schizonepeta tenuifolia	jīngjiè	50–500	>197	2500–2757	606–1000
Scutellaria baicalensis	huángqín	300–1000	~160	2600–3100	402–883
Trichosanthes kirilowii	guālóu	sea level to 200	190–220	2300–2800	520–680
Trollius chinensis	jīnliánhuā	1200–2000	>135	2600–2700	402–883
Tussilago farfara	kuǎndōnghuā	600–2800	>128	2800–2950	300–500
Vaccaria segetalis	wángbùliúxíng	20–500	>178	1998–2956	500–800

* Frost-free period data is not available for these herb; temperatures listed are the average annual temperature range.

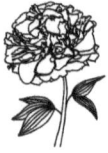

Appendix III
Ecological Conditions
Organized by Chinese Pinyin Name

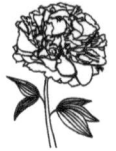

Chinese Name	Botanical Latin Binomial	Elevation (m)	Frost-Free Period (days)	Photo Period (lx)	Annual Rainfall (mm)
bǎihé	Lilium lancifolium	100–800	14.2–16.1°C*	n/a	1300–1800
báizhǐ	Angelica dahurica	50–500	>190	2500–2757	500–1000
báizhú	Atractylodes macrocephela	500–800	200–260	~2000	1200–1500
cāngzhú	Atractylodes lancea	100–1000	~220	~2000	~1000
cháihú	Bupleurum chinensis & B. scorzonerifolium	260–1500	181–204	1998–2957	331–1032
dāngguī	Angelica sinensis	2000–2500	4.5–5.7°C*	n/a	570–650
dǎngshēn	Codonopsis pilosula	1000–3200	157–182	1800–1900	500–1000
dānpí	Paeonia suffruticosa	50–300	~258	n/a	>1200
dānshēn	Salvia miltiorrhiza	60–1000	170–220	2290–2890	550–950
dìhuáng	Rehmannia glutinosa	150–300	>210	n/a	550–700
gāncǎo	Glycyrrhiza uralensis	1000–1500	6–8°C*	n/a	150–300
guālóu	Trichosanthes kirilowii	sea level to 200	190–220	2300–2800	520–680
hónghuā	Carthamus tinctorius	100–1000	8–12°C*	n/a	150–300
huánglián	Coptis chinensis	1100–1800	170–220	1100–1400	1300–1600
huángqí	Astragalus membracaceus var. mongholicus	1000–1500	>95	2500–3100	250–350
huángqín	Scutellaria baicalensis	300–1000	~160	2600–3100	402–883
jīngjiè	Schizonepeta tenuifolia	50–500	>197	2500–2757	606–1000
jīnliánhuā	Trollius chinensis	1200–2000	>135	2600–2700	402–883
júhuā	Chrysanthemum morifolium	50–500	>197	2500–2757	500–1000
kuǎndōnghuā	Tussilago farfara	600–2800	>128	2800–2950	300–500
liánqiáo	Forsythia suspensa	300–2200	>196	1916–3216	300–800
lóngdǎn	Gentiana rigescens	1700–2500	7–21°C*	n/a	800–1400
mùxiāng	Aucklandia lappa	2700–3300	150–180	n/a	800–1000
niúxī	Achyranthes bidentata	50–500	>197	2500–2757	500–1000
qúmài	Dianthus superbus & D. chinensis	50–500	~197	2500–2757	500–1000
ròucōngróng	Cistanche deserticola	800–1400	120–180	3000–3700	80–220
sānqī	Panax notoginseng	1400–1800	>300	1516–2016	900–1300
shānyao	Dioscorea opposita	150–300	~210	n/a	550–700
shāshēn	Glehnia littoralis	50–500	>197	2500–2757	500–800
shègān	Belamcanda chinensis	100–1000	~200	1516–2016	300–1200
táizǐshēn	Pseudostellaria heterophylla	650–1300	255–294	1060–1350	1000–1200
tiānmá	Gastrodia elata	1400–2300	7.9–12.5°C*	n/a	972–1125
wángbùliúxíng	Vaccaria segetalis	20–500	>178	1998–2956	500–800
yínhuā	Lonicera japonica	50–1500	150–230	2290–2890	550–950
yínyánghuò	Epimedium wushanense	300–1700	>270	200–1500	~1000
yuǎnzhì	Polygala tenuifolia	50–500	>197	2500–2757	500–1000
yùjīn	Curcuma phaeocaulis	450–550	>290	1100–1200	950–1000
zhīmǔ	Anemarrhena asphodeloides	100–1000	8–12°C*	n/a	150–300
zǐwǎn	Aster tataricus	50–500	>197	2500–2757	500–1000

* Frost-free period data are not available for these herbs; temperatures listed are the average annual temperature range.

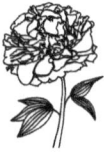

Appendix IV
Ecological Conditions
Organized by Elevation in Meters

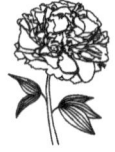

Elevation (m)	Chinese Name	Botanical Latin Binomial	Frost-Free Period (days)	Photo Period (hours)	Annual Rainfall (mm)
0–200	guālóu	Trichosanthes kirilowii	190–220	2300–2800	520–680
20–500	wángbùliúxíng	Vaccaria segetalis	>178	1998–2956	500–800
50–300	dānpí	Paeonia suffruticosa	~258	n/a	>1200
50–500	niúxī	Achyranthes bidentata	>197	2500–2757	500–1000
50–500	báizhǐ	Angelica dahurica	>190	2500–2757	500–1000
50–500	zǐwǎn	Aster tataricus	>197	2500–2757	500–1000
50–500	júhuā	Chrysanthemum morifolium	>197	2500–2757	500–1000
50–500	qúmài	Dianthus superbus & D. chinensis	~197	2500–2757	500–1000
50–500	shāshēn	Glehnia littoralis	>197	2500–2757	500–800
50–500	yuǎnzhì	Polygala tenuifolia	>197	2500–2757	500–1000
50–500	jīngjiè	Schizonepeta tenuifolia	>197	2500–2757	606–1000
50–1500	yínhuā	Lonicera japonica	150–230	2290–2890	550–950
60–1000	dānshēn	Salvia miltiorrhiza	170–220	2290–2890	550–950
100–800	bǎihé	Lilium lancifolium	14.2–16.1°C*	n/a	1300–1800
100–1000	zhīmǔ	Anemarrhena asphodeloides	8–12°C*	n/a	150–300
100–1000	cāngzhú	Atractylodes lancea	~220	~2000	~1000
100–1000	shègān	Belamcanda chinensis	~200	1516–2016	300–1200
100–1000	hónghuā	Carthamus tinctorius	8–12°C*	n/a	150–300
150–300	shānyao	Dioscorea opposita	~210	n/a	550–700
150–300	dìhuáng	Rehmannia glutinosa	>210	n/a	550–700
260–1500	cháihú	Bupleurum chinensis & B. scorzonerifolium	181–204	1998–2957	331–1032
300–1000	huángqín	Scutellaria baicalensis	~160	2600–3100	402–883
300–1700	yínyánghuò	Epimedium wushanense	>270	200–1500	~1000
300–2200	liánqiáo	Forsythia suspensa	>196	1916–3216	300–800
450–550	yùjīn	Curcuma phaeocaulis	>290	1100–1200	950–1000
500–800	báizhú	Atractylodes macrocephala	200–260	~2000	1200–1500
600–2800	kuǎndōnghuā	Tussilago farfara	>128	2800–2950	300–500
650–1300	táizǐshēn	Pseudostellaria heterophylla	255–294	1060–1350	1000–1200
800–1400	ròucōngróng	Cistanche deserticola	120–180	3000–3700	80–220
1000–1500	huángqí	Astragalus membracaceus var. mongholicus	>95	2500–3100	250–350
1000–1500	gāncǎo	Glycyrrhiza uralensis	6–8°C	n/a	150–300
1000–3200	dǎngshēn	Codonopsis pilosula	157–182	1800–1900	500–1000
1100–1800	huánglián	Coptis chinensis	170–220	1100–1400	1300–1600
1200–2000	jīnliánhuā	Trollius chinensis	>135	2600–2700	402–883
1400–1800	sānqī	Panax notoginseng	>300	1516–2016	900–1300
1400–2300	tiānmá	Gastrodia elata	7.9–12.5°C*	n/a	972–1125
1700–2500	lóngdǎn	Gentiana rigescens	7–21°C	n/a	800–1400
2000–2500	dāngguī	Angelica sinensis	4.5–5.7°C*	n/a	570–650
2700–3300	mùxiāng	Aucklandia lappa	150–180	n/a	800–1000

* Frost-free period data are not available for these herbs; temperatures listed are the average annual temperature range.

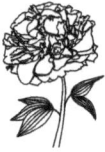

Appendix V
Ecological Conditions
Organized by Frost-Free Period in Days

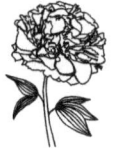

Frost-Free Period (days)	Chinese Name	Botanical Latin Binomial	Elevation (m)	Photo Period (lx)	Annual Rainfall (mm)
>95	huángqí	Astragalus membracaceus var. mongholicus	1000–1500	2500–3100	250–350
120–180	ròucōngróng	Cistanche deserticola	800–1400	3000–3700	80–220
>128	kuǎndōnghuā	Tussilago farfara	600–2800	2800–2950	300–500
>135	jīnliánhuā	Trollius chinensis	1200–2000	2600–2700	402–883
150–180	mùxiāng	Aucklandia lappa	2700–3300	n/a	800–1000
150–230	yínhuā	Lonicera japonica	50–1500	2290–2890	550–950
157–182	dǎngshēn	Codonopsis pilosula	1000–3200	1800–1900	500–1000
~160	huángqín	Scutellaria baicalensis	300–1000	2600–3100	402–883
170–220	huánglián	Coptis chinensis	1100–1800	1100–1400	1300–1600
170–220	dānshēn	Salvia miltiorrhiza	60–1000	2290–2890	550–950
>178	wángbùliúxíng	Vaccaria segetalis	20–500	1998–2956	500–800
181–204	cháihú	Bupleurum chinensis & B. scorzonerifolium	260–1500	1998–2957	331–1032
>190	báizhǐ	Angelica dahurica	50–500	2500–2757	500–1000
190–220	guālóu	Trichosanthes kirilowii	0–200	2300–2800	520–680
>196	liánqiáo	Forsythia suspensa	300–2200	1916–3216	300–800
>197	niúxī	Achyranthes bidentata	50–500	2500–2757	500–1000
>197	zǐwǎn	Aster tataricus	50–500	2500–2757	500–1000
>197	júhuā	Chrysanthemum morifolium	50–500	2500–2757	500–1000
~197	qúmài	Dianthus superbus & D. chinensis	50–500	2500–2757	500–1000
>197	shāshēn	Glehnia littoralis	50–500	2500–2757	500–800
>197	yuǎnzhì	Polygala tenuifolia	50–500	2500–2757	500–1000
>197	jīngjiè	Schizonepeta tenuifolia	50–500	2500–2757	606–1000
~200	shègān	Belamcanda chinensis	100–1000	1516–2016	300–1200
200–260	báizhú	Atractylodes macrocephela	500–800	~2000	1200–1500
~210	shānyao	Dioscorea opposita	150–300	n/a	550–700
>210	dìhuáng	Rehmannia glutinosa	150–300	n/a	550–700
~220	cāngzhú	Atractylodes lancea	100–1000	~2000	~1000
255–294	táizǐshēn	Pseudostellaria heterophylla	650–1300	1060–1350	1000–1200
~258	dānpí	Paeonia suffruticosa	50–300	n/a	>1200
>270	yínyánghuò	Epimedium wushanense	300–1700	200–1500	~1000
>290	yùjīn	Curcuma phaeocaulis	450–550	1100–1200	950–1000
>300	sānqī	Panax notoginseng	1400–1800	1516–2016	900–1300
4.5–5.7°C*	dāngguī	Angelica sinensis	2000–2500	n/a	570–650
6–8°C*	gāncǎo	Glycyrrhiza uralensis	1000–1500	n/a	150–300
7–21°C*	lóngdǎn	Gentiana rigescens	1700–2500	n/a	800–1400
7.9–12.5°C*	tiānmá	Gastrodia elata	1400–2300	n/a	972–1125
8–12°C*	hónghuā	Carthamus tinctorius	100–1000	n/a	150–300
8–12°C*	zhīmǔ	Anemarrhena asphodeloides	100–1000	n/a	150–300
14.2–16.1°C*	bǎihé	Lilium lancifolium	100–800	n/a	1300–1800

* Frost-free period data are not available for these herbs; temperatures listed are the average annual temperature range.

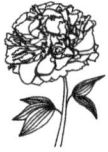

Appendix VI
Ecological Conditions
Organized by Photo Period in Lux

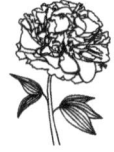

Photo Period (lx)	Chinese Name	Botanical Latin Binomial	Elevation (m)	Frost-Free Period (days)	Annual Rainfall (mm)
200–1500	yínyánghuò	Epimedium wushanense	300–1700	>270	~1000
1060–1350	táizǐshēn	Pseudostellaria heterophylla	650–1300	255–294	1000–1200
1100–1200	yùjīn	Curcuma phaeocaulis	450–550	>290	950–1000
1100–1400	huánglián	Coptis chinensis	1100–1800	170–220	1300–1600
1516–2016	shègān	Belamcanda chinensis	100–1000	~200	300–1200
1516–2016	sānqī	Panax notoginseng	1400–1800	>300	900–1300
1800–1900	dǎngshēn	Codonopsis pilosula	1000–3200	157–182	500–1000
1916–3216	liánqiáo	Forsythia suspensa	300–2200	>196	300–800
1998–2957	cháihú	Bupleurum chinensis & B. scorzonerifolium	260–1500	181–204	331–1032
1998–2956	wángbùliúxíng	Vaccaria segetalis	20–500	>178	500–800
~2000	cāngzhú	Atractylodes lancea	100–1000	~220	~1000
~2000	báizhú	Atractylodes macrocephela	500–800	200–260	1200–1500
2290–2890	yínhuā	Lonicera japonica	50–1500	150–230	550–950
2290–2890	dānshēn	Salvia miltiorrhiza	60–1000	170–220	550–950
2300–2800	guālóu	Trichosanthes kirilowii	0–200	190–220	520–680
2500–2757	niúxī	Achyranthes bidentata	50–500	>197	500–1000
2500–2757	báizhǐ	Angelica dahurica	50–500	>190	500–1000
2500–2757	zǐwǎn	Aster tataricus	50–500	>197	500–1000
2500–3100	huángqí	Astragalus membracaceus var. mongholicus	1000–1500	>95	250–350
2500–2757	júhuā	Chrysanthemum morifolium	50–500	>197	500–1000
2500–2757	qúmài	Dianthus superbus & D. chinensis	50–500	~197	500–1000
2500–2757	shāshēn	Glehnia littoralis	50–500	>197	500–800
2500–2757	yuǎnzhì	Polygala tenuifolia	50–500	>197	500–1000
2500–2757	jīngjiè	Schizonepeta tenuifolia	50–500	>197	606–1000
2600–2700	jīnliánhuā	Trollius chinensis	1200–2000	>135	402–883
2600–3100	huángqín	Scutellaria baicalensis	300–1000	~160	402–883
2800–2950	kuǎndōnghuā	Tussilago farfara	600–2800	>128	300–500
3000–3700	ròucōngróng	Cistanche deserticola	800–1400	120–180	80–220
n/a	zhīmǔ	Anemarrhena asphodeloides	100–1000	8–12°C*	150–300
n/a	dāngguī	Angelica sinensis	2000–2500	4.5–5.7°C*	570–650
n/a	mùxiāng	Aucklandia lappa	2700–3300	150–180	800–1000
n/a	hónghuā	Carthamus tinctorius	100–1000	8–12°C*	150–300
n/a	shānyao	Dioscorea opposita	150–300	~210	550–700
n/a	tiānmá	Gastrodia elata	1400–2300	7.9–12.5°C*	972–1125
n/a	lóngdǎn	Gentiana rigescens	1700–2500	7–21°C	800–1400
n/a	gāncǎo	Glycyrrhiza uralensis	1000–1500	6–8°C	150–300
n/a	bǎihé	Lilium lancifolium	100–800	14.2–16.1°C*	1300–1800
n/a	dānpí	Paeonia suffruticosa	50–300	~258	>1200
n/a	dìhuáng	Rehmannia glutinosa	150–300	>210	550–700

* Frost-free period data are not available for these herbs; temperatures listed are the average annual temperature range.

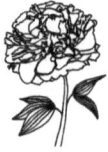

Appendix VII
Ecological Conditions
Organized by Annual Rainfall

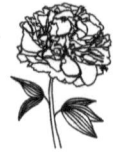

Annual Rainfall (mm)	Chinese Name	Botanical Latin Binomial	Elevation (m)	Frost-Free Period (days)	Photo Period (lx)
80–220	ròucōngróng	Cistanche deserticola	800–1400	120–180	3000–3700
150–300	zhīmǔ	Anemarrhena asphodeloides	100–1000	8–12°C*	n/a
150–300	hónghuā	Carthamus tinctorius	100–1000	8–12°C*	n/a
150–300	gāncǎo	Glycyrrhiza uralensis	1000–1500	6–8°C	n/a
250–350	huángqí	Astragalus membracaceus var. mongholicus	1000–1500	>95	2500–3100
300–500	kuǎndōnghuā	Tussilago farfara	600–2800	>128	2800–2950
300–800	liánqiáo	Forsythia suspensa	300–2200	>196	1916–3216
300–1200	shègān	Belamcanda chinensis	100–1000	~200	1516–2016
331–1032	cháihú	Bupleurum chinensis & B. scorzonerifolium	260–1500	181–204	1998–2957
402–883	huángqín	Scutellaria baicalensis	300–1000	~160	2600–3100
402–883	jīnliánhuā	Trollius chinensis	1200–2000	>135	2600–2700
500–800	shāshēn	Glehnia littoralis	50–500	>197	2500–2757
500–800	wángbùliúxíng	Vaccaria segetalis	20–500	>178	1998–2956
500–1000	niúxī	Achyranthes bidentata	50–500	>197	2500–2757
500–1000	báizhǐ	Angelica dahurica	50–500	>190	2500–2757
500–1000	zǐwǎn	Aster tataricus	50–500	>197	2500–2757
500–1000	júhuā	Chrysanthemum morifolium	50–500	>197	2500–2757
500–1000	dǎngshēn	Codonopsis pilosula	1000–3200	157–182	1800–1900
500–1000	qúmài	Dianthus superbus & D. chinensis	50–500	~197	2500–2757
500–1000	yuǎnzhì	Polygala tenuifolia	50–500	>197	2500–2757
520–680	guālóu	Trichosanthes kirilowii	0–200	190–220	2300–2800
550–700	shānyao	Dioscorea opposita	150–300	~210	n/a
550–700	dìhuáng	Rehmannia glutinosa	150–300	>210	n/a
550–950	yínhuā	Lonicera japonica	50–1500	150–230	2290–2890
550–950	dānshēn	Salvia miltiorrhiza	60–1000	170–220	2290–2890
570–650	dāngguī	Angelica sinensis	2000–2500	4.5–5.7°C*	n/a
606–1000	jīngjiè	Schizonepeta tenuifolia	50–500	>197	2500–2757
800–1000	mùxiāng	Aucklandia lappa	2700–3300	150–180	n/a
800–1400	lóngdǎn	Gentiana rigescens	1700–2500	7–21°C	n/a
900–1300	sānqī	Panax notoginseng	1400–1800	>300	1516–2016
950–1000	yùjīn	Curcuma phaeocaulis	450–550	>290	1100–1200
972–1125	tiānmá	Gastrodia elata	1400–2300	7.9–12.5°C*	n/a
~1000	cāngzhú	Atractylodes lancea	100–1000	~220	~2000
~1000	yínyánghuò	Epimedium wushanense	300–1700	>270	200–1500
1000–1200	táizǐshēn	Pseudostellaria heterophylla	650–1300	255–294	1060–1350
>1200	dānpí	Paeonia suffruticosa	50–300	~258	n/a
1200–1500	báizhú	Atractylodes macrocephela	500–800	200–260	~2000
1300–1600	huánglián	Coptis chinensis	1100–1800	170–220	1100–1400
1300–1800	bǎihé	Lilium lancifolium	100–800	14.2–16.1°C*	n/a

* Frost-free period data are not available for these herbs; temperatures listed are the average annual temperature range.

Editors of the Original Chinese Text

Guo Lan-ping, PhD is a Professor and graduate student advisor at the China Academy of Chinese Medicinal Sciences. She did her graduate work at Chinese Academy of Forestry Sciences and was a visiting scholar of Universität Innsbruck (Austria). She is the winner of the first National Innovation prize and received the state council special allowance. Professor Guo is the Director of National Resource Center for Chinese Materia Medica and Daodi Herbs at the China Academy of Chinese Medical Sciences. She is also the Director of Key laboratory of Investigation and Zoning of Traditional Chinese Medicine Resources and Head of Key Disciplines of Medicinal Plants, which are both part of the State Administration of Traditional Chinese Medicine (SATCM). Professor Guo is also the Vice group leader of National Survey of Chinese Medicinal Material Resources Dynamic Monitoring Group and the head of "Innovation Team for Ecological Agriculture of Chinese Materia Medica" in key field of MOST of China. Professor Guo is mainly engaged in the research of Chinese medicinal materials resource ecology, particularly eco-agriculture of Chinese medicinal materials and the influences of environmental stress on plants growth, with a special focus on secondary metabolite accumulation under different environmental influences. Undertook more than 20 national and provincial research projects, published more than 400 academic papers, was author and editor of 14 books. Won 3 times the second prize of state science and technology progress award and 8 provincial and ministerial awards, owned 12 patents and software databases, established 3 ISO standards, established or participated in more than 200 standards. In 2017, she won the first National Innovation prize and was granted the winner of the 2017 ISSCNL Awards for the use of ecological agriculture in growing medicinal plants.

Huang Lu-qi, academician of Chinese Academy of Engineering and received PhD from Peking University health science center. He is the current president of China Academy of Chinese Medical Sciences, leading researcher, group leader of the experts guiding group for the 4th National Survey on Chinese Medicinal Material Resources, head of Chinese Medicinal Material Resources innovation team of key area issued by Ministry of science and technology, director of State Key Laboratory of Daodi Herbs that was established by both Ministry of Science and Technology and State Administration of Traditional Chinese Medicine, chief scientist of the National Technology System of TCM Materials Industry, director of National Center for TCM Materials Industry Technical Guidance for Poverty Alleviation, group leader of TCM Materials Industry Technical Guidance team poverty alleviation, and previously served as the chief scientist of national 973 plan project. He put forward and developed the theories of "molecular pharmacognosy" and daodi herbs formation and established 5 protection modes on rare and endangered TCM resources which are commonly used. He has won 4 second prizes of state science and technology progress award. He is the winner of "National Outstanding Youth Fund," "China standard innovation outstanding contribution award," and the award for "Supervisor of the National Outstanding Doctoral Dissertations." Professor Huang is a permanent member of the 13th National Committee of the Chinese people's political consultative conference, member of the 15th Beijing municipal people's congress, and the 9th national committee of China association for science and technology.

Xiaoliang Xie, PhD, is a researcher, state council special allowance expert, member of the guidance group of experts on traditional Chinese medicine of Ministry of Agriculture and Rural Affairs. He is currently the director of Medical Plant Research Center of Hebei Academy of Agriculture and Forestry Sciences, the chairman of the Technical Committee of Standardization of Chinese Medicinal Materials of Hebei Province, the director of the Engineering Technical Research Center of Medicinal Plants of Hebei Province, and the chief expert of the technical system of Hebei Chinese Medicinal Materials Industry. He has presided over the cultivation of 12 new varieties of Chinese medicinal materials, formulated more than 80 series standards for Chinese medicinal materials, won 11 scientific research awards at or above the provincial or ministerial levels, obtained 13 national invention patents, and compiled 10 books such as "Pollution-free Production Technology of Chinese Medicinal Materials," "Rare and Endangered Medicinal Plant Resources in Hebei," "Chinese Medicine Ingredients and Diet Health," and other works.

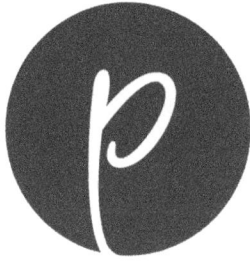

Passiflora
Press

www.passiflora-press.com

www.ingramcontent.com/pod-product-compliance
Lightning Source LLC
Chambersburg PA
CBHW052337210326
41597CB00031B/5285